Clinical management of
articulation disorders

Clinical management of
articulation disorders

CURTIS E. WEISS, Ph.D.

Professor of Speech-Language Pathology,
Department of Communicative Arts and Sciences;
Director of Speech, Language and Hearing Clinic,
Eastern New Mexico University, Portales, New Mexico

HEROLD S. LILLYWHITE, Ph.D.

Professor Emeritus of Speech Pathology, Department of Pediatrics,
University of Oregon Health Sciences Center,
Portland, Oregon

MARY E. GORDON, M.S.

Assistant Professor of Speech Pathology and Chairperson,
Department of Speech Communication, Portland State University,
Portland, Oregon

with 44 illustrations

The C. V. Mosby Company

ST. LOUIS • TORONTO • LONDON   1980

The C. V. Mosby Company
11830 Westline Industrial Drive, St. Louis, Missouri 63141

Library of Congress Cataloging in Publication Data

Weiss, Curtis E   1936-
   Clinical management of articulation disorders.

   Bibliography: p.
   Includes index.
   1. Articulation disorders. 2. Speech therapy.
I. Lillywhite, Herold S., joint author. II. Gordon,
Mary Ellen, 1943-   joint author. III. Title.
[DNLM: I. Articulation disorders. WV500 W427c]
RC424.7.W44   616.85′5   80-17348
ISBN 0-8016-5391-6

VT/CB/CB 9 8 7 6 5 4 3   02/A/265

Preface

All too often instructors and students of undergraduate training programs in speech-language pathology and audiology have great difficulty finding textbooks and reference materials dealing with articulation and its disorders in a direct, organized, practical, and comprehensive manner. Authors almost without exception have chosen to discuss articulation as just one part, and often a minor part, of the entire field of communication and its disorders. There has been a tendency to research and write about the more "exotic" communication disorders, such as those occurring with cleft palate, cerebral palsy, dysphasia, stuttering, and language disorders, and to neglect articulation. The result is that instructors and students have had to search too long, pay too much, and receive too little about articulation or get more than they want about too many other areas of communication at the particular time they would like to concentrate on articulation disorders.

Yet there is a fairly certain chance that when the student becomes a clinician up to 90% of the case load will be comprised of articulation disorders. This is because nearly all other types of communication disorders, especially those occurring because of organic deviations such as cleft palate, cerebral palsy, dysphasia, and other central nervous system damage, will include articulation disorders, often as the principal problem. Also, at least 75% of all job openings are in public elementary and secondary schools, which is where most clinicians will be employed. It follows then that almost the total case load of many school clinicians will involve problems of articulation. And the same is true, to a somewhat lesser ex-

tent, of clinicians working in private speech and hearing clinics and in college and university settings. Problems in these clinics may involve greater diversity, but most of them will include many articulation disorders. Thus the importance of thorough, practical information and training in articulation becomes evident.

To meet this end this book concentrates on articulation development and disorders and their management, not to the exclusion of other disorders, but only insofar as they may present articulation problems. It is our intention to discuss articulation and its disorders thoroughly but at the same time to keep the material as uncluttered, direct, and pertinent as possible. Special stress is placed on assessment, using a new and promising articulation test developed by Dr. Weiss and published separately by Teaching Resources Corporation. Emphasis is also placed on the many approaches and techniques of treatment embodying the latest reliable information from research and clinical practice available in the field.

The word "clinical" was purposely included in the title to emphasize to clinicians, regardless of setting, the importance of assuming a "clinical" approach or philosophy in diagnosis and treatment. To us the term denotes the concepts of thoroughness and individuality essential to success in all settings. Clinical management, as used in this book, implies optimum management of all clients with articulation disorders in all possible settings rather than management of clients only in a "clinical" setting.

We bring to this book a variety of training and experience, covering a combined total of 80 years of working clinically, doing research, and teaching in the field of communication and its disorders. We have had experience as teachers in public schools at almost all levels, as speech-language pathologists in public schools, private clinics, and university clinics, and as professors in clinical, academic, and research environments. We hope that we have successfully combined our experience and expertise to bring instructors, students, and clinicians the kind of assistance in articulation management they have been seeking.

Curtis E. Weiss
Herold S. Lillywhite
Mary E. Gordon

Contents

CHAPTER ONE

Introduction

The significance of articulation and its disorders

"Only the feet that move in order dance.
Only the words that move in order sing."
ALFRED NOYES

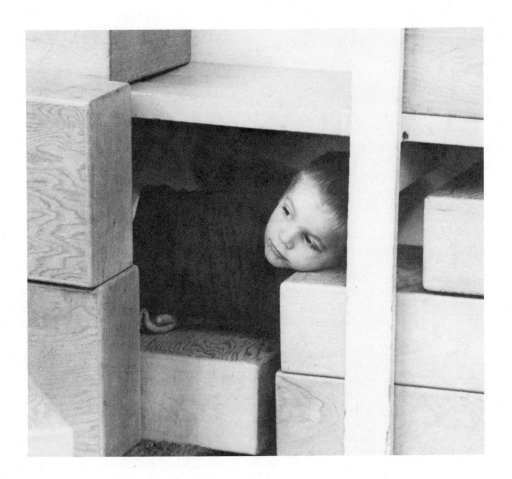

It has been said, "Every time you say a word you perform a miracle." Yet those of us who use words so freely and so easily come to take them for granted, forgetting that oral communication probably is the most important and most complex of all human behaviors. Hoy and Somer (1974) have expressed it this way, "Like the phenomenon of birth, with which it shares many similarities, language is both a very common and a very rare behavior. Almost everyone is capable of procreation, just as almost everyone has acquired a native tongue. The birth of an individual child is perhaps the most marvelous physical miracle permitted man, just as the acquisition of language is man's greatest cerebral miracle."*

Oral communication is important because it is the primary means for interacting with others, for expressing feelings and ideas, for venting anxieties and frustrations, for effecting change, and for enabling one person to find out what another person is perceiving and thinking. Oral communication is complex because it involves understanding and using abstract, arbitrary symbols; it utilizes many different combinations of phonemes, morphemes, words, and inflections; it integrates millions of neurons, nerve fibers, and multiple synaptic connections of the neurologic system; and it simultaneously encompasses virtually all of the bodily systems in its feedback functions.

Oral communication is complex also from another standpoint and because of this is quite unstable as a human process. All of the organs used in the process of oral communication have a more demanding priority than producing speech, or indeed of hearing and processing it as well. That priority is the preservation of the human organism in the face of any kind of threat, be it real or imagined, overt or covert. Thus the communication process may be altered or stopped, temporarily or permanently, by illness, physical threat, psychologic trauma,

or many other conditions that may occur. The secondary nature of oral communication has been called an "overlaid" or "assumed" function.

In a large measure this is true even though there is a strong claim made by psycholinguists (Lenneberg, 1967; Dale, 1972) and others that there is an innate capacity for the development of language in the human being at birth. They point to "small but important differences" in the structure and function of the organs used for speech that are not found in other animals. Because muscles of the tongue and lips are more highly developed and agile, the human being can alter respiration to produce speech by a different interplay of muscles than for normal breathing without speech. Perkins (1971) agrees with Langer (1951) that another highly significant difference in man from other animals is that man is born with a brain that is a "symbol-producing mechanism" or a "symbolic transformer" more highly specialized than that of any other animal and therefore able to accommodate the learning of language.

It is difficult to disagree with any of the preceding, but it does not alter the fact that the so-called speech mechanism is first and foremost a vegetative mechanism with priority always given to the biologic function if a choice must be made. It may be that the finer muscle development of the articulators and the ability to alter respiration for speaking are results of learning to speak rather than causes. In any event language and speech are not instinctive processes inherent with human birth as is the capacity to crawl, walk, and eat. Therefore, oral communication must be learned and taught, but the fact that humans can accomplish this incredible feat, using organs designed biologically for other functions, approaches the miraculous. As Hoy and Somer (1974) say, "The creative power of language is the very essence of that which distinguishes us from other animals. We are human precisely because we have the ability to say we are human."

Just how, when, and where this distinctly

---

*From Hoy, J., and Somer, J., editors: The language experience, New York, 1974, Dell Publishing Co., p. 1.

human attribute might have come about in the evolution of man is as much a mystery as the emergence of life itself. Scholars, scientists, and clinicians have marveled, theorized, studied, experimented, and conjectured for centuries about the emergence, intricacies, and complexities of oral communication (Berry, 1969; West, 1957; Ingram, 1976; Piaget, 1962; Compton, 1970). They have been intrigued, frustrated, and often awed by the potential power of language to effect both positive and negative changes. Not only is oral communication an invaluable asset for those persons who have mastered it, but an enormous liability for those who have not. This unstable, "borrowed" achievement shapes human behavior and is shaped by it. It offers freedom for great achievement but also a heavy responsibility for personal and social conduct, and it can mean success or failure to the individual. Our concern in this book is with the individual and with the particular aspects of oral communication that are most unstable and vulnerable yet that carry the greatest responsibility for making ourselves understood and for being understood by others.

The principal vehicle for conveying meanings, thoughts, ideas, concepts, and attitudes through sounds, words, phrases, and sentences is articulation. An oversimplified definition of articulation is: the adjustments and movements of speech structures and vocal tract necessary for modifying the breath stream for producing the phonemes of speech (see Chapter 2 for detailed discussion of the articulation process).

Psycholinguistic literature suggests that articulation is the mastery of phonologic rules and contrastive features that govern the perception and production of speech; that is, the readily distinguishable speech mechanism adjustments that produce different speech sounds. Perkins (1977) describes articulation in terms of (1) how intelligible the speaker is, (2) how well the speaker's speech meets the cultural standards, (3) how appropriate the speech is in regard to the vocational goals, and (4) how satisfied the speaker is with his speech.

The anatomic and neurophysiologic mechanisms that mediate perception, respiration, phonation, resonation, and articulation help to make oral expression possible (Zemlin, 1968). Although inextricably interwoven and interrelated, these mechanisms will be discussed as separate entities for academic purposes only. Of these mechanisms, articulation will be stressed, since it is one of the major aspects of oral communication and the reason for this textbook. The other parameters of speech—voice, fluency, rate, and other prosodic and pragmatic features—will be discussed only as they relate to articulation.

Articulation disorders, commonly referred to as the most treatable of communicative disorders, may also be the most commonly underestimated disorders in regard to ease of remediation. Not only are articulation disorders the most prevalent communication disorders, but they also are deceptively variable across etiologic modalities. Articulation disorders associated with cleft palate are quite different from articulation disorders associated with cerebral palsy. Misarticulations associated with verbal dyspraxia present a completely different articulation pattern than those associated with functional infantile perseveration ("baby talk"). The treatment approaches likewise are different.

Unfortunately neither the diagnostic procedures nor the treatment procedures have traditionally incorporated a differential or individualistic approach or philosophy. Clinicians have historically used the same traditional diagnostic tools and the same basic treatment approaches regardless of the etiology and symptomatology. Psycholinguistic researchers (Ferguson and Farwell, 1975; Ingram, 1976; Jakobson, 1968; Smith, 1973; Moskowitz, 1970) have begun to change these traditions by applying recent developments in phonologic theory and analysis.

As with any deviation of human behavior, generalizations about articulation disorders should be made with caution, if at all. What initially might appear to be a "simple" articulation disorder may prove to be an exceedingly "difficult" articulation disorder. The common interdental lisp may be common because it is not readily amenable to treatment because of its possible multiple etiology. The functional articulation disorder may turn out to be organically based requiring multidisciplinary assistance. Knowledge of the anatomy and neurophysiology of speech, phonetics, acoustics, phonology, scientific method, and learning theory is an indispensable requisite if the clinician is to treat successfully articulation disorders.

Perhaps certain types of articulation disorders are quickly and effectively remedied, but just as certainly there are articulation disorders that may not be alleviated with present-day techniques. The challenge to the student, the future clinician, remains—to master the science and art of clinically managing persons with articula-

tion disorders. Implicit in this challenge is the need for creating, developing, and exploring new, different, and hopefully better diagnostic and therapeutic techniques.

If articulation is defective, oral communication is impaired. The extent to which oral communication is impaired depends on a number of variables, including the person who has the impairment. No two persons with a similar articulation disorder may experience the same degree of handicap. Likewise one listener may be unaware of the presence of an articulation disorder, whereas another may be quite aware of the disorder and may be highly distracted by it. A third person may ask, "So what if articulation is defective; haven't we all seen and heard teachers, movie stars, community leaders, and politicians with defective articulation?" Such different attitudes may also exist among those persons having defective articulation. However, clinical experience

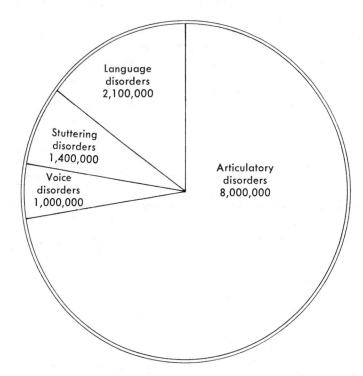

Fig. 1-1. Estimated prevalence of communication disorders. (From Perkins, W. H.: Speech pathology: an applied behavioral science, St. Louis, 1971, The C. V. Mosby Co.)

shows that most adolescents and adults with articulation disorders are acutely aware of and bothered by their deviant articulation.

The effects of an articulation disorder may not be readily apparent to the listener, but they could have far-reaching repercussions on the person's social-emotional well-being, occupation, and, of course, interpersonal relations. As Van Riper (1972) so aptly stated, "The essence of human behavior is speech. Those of us who have spoken so much, so easily, so well, for so long find it difficult to comprehend the remarkable complexities of communication." Have we taken communication for granted? Other communicative disorders may be equally devastating, but as Fig. 1-1 shows, almost 75% of all communicative disorders are disorders of articulation, and this is a very conservative estimate. The fact that articulation constitutes such a large percentage of communicative disorders makes it the cause of more human distress and suffering than any other communicative disorder. Because articulation is so visible and audible, it invites judgments and penalties by listeners far out of proportion to the severity of the actual deviation. It has always been so. There is a biblical account (Judges **12**:5-6) of such a judgment and resulting penalty. The Gileadites had taken a place at the crossing of the River Jordan to prevent the Ephraimites from crossing the river. The account says, "And it was so, that when one of those Ephraimites which had got away said, 'Let me go over' that the men of Giliad said to him, 'Are you an Ephraimite?' If he said, 'Nay,' then they said to him, 'Say now Shibboleth,' and he said 'Sibboleth,' for he was not able to give it the right sound. Then they took him and put him to death there by the Jordan. And there were forty and two thousand Ephraimites put to death at that time."

Modern man does not exact such severe punishment on another because of the inability to articulate a word correctly, but many less severe and sometimes devastating penalties are exacted.

SOCIAL-EMOTIONAL EFFECTS OF ARTICULATION DISORDERS

Beginning in childhood, the person with defective articulation may experience unfavorable comments, teasing, ostracism, exclusion, labeling, and frustration. Such experiences may result in a low sense of personal worth with the accompanying attitudes of feeling different, incompetent, stupid, socially inept, or disliked. As these unfavorable attitudes continue to develop, they may affect academic performance and behavior. The person with atypical articulation may begin to "play the part" of an atypical person. Grades may begin to drop, and disruptive behavior may become commonplace.

Some instances of truancy and delinquency may have their roots in atypical articulation development, and there is some evidence of a higher incidence of communicative disorders among prisoners (Taylor, 1969; Walle, 1972; Bountress and Richards, 1979). The latter investigators compared the incidence and prevalence of types of communicative disorders of prisoners with those of nonprisoners. In a medium-security penal institution in Virginia they found a higher prevalence of articulation, voice, and hearing disorders as well as more deficiencies in receptive vocabulary skills than among nonprison populations; strangely they found a slightly lower incidence of stuttering. After reviewing all available research on this topic, they issued a report stating that "a strong relationship exists between communicative disorders and antisocial and criminal behaviors." As with nonprison populations, articulation is most often found to be the disorder in question.

If social-emotional problems can develop and progress to such a level possibly because of defective articulation, speech-language pathologists have a great responsibility for alleviating such disorders early in the child's life. From the standpoint of social-emotional well-being, safety, protection of society, and simple economics, preventing articulation problems and successfully treating them early in life would seem to be the best clinical approach (Weiss and Lillywhite, 1976).

It is almost ironical that unacceptable speech causes unacceptable social-emotional adjustment, which in turn is treated through effective speech. Psychoanalysis and certain other forms of psychiatric intervention rely on effective speech for treating patients whose problems may have stemmed from disordered speech early in life. The fact that defective articulation may no longer be present in adulthood tends to minimize the relationship, or at least the awareness of a relationship, between disordered articulation and social-emotional problems. Disordered articulation as a cause of adjustment problems may be obscured or not even be considered because it is not present when the psychologic problem becomes manifest. Determining cause and effect of human psychopathology is not easy. Behavioral scientists would be the first to admit that making an accurate differential diagnosis relative to etiology is a challenging and complex task. More research is needed to determine the effect that disordered articulation has on social-emotional adjustment. The cumulative effects of a "mild," not to mention "severe," articulation disorder on psychosocial development may be surprising.

OCCUPATIONAL EFFECTS OF ARTICULATION DISORDERS

It has been said that the average person is capable of performing successfully 7000 different jobs. This estimate obviously presupposes that the person has normal oral communication skills. The presence of an articulation disorder would probably reduce the number of job possibilities by as much as 80%. After all, how many occupations are there that do not require intelligible articulation? Even if the actual job has a low communication demand, the potential employee with defective articulation may not be able to speak well enough during the interview to avoid rejection. It is still true that many people, including employers, associate disordered or "different" speech

with ignorance, incompetence, and even lack of intelligence. In this verbal society a person probably is judged, or misjudged, more by the type of speech used than by any other factor or combination of factors.

In the United States society today competition in most aspects of life is keener than it has ever been. There are many applicants for every job, many buyers for every home, and many customers for every vacation property. In this culture in which many aspects of human beings are relegated to numerical codes—zip codes, area codes, identification numbers, parcel pickup numbers, social security numbers, checking account numbers, loan numbers, post office numbers, welfare numbers, retirement numbers, credit card numbers, check-cashing card numbers, and so on, the need for recognition and identification becomes increasingly important. One of the most important and most effective ways to gain this recognition and identification is through articulate oral communication. Thus effective speech becomes an important factor in establishing oneself, in convincing the prospective employer of one's qualifications, and of relating to society at levels somewhat higher than numerical codes.

As Van Riper (1972) has pointed out, the degree and type of penalty suffered by the communicatively handicapped person are dependent on several factors. These factors are indicated in hierarchical order of handicapping effect in Fig. 1-2 and are described as follows:

1. *Articulation demand:* The more a communicatively handicapped person has to talk, the greater the potential penalty.
2. *Offsetting personal assets:* The more positive behaviors and attributes present in an individual, the less that person may be bothered by defective articulation.
3. *Overprotection:* The greater the overprotection, the more vulnerable that person becomes to penalty from the speech handicap.
4. *Stereotyped or preconceived listener attitudes:* The more distracted listeners are by disordered articulation, the greater the penalty. The worst penalties come from persons who

Level 7	Degree of unintelligibility
Level 6	Conspicuousness of speech disorder
Level 5	Attitudes of impaired speaker
Level 4	Stereotyped or preconceived listener attitudes
Level 3	Overprotection
Level 2	Offsetting personal assets
Level 1	Articulation demand

Fig. 1-2. A hierarchy of handicapping characteristics associated with disordered articulation.

are most sensitive about some difference of their own, that is, defective articulation.

5. *Attitudes of impaired speaker:* A negative attitude by the speaker is often transferred to and assumed by the listener.
6. *Conspicuousness of speech disorder:* The more unusual the speech in terms of acoustic, physiologic, and cosmetic distortions, the greater the penalty.
7. *Degree of unintelligibility:* The more unintelligible the speech, the greater the penalties. The penalties are great when persons listen but cannot understand.

These handicapping effects may assume different levels within this hierarchy depending on the person with disordered articulation, the situation, and the overall environment. Regardless of the assets and potential a person may have, if articulation is defective, penalties imposed by society or by communicatively handicapped persons on themselves will present barriers that interfere with self-actualization.

INTERPERSONAL EFFECTS OF ARTICULATION DISORDERS

Closely related to social-emotional adjustment and occupational employment are interpersonal skills. Obviously none of these topics is mutually exclusive because

they all deal with communication and other similar aspects of human behavior. For these reasons, one area can hardly be affected without affecting the other areas.

Different societies and cultures have different value systems. Some cultures stress physical attributes, some emphasize material possessions, some place high premiums on educational achievements, and some regard artistic accomplishments highly. A large segment of the culture of the United States considers articulate communication important. In fact disordered articulation in this society is one of the more serious handicaps a person can have. Van Riper (1972) mentioned a number of autobiographic testimonies of persons with communication disorders. The poignant experiences these communicatively handicapped persons related emphasize the effect that disordered communication can have on interpersonal relations (Duncan, 1955). Their testimonies included experiencing a number of covert and overt penalties (Fig. 1-3). Many normal-speaking persons may not be cognizant of the types and extent of penalties that are faced daily by communicatively handicapped persons. Awareness of the problems of these persons is an important first step; acceptance of their problems is a giant second step; and effective professional intervention in their problems is the final step.

Penalties experienced by communicatively handicapped persons vary according to the seven levels of handicapping conditions mentioned earlier. People use a great variety of ways, usually with good intentions, to penalize others whose behavior deviates from their own standards or from what is generally considered acceptable. As pointed out previously, almost any type of communication disorder may stimulate penalizing behavior by a "normal" speaker toward one with deviant speech. There are two characteristics of defective articulation that attract the most attention and thereby draw the most penalties—conspicuousness of the articulation disorder and degree of unintelligibility. Either one may result in

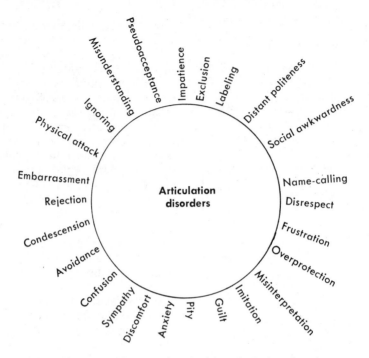

Fig. 1-3. Penalties associated with articulation disorders.

the person experiencing a number of overt and covert penalties (Fig. 1-3).

An occurrence that is fairly common among children and not that uncommon among adults is to attach labels, usually negative ones, to a person who exhibits any kind of behavior that they do not understand or that is considered to be "different," such as disordered articulation. The child with a pronounced lateral lisp, a conspicuously defective /r/, or atypically indistinct speech, may be labeled, teased, and sometimes ridiculed. In the early years this can be quite direct and persistent. During adolescence and adulthood labeling may be more subtle and less obvious, but either way it can be devastating.

If a handy label cannot be found or if name-calling does not seem to fit, mocking imitation of the deviant speech often occurs, resulting in embarrassment, frustration, or other discomfort to the individual with the disorder. An interdental lisp, for example, invites imitation, and the substitution of /w/ for /r/ or /l/, such as in "witto wed widing

hood," can hardly be resisted. In fact many parents and others often find it so difficult to resist that they also imitate the articulation errors, much to the detriment of the child. It should be noted that this kind of imitation is different from imitating and stimulating an infant's baby sounds or babbling, which is desirable in helping the child learn to talk (Weiss and Lillywhite, 1976). Imitation that can be cruel and damaging is that which occurs after a child is past the stage when a sound should be used correctly, but for some reason is not. Ridicule of this kind of deviation by a parent, sibling, classmate, or other person can have a long-lasting negative influence on the child's communication development and emotional health.

Other forms of unfavorable attention, whereas less direct and sometimes more esoteric, can be equally damaging. Some of these are anxiety, overprotection, pity, and condescension. Parents in particular may show undue anxiety and sometimes overprotect the child with a speech problem. Fortunately most schools now have clinical services for speech handicapped children, and the good clinician will make certain that attitudes at home are as advantageous as possible for the child with a speech problem. However, sometimes this is not feasible or may be neglected by the clinician. More difficult still is to control the penalties of pity and condescension, because these may be covertly exhibited by anyone at any time or place. It is essential to help the child to react in a mature, unemotional manner to such attitudes.

Impatience, avoidance, rejection, and exclusion—characteristics that may be exhibited at times by children or adults—are difficult to control. A surprising number of parents, other adults, and sometimes teachers may show impatience at not being able to understand a child with a severe articulation problem. They may misunderstand and then misjudge the child. Such a penalty only reinforces the child's feelings of inadequacy and amplifies the disorder. Avoidance, rejection, or outright exclusion is more likely to be used by children. Fortunately these drastic behaviors are not exhibited in most cases, but the child with dysarthria (p. 35), dyspraxia (p. 91), or severe dyslalia (p. 91) who cannot be understood or who may even sound and look somewhat grotesque to peers when trying to speak quite possibly will be avoided, rejected, or excluded from games, conversations, clubs, and parties. When negative behaviors reach such proportions, the results can be most serious.

The child with a speech disorder who suffers from one of these unfavorable experiences may react in any of a number of ways. Embarrassment and frustration may be the most common reactions and perhaps the least serious. Feelings of guilt and shame may also occur, especially if the child has been teased or ridiculed at home or at school or has been made to feel inadequate because of the speech problem. In the very young child confusion may result and the entire process of communication development may be seriously disrupted or delayed.

The most effective safeguard for the child is to prevent articulation disorders from occurring or from developing further, but this may not always be possible. However, many of the penalties discussed previously can be avoided or reduced in number and severity by an awareness, understanding, and acceptance of the speech problems by parents, teachers, and others most directly involved with the child. The surest and most efficient way to eliminate negative experiences altogether when articulation disorders are present is to have the problems treated at the earliest opportunity by a competent speech-language pathologist.

A pertinent point made by Celler (1956) must be foremost in the minds of clinicians who work with speech-handicapped children—they may be helpless, but not hopeless. From this premise of hope we shall proceed to discuss the many etiologies, remedial approaches, and overall clinical management of articulation disorders among those persons who need, although sometimes seemingly do not want, the professional help of speech-language pathologists.

SUMMARY

A number of penalties caused by defective articulation, the most common disorder of communication, have been mentioned in this chapter. Social-emotional and occupational effects of disordered articulation were also discussed. The degree and type of penalty a particular person with a communication disorder experiences depend on seven factors: (1) articulation demand, (2) offsetting personal assets, (3) overprotection, (4) stereotyped or preconceived listener attitudes, (5) attitudes of impaired speaker, (6) conspicuousness of speech disorder, and (7) degree of unintelligibility. The most effective safeguard is prevention of articulation disorders from occurring, or from becoming worse, whenever possible.

STUDY SUGGESTIONS

1. Explore the statement, "Articulation disorders may be the most commonly underestimated disorders in regard to ease of remediation." Why? In what ways? Under what circumstances?

2. How can a functional articulation disorder turn out to be organically based?
3. How is it possible that "some instances of truancy and delinquency may have roots in atypical articulation development"? Under what circumstances could this happen? Why only in "some instances and not all"?
4. Relate frequency of occurrence of various phonemes in speech to degree and type of penalties if articulation is defective.
5. Develop a list of measures that can be taken by parents and siblings to help prevent articulation disorders.

REFERENCES

Berry, M.: Language disorders of children: the basis and diagnoses, New York, 1969, Appleton-Century-Crofts.

Bountress, N., and Richards, I. J.: Speech language and hearing disorders in an adult penal institution, J. Speech Hear. Disord. **44-3:**293-298, 1979.

Celler, J.: Helpless, not hopeless, Ment. Hyg. **60:**535-550, 1956.

Compton, A.: Generative studies of children's phonological disorders, J. Speech Hear. Disord. **35:**315-339, 1970.

Dale, P. S.: Language development structure and function, Hinsdale, Ill., 1972, Dryden Press, pp. 160 and 161.

Duncan, M.: Emotional aspects of the communication problem in cerebral palsy, Cerebral Palsy Rev. **86:**19-23, 1955.

Ferguson, C., and Farwell, C.: Words and sounds in early language acquisition: English initial consonants in the first 50 words, Language **51:**1-61, 1975.

Hoy, J., and Somer, J., editors: The language experience, New York, 1974, Dell Publishing Co., p. 1.

Ingram, D.: Phonological disability in children, London, 1976, Edward Arnold.

Jakobson, R.: Child language, aphasia, and phonological universals, The Hague, 1968, Mouton.

Johnson, W., and associates: Speech handicapped school children, ed. 3, New York, 1967, Harper & Row, Publishers.

Langer, S.: Philosophy in a new key, New York, 1951, Mentor Books.

Lenneberg, E. H.: Biological foundations of language, New York, 1967, John Wiley & Sons, Inc.

Moskowitz, H.: The two-year-old stage in the acquisition of English phonology, Language **46:**426-441, 1970.

Perkins, W. H.: Speech pathology: an applied behavioral science, ed. 2, St. Louis, 1977, The C. V. Mosby Co., pp. 100 and 101.

Piaget, J.: Play, dreams, and imitation in childhood, New York, 1962, W. W. Norton and Co., Inc.

Smith, N.: The acquisition of phonology: a case study, New York, 1973, Cambridge University Press.

Taylor, J.: Incidence of communication disorders among prisoners, Dissertation completed at University of Missouri, Columbia (1969).

Van Riper, C.: Speech correction principles and methods, ed. 5, Englewood Cliffs, N.J., 1972, Prentice-Hall, Inc.

Walle, E.: The prison speech and hearing clinic, Envoy **1:**1972.

Weiss, C. E., and Lillywhite, H. S.: Communicative disorders: a handbook for prevention and early intervention, St. Louis, 1976, The C. V. Mosby Co.

West, R.: The neurophysiology of speech. In Travis, L., editor: Handbook of speech pathology, New York, 1957, Appleton-Century-Crofts.

Zemlin, W.: Speech and hearing science, Englewood Cliffs, N.J., 1968, Prentice-Hall, Inc.

GLOSSARY

acoustic The study of sound and the properties and environments of sound as they relate to hearing.

articulation The processes of speech production; the vocal tract movements and positions interrelating and integrating to produce speech sounds.

clinical management The total process of detection, assessment, treatment, follow-up, and related aspects of communication disorders.

covert penalties Disguised, hidden, or surreptitious attitudes, feelings, and actions that may penalize persons having communication disorders.

overt penalties Obvious, open attitudes, feelings, and actions that may penalize persons with communication disorders.

phonation Production of voice or voiced sounds by action of the vocal cords in relation to the airstream moving upward from the lungs.

physiologic The functioning of organs and organ systems of the body.

resonation Shaping and modification of the voiced airstream moving upward from the larynx, by the cavities of the pharynx, nose, and sinuses.

respiration The processes of breathing; of concern here, especially the expiratory process related to voice, resonation, and articulation.

CHAPTER TWO

Anatomy and physiology of speech

"Death and life are in the hands of the tongue."
PROVERBS

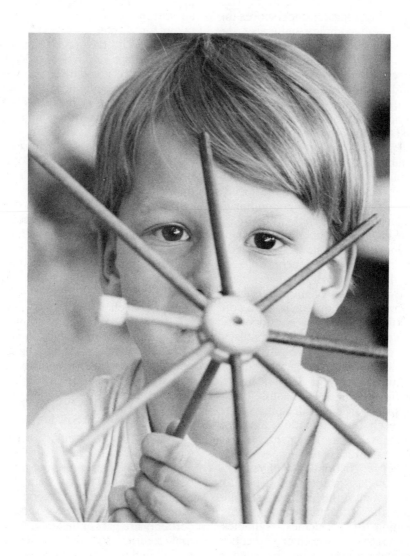

The speech mechanism is composed of two basic components, the anatomic structures and the physiologic functions of the innervation and bodily systems. Since these systems were innately intended to provide life-sustaining functions, the speech mechanism can be considered a borrowed mechanism, one that is inextricably superimposed on the existing biologic functions. Utilization of these different systems in oral communication clearly implicates speech as an "overlaid" or borrowed function. This sharing of functions further underscores the extraordinary and complex nature of the speech mechanism.

Included as part of the speech mechanism are the innervation systems (central, peripheral, and autonomic nervous systems), eleven bodily systems, approximately 100 muscles, and about fifteen movable and immovable structures that comprise the articulators. This composite of structures and systems enables the speech mechanism to carry out many complex and dynamic functions. Since it includes the brain, the speech mechanism is capable of programming or preplanning what is to be spoken; that is, it provides the linguistic or cognitive planning necessary for oral communication. Then the mechanism is involved in oral speech production or the actual utterance, which requires the integration of the central nervous system, presence of psychologic controls over the physiologic and acoustic processes, conduction of nerve impulses, movement of muscles and structures, changes in air pressures and airflows, and occurrence of a variety of acoustic waveforms (Minifie, Hixon, and Williams, 1973). Finally the speech mechanism enables us to perceive speech (discrimination, recognition, and comprehension), which is essentially the reverse process of the speech production sequence. Anatomy and physiology of speech encompass many of the structures and bodily systems, the neurophysiologic integration of these structures and systems, the production of phonemes, syllables, words, and sentences and their respective suprasegmental features, and the accompanying acoustic, psychologic, and perceptual correlates involved in oral speech.

The difficulty involved in trying to review simply and concisely the anatomy and physiology of speech can be readily appreciated. A simple explanation is not possible, because speech is not a simple process. For example, the neurophysiology of speech is a complex process that continues to mature until about age 12 years, even though speech itself spontaneously changes very little after age 7 years. Since speech is such an extremely complex event, it cannot be taken for granted and should be generally understood by the speech-language pathologist. Perhaps one reason why the speech processes are not entirely understood, besides the fact that they are tremendously complex, is that in the phylogenetic (biologic history of a race) and ontogenetic (history of the individual organism) development, speech was acquired comparatively late. It is a recent development in the history of human evolution, probably less than 50 thousand years ago; it is still a phylogenetic neophyte (Lillywhite, 1963). Because of the late development of speech and the fact that it is an "overlaid" function of the organs involved, it is relatively unstable and vulnerable to any condition that threatens the welfare of the human organism. However, with some understanding of the speech system and its relation to other systems of the body, clinicians should be better able to develop and use scientifically and clinically sound behavioral procedures for evaluating and treating persons with articulation disorders (Sperry, 1964).

ANATOMY AND PHYSIOLOGY OF INNERVATION SYSTEMS

Among the structures of the innervation systems are the brain, cerebellum, brain stem, twelve paired cranial nerves, thirty-one paired spinal nerves, innumerable autonomic nerves, and their accompanying neurons and neural pathways. Other structures certainly are part of the innervation systems that mediate speech, but space does not permit inclusion of all of them. The purpose of this chapter is merely to review the structures and functions that mediate speech. Additional information can be found in the following sources: Gardner, 1975; Minifie, Hixon, and Williams, 1973; Carpenter, 1978; and Zemlin, 1968.

The central nervous system is composed of the spinal cord and brain, which includes the cerebrum (the center of all neural and speech activity), brain stem, and cerebellum (Fig. 2-1). The *cerebrum* is perhaps the most intricate structure in the human body. It is comprised of approximately 14 billion highly specialized neurons (nerve cells) in the cortex (outside covering of gray matter) and 200 million incoming and outgoing projectional nerve fibers embedded in the white matter of the brain. The cortex has a convoluted surface with gyri (elevations) and sulci (valleys), many of which are named (Fig. 2-2). This convoluted surface provides a maximum amount of cortical surface in a relatively small space. Aggregates of motor neurons form the basal ganglia (motor nuclei areas) that lie deep in each of the two cerebral hemispheres, as does the thalamus (structure for receiving and relaying sensations to the cortex) and the reticular formation (sorting and alerting mechanism through which incoming stimuli

pass). Connecting the two cerebral hemispheres are a collection of nerve fibers called the corpus callosum (Fig. 2-2). Joining the hemispheres inferiorly with the brain stem are nerve tracts called the cerebral peduncles. The cerebellum, which functions in motor coordination such as in walking, is located posteriorly to the brain stem (midbrain, pons, and medulla oblongata) (Fig. 2-1). All of these structures are interconnected by dendrites and axons (neural fibers) that provide multiple synaptic contacts or connections and excite hundreds of thousands of other neurons (Eccles, 1953). It is the excitation of these neurons that provides innervation to the speech musculature for speech production.

The cerebrum may be anatomically divided as follows: frontal, parietal, temporal, occipital, and limbic lobes (Barr, 1974) (Fig. 2-3). The cerebrum can also be divided into regions: forebrain, midbrain, and hindbrain, exclusive of the spinal column; or into regions such as telencephalon, diencephalon, mesencephalon, metencephalon, and myelencephalon. Different authors use somewhat different anatomic divisions (Chusid and McDonald, 1967; Gardner, 1975; Carpenter, 1978; Crafts, 1966; and Gray, 1959). We prefer the division by

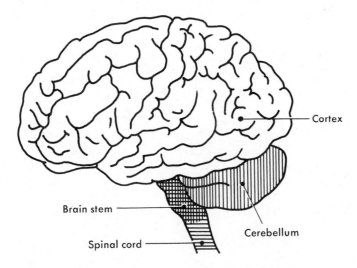

Fig. 2-1. Brain, brain stem, and cerebellum.

lobes. Total weight of the cerebrum is approximately 1200 gm (2½ pounds) in adult females and 1400 gm (3 pounds) in adult males (Coppoletta and Wolbach, 1933; Kaplan, 1971). The magnitude of functions this tiny mass of nervous tissue performs is truly amazing.

Functionally the cerebrum may be described as a symbolic receiver and transformer (Perkins, 1977) because it receives and transforms sensory-motor experiences into ideational symbols or oral communication. The cerebrum is also concerned with voluntary control of the speech mechanism

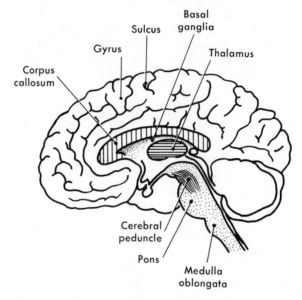

Fig. 2-2. Structures and landmarks of the brain and brain stem.

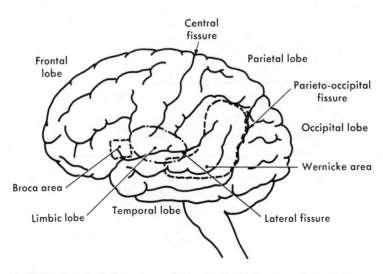

Fig. 2-3. Lobes, fissures, and communication areas of the brain.

capable of telling the articulators when, where, and how to move. It is the highest level of neuromuscular (sensory-motor) integration.

Although all five lobes are interrelated, the primary structures and functions of each one will be discussed separately.

Frontal lobe

This lobe extends from the most anterior part of the cerebrum to the central fissure (fissure of Rolando) and inferiorly to the lateral fissure (fissure of Sylvius) (Fig. 2-3). Located in this lobe is the motor cortex and the site of Broca's motor speech area. The motor cortex is made up of large, pyramidal-shaped motor or Betz nerve cells necessary for motoric functions. The area anterior to the precentral gyrus is called the primary or premotor cortex including a large representational area for coordination of motor function. Parenthetically the larger the representational area on the cortex for a particular structure, such as the tongue, the greater the amount of nerve supply to that structure, which may or may not suggest greater sensitivity of that structure. Excellent illustrations of sensory and motor representations indicating the size

and location of various body parts can be found in Penfield and Rasmussen (1950). It is in this lobe that speech production movements are programmed or planned.

Motor fibers descend from the motor cortex of the frontal lobe via the *corticobulbar tract* (also called extrapyramidal tract system with fibers from the cortex to the medulla oblongata) through various pathways and structures (internal capsule, cerebral peduncles, midbrain, and brain stem) (Fig. 2-4). These motor fibers continue to the medulla oblongata of the brain stem where approximately 90% of them cross (decussate) to the other side of the brain stem (Fig. 2-5). This explains, for example, why paralysis of the right side of the body indicates injury to the left hemisphere of the brain and vice versa. Neural impulses from the motor cortex are also conducted through these motor pathways to the motor cells of the cranial nerves at the base of the brain where they synapse (connect) and are transmitted to the respective articulators for speech production and vegetative functions. However, as Abbs (1971) suggested, the muscle spindle system is also a necessary mechanism for controlling speech movements through sensory feedback. The

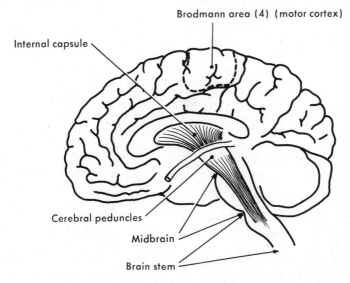

Brodmann area (4) (motor cortex)

Internal capsule

Cerebral peduncles

Midbrain

Brain stem

Fig. 2-4. Internal capsule, cerebral peduncles, and brain stem.

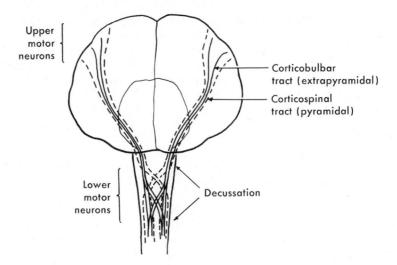

Fig. 2-5. Motor pathways from the cortex.

other major motor pathway that descends from the motor cortex to the spinal cord is called the *corticospinal pathway* or pyramidal tract system. This neural pathway conducts motor impulses to the body. These fibers also interrelate with the extrapyramidal fibers.

Since the twelve cranial nerves exit the brain above the level of the medulla oblongata, most are not involved in decussation and therefore innervate the speech musculature on the same (ipsilateral) side, unlike the corticospinal fibers, which innervate structures of the body of the opposite (contralateral) side. For example, if the left hypoglossal nerve (XII) is impaired, the left side of the tongue is impaired; however, if a peripheral nerve on the left side is impaired, the right or opposite side of the body is impaired.

Motor pathways may be designated as having upper or lower motor neurons, or as being upper motor pathways and lower motor pathways (Fig. 2-5). Darley, Aronson, and Brown (1975) have suggested a hierarchical order of these motor pathways. The first three levels would appear to be part of the lower motor pathways and the last three levels part of the upper motor pathways, as follows:

Level one: Bulbar level (functions reflexly in relation to motor speech)

Level two: Vestibular-reticular level (regulates reflex activity)

Level three: Extrapyramidal level (involved with subconscious, automatic aspects of motor performance)

Level four: Cerebral motor cortex level (concerned with voluntary movements)

Level five: Cerebellar level (controls accuracy of responses initiated at the four lower levels but does not initiate movement)

Level six: Conceptual-programming level (plans and programs aspects of movement including the total conceptual plan, sequence of movement, and programming details)

A lesion or injury of the upper motor neuronal pathway often results in excessive muscle tone, that is, spasticity or hypertonia. Lower motor neuronal pathways are the final communication pathway and as such begin at the level of the cranial nerve nuclei in the lower brain stem and synapse with various spinal nerves. A lesion at the level of the lower motor neuron often results in excessively decreased muscle tone, that is, flaccidity or hypotonia (Espir and Rose, 1970). A lesion in the frontal lobe could result in expressive or motor dysphasia (Broca aphasia); motor speech problems; changes in personality, intellect, temperament, and emotional control; paresis or paralysis; and impairment of writing ability.

Parietal lobe

The parietal lobe extends posteriorly from the central fissure to the parieto-occipital fissure and laterally to the lateral fissure (Fig. 2-3). The primary receptive areas for general sensory stimuli, excluding audition, vision, smell, and taste, are in the parietal lobe. Functionally afferent (toward the brain) sensory impulses emanate from end-organs in various parts of the body and are relayed by the spinal and cranial nerves through the brain stem, thalamus, and on to the appropriate receptive sensory area and association area of the cortex (Fig. 2-2). Parietal lobe lesions may result in various types of disorders indirectly relating to communication such as agnosia, impairment of sensation on the opposite side of the body, disorientation, and astereognosis.

Temporal lobe

The temporal lobe is located below the fissure of Sylvius and extends back to the parieto-occipital fissure and occipital lobe. This lobe is primarily responsible for assimilating and interpreting phonemes, words, and other communication symbols for receptive speech and language (Penfield and Rasmussen, 1950). The temporal lobe (usually the left) is responsible for comprehending oral communication. Lesions in this lobe may result in receptive dysphasia (Wernicke aphasia), loss of memory—usually recent memory (amnesia) located in the deeper structures of this lobe (that is, hippocampus), and inability to smell.

Occipital lobe

This pyramidal-shaped lobe occupies the area behind the parieto-occipital fissure. It is mainly concerned with vision. Lesions in this lobe may result in various types of visual impairments such as hemianopia (vision of half the visual field), double vision, tunnel vision, and quadrantic vision (vision in one quarter of the visual field). A lesion in this lobe may also result in visual disorientation and problems in spatial orientation, visual hallucinations, and visual agnosia—inability to recognize visual stimuli. Visual impairment can cause delay in the development of speech and faulty articulation.

Limbic lobe

This lobe, which is not always included as one of the lobes of the brain, was named and described by Broca in 1878. Phylogenetically it is the old portion of the cerebral hemisphere situated in the medial aspect of the brain (Fig. 2-3). Initially this lobe was thought to be involved only with smell (olfaction) and taste (gustation), but now its functions are thought to include control of emotions of anger and fear, hyperactivity and restlessness, sexual behavior, motivation, metabolism, recent memory, and purposive motor responses (Berry, 1969; and Zemlin, 1968). A lesion in this lobe could affect the voluntary and emotional (suprasegmental or nonsegmental) aspects of speech.

Another important structure of the central nervous system is the *brain stem*. This stemlike midbrain structure is the most inferior integrating and neural pathway structure of the central nervous system. It includes the pons and medulla oblongata (Fig. 2-2). Gardner (1975) also includes the diencephalon (thalamus and hypothalamus) as part of the brain stem. Lesions in the brain stem could cause paralysis of upward movements of the eyes, squinting, strabismus, double vision, nystagmus, ptosis or drooping of the eyelid, limited eye movement, and dizziness. If this integrating mechanism is impaired, speech might be affected.

The *pons* lies ventral to the cerebellum and above the medulla oblongata (Fig. 2-2). It is made up of a number of motor pathway fibers, cranial nerve nuclei, and some of the cranial nerves. It also includes part of the reticular formation concerned with motor and autonomic functions, that is, wakefulness, conscious states, and attention. Like the other brain stem structures, the pons is important in integrating and interconnecting neural impulses and nervous system structures. Lesions in the pons may cause alternating visual and facial hemiplegia, paralysis of jaw muscles and muscles of facial expression, nystagmus, tinnitus, progressive deafness, paralysis of tongue, vertigo, and hypotonia.

The *medulla oblongata* is the pyramidal-shaped portion of the brain stem. It is contiguous with the pons above and the spinal cord below (Fig. 2-2). This structure contains cranial nerve nuclei, the site of decussation of the corticobulbar tract fibers, and part of the reticular formation. Lesions in the medulla oblongata may cause deviations in posture and righting reflexes, hypotonic paralysis of tongue, soft palate, and pharynx; problems in swallowing, respiration, and cardiovascular control; problems with gag, taste, aphonia or dysphonia, and sensation and perception; and, of course, motor speech problems.

The *spinal cord* extends inferiorly from the medulla oblongata beginning at the first cervical vertebra and ending at approximately the lower border of the first lumbar vertebra. It does not occupy the entire length of the spinal column (vertebral canal). It is surrounded and protected by vertebrae along its entire length. A transverse section of the spinal cord (Fig. 2-6) shows, in contrast to the composition of the cerebral hemisphere, a central core of gray matter (shaped like an H) surrounded by white matter. Gray matter contains nerve cell bodies involved with sensory and motor impulses, muscle activity, and functions of viscera, glands, and blood vessels. White matter, arranged into cords (funiculi) contains nerve fibers connecting dorsal and ventral root fibers with other parts of the spinal cord and brain. Lesions to the spinal cord, which are usually traumatic in origin, can result in motor loss to the body manifested by muscle weakness or paralysis, deviations in posture and skin, joint changes, contractures, limited motion, muscle atrophy, and changes in reflex. Lesions may

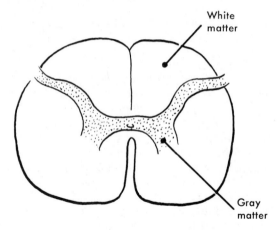

Fig. 2-6. Transverse section of the spinal cord.

also cause sensory deficits related to pain, temperature sense, vibration, pressure, proprioception, and numbness. Severing the spinal cord could result in bilateral paralysis of both arms or both legs or all four depending on where the spinal cord was severed.

The *cerebellum,* oval in shape, is situated behind the pons and medulla oblongata (Fig. 2-1). Because of its embryonic origin, the cerebellum sometimes is considered part of the hindbrain, along with the medulla oblongata and pons. This structure has two deeply fissured hemispheres joined by the vermis (connecting tissue) and with the brain stem by paired peduncles or projectional fibers. The cerebellum is interconnected with the other structures of the brain, brain stem, and spinal cord and functions integrally with them. It is composed of gray and white matter and functions primarily in controlling muscular activity and in orienting the body in space. Lesions in the cerebellum may cause lack of coordinated (asynergistic) muscular movements and spacial disorientation as in ataxic cerebral palsy (McDonald and Chance, 1964).

Before completing the discussion on the central nervous system, some mention should be made of the functional properties of *neurons.* The neuron is the basic functional unit of structure of the nervous system and consists of a cell body, a single

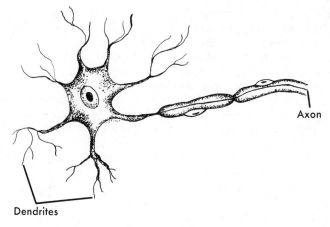

Axon

Dendrites

Fig. 2-7. Neuron.

axon, and long dendrites (Fig. 2-7). Axons generally conduct impulses away from the cell body, and dendrites conduct impulses to it. Neurons produce electrical current (spikes) and chemical changes as they synapse with other nerves. Nerves are also fatigable, differ in their excitability, and vary in their speed of conduction, depending on the size and state of the nerve fibers.

Another property of neurons is that their axons respond to stimuli maximally or not at all, regardless of the strength of the stimuli. This all-or-none response of axons does not apply to receptors or to the other parts of neurons; it relates only to the axon. The all-or-none response of the axon may have implications with respect to articulation treatment by way of explaining unexpected responses or lack of responses to stimuli.

Nerve cells continually die and are not replaced, so that by the time of advanced age (around 80 years of age), about one fourth of all nerve cells have died (Noback, 1967). The rate at which nerve cells die, however, varies considerably from one person to another. Also, if cell processes are destroyed, cell bodies may survive, but they do undergo changes. Nerve cells cannot replace themselves once destroyed. If recovery of central nervous system function occurs after being impaired, it probably happens because cells were not completely destroyed or because other cells have taken over their function. In muscles partially denervated, some muscle fibers will respond to direct stimulation (actually touching or moving them) and others to nerve impulses. These neuronal properties have broad implications with respect to articulation assessment and treatment, especially when there is evidence of previous or present nervous system damage.

Synapses, functional connections between axons of one neuron and dendrites or cell bodies of another, are especially important to functions of long-term memory. This system of conduction is one of the most highly specialized functions of the nervous system. It not only carries nerve impulses to and from the brain, but it is also responsible for neural imprinting or learning. Deterioration in synaptic junctions correlates closely with the aging process.

Another major component of the innervation systems is the *peripheral nervous system.* This system consists of an intricate conduction process important to speech, lies outside the body confines of the central nervous system, and innervates much of the body (Zemlin, 1968). It is made up of thirty-one paired spinal nerves, roots, and branches, twelve paired cranial nerves, and the autonomic nerves.

The *spinal nerves,* which originate and emerge from the spinal cord, are distributed accordingly: eight nerves in the cervical region, twelve nerves in the thoracic region, five nerves in the lumbar region, five nerves in the sacral region, and one (sometimes two) nerves in the coccygeal region. These nerves have dorsal roots (carry afferent impulses to the spinal cord) and ventral roots (carry efferent impulses from the spinal cord). Destruction of the efferent nerves results in paralysis of the organs innervated by them.

Twelve paired *cranial nerves*, referred to by names and by Roman numerals, follow complicated pathways to their peripheral structures of the head, face, and neck. They originate at the base of the brain and include:

I	Olfactory
II	Optic
III	Oculomotor
IV	Trochlear
V	Trigeminal
VI	Abducent
VII	Facial
VIII	Acoustic
IX	Glossopharyngeal
X	Vagus
XI	Accessory
XII	Hypoglossal

Of the twelve cranial nerves, seven—cranial nerves V, VII, VIII, IX, X, XI and XII—are more directly related to speech than the others. Cranial nerve I is concerned with smell, and cranial nerves II, III, IV, and VI mediate visual functions. Therefore, only the nerves involved in speech will be discussed.

Cranial nerve V (trigeminal), the largest of the cranial nerves, is both sensory and motor and consists of three divisions: ophthalmic, maxillary, and mandibular, the largest and most important branch to speech. It is important to speech because it provides sensation to the deep structures of the face, mouth, and mandible; superficial sensation to the mucosa of the anterior two thirds of the tongue, cheeks, hard palate, and lips; and motor impulses to the muscles of chewing, soft palate (levator), and two suprahyoid (above the hyoid bone) muscles (di-

gastric and mylohyoid). A lesion of this nerve may affect articulation because of impaired tactile sensation of the anterior two thirds of the tongue and paralysis of the muscles of mastication that control jaw movements. Resonance may also be impaired because of soft palate involvement. Hearing may be impaired by paralysis of the tensor tympani muscle, which it innervates. Damage to this nerve often results in articulation and resonance problems common to several types of cerebral palsy, dyspraxia, and other forms of paresis and velopharyngeal inadequacy.

Cranial nerve VII (facial), which communicates with four other cranial nerves, has a long and circuitous course. Being both sensory and motor, this nerve supplies motor impulses to the stapedius muscle of the middle ear and superficial muscles of the face and scalp. Sensory innervation includes taste for the anterior two thirds of the tongue (secretive motor) and parotid gland, soft palate, and deep pressure and position sense (proprioception or kinesthesis) to the facial muscles. Involvement of this nerve may cause one or more of the following conditions: paralysis of the muscles of facial expression (Bell's palsy), pain behind and in the ear, hearing loss because the stapedius muscle of the middle ear is paralyzed, loss of taste, loss of lacrimation during eating, unilateral twitching of facial muscles, drooling, and grimaces. Pathology of this nerve also affects the nonverbal aspects of speech, such as facial expressions. It has been said that 93% of all communication is nonverbal (Egolf and Chester, 1973). This estimate underscores the importance of facial expressions in the emotional, affective, or cosmetic aspects of communication. When these nonverbal characteristics are defective, communication is seriously impaired.

Cranial nerve VIII (acoustic) consists of two separate sensory parts that are concerned with hearing and balance, both important to speech. The cochlear part supplies the auditory mechanism in the inner ear, and the vestibular part supplies the balance mechanism in the inner ear. Pathology affecting this nerve may result in auditory acuity deafness, word deafness, auditory hallucinations, ringing in the ears (tinnitus), dizziness (vertigo), and nystagmus. Impairment of this nerve may seriously affect the development and maintenance of speech.

Cranial nerve IX (glossopharyngeal) is both sensory and motor. It supplies sensation to the pharynx, soft palate, posterior one third of the tongue, uvula, pillars of fauces, tonsils, eustachian tube, and tympanic cavity as well as motor impulses to pharyngeal and stylopharyngeus muscles. A lesion affecting this nerve could result in loss of gag reflex, loss of sensation to the pharynx, tonsils, fauces, and back of tongue; loss of constriction of the posterior pharyngeal wall movement; increased salivation; deviation of the uvula; and difficulty in swallowing (dysphagia). The effect on speech would be hypernasality and nasal air flow associated with inadequate velopharyngeal closure related to defective sensory and motor functioning of the velopharyngeal structures. Articulation might also be somewhat impaired because the back of the tongue would be involved.

Cranial nerve X (vagus), which is both sensory and motor, also assumes a long, circuitous route as it interrelates with cranial nerves IX and XI. It supplies sensation to the external auditory ear canal and to various structures in the pharynx and larynx as well as motor impulses to the pharynx, larynx, and base of the tongue. Involvement of this nerve may cause loss of voice, impaired voice, changes in vocal cord position, dysphagia, loss of gag reflex, pain, abnormal spontaneous sensation (paresthesia) in the pharynx, larynx, and external auditory ear canal, and lack of sensitivity of the lower pharynx and larynx. These effects on speech would mainly be in voice production and voice quality but could mildly affect articulation as well.

Cranial nerve XI (accessory) is a motor nerve with two separate branches. It innervates the intrinsic muscles of the upper larynx, pharynx, uvula, and muscles of the neck, primarily the trapezius and sternocleidomastoid. As its name implies, it is an accessory or assisting nerve to other nerves in this area of the back of the mouth and throat, specifically cranial nerves IX and X. For this reason, determining its exact functions is difficult. A lesion of this nerve may affect phonation, resonation, rotating the head, shrugging the shoulder, and raising the chin. The effect on phonation would be the result of the intrinsic muscles of the larynx being unable to make fine adjustments, whereas the adverse effect on resonation would relate to lack of pharyngeal constriction. Speech could be affected because of faulty resonation and the presence of adverse postural positions of the neck and head.

Cranial nerve XII (hypoglossal), which is both sensory and motor, is perhaps the most important nerve to articulation. It provides for proprioceptive or kinesthetic feedback from the tongue. Van Riper and Irwin (1958) have postulated that this feedback is probably the most important sensory information for maintaining normal articulation but not necessarily for learning normal articulation. Motor supply is to the intrinsic and extrinsic muscles of the tongue, mediating the production of both consonants and vowels. Since it provides both motor and sensory information to the tongue, a lesion of this nerve could result in unilateral or bilateral paralysis or paresis of the tongue. Unilateral upper motor neuronal involvement (spastic paralysis) would cause the tongue to deviate to the side opposite the lesion (toward the undamaged side), degeneration, and atrophy of the tongue. Unilateral lower motor neuronal involvement (flaccid paralysis) would cause the tongue to deviate to the side of the lesion (toward the damaged side), sensory disturbances, chewing difficulty, arrhythmic tongue movement, and, most importantly, dysarthria. The results of hypoglossal nerve involvement could range from mild dysarthria to complete anarthria, or inability to move the tongue for purposes of articulation, chewing, and swallowing.

An attempt was made to relate specific cranial nerves to the production of specific phonemes (West and Ansberry, 1968). Although such exact neuromuscular correlates of speech apparently do not exist, we should constantly strive to relate innervation with speech production in order to determine etiology or site of lesion or when site of lesion is known, we can anticipate type of speech abnormality. Perhaps we can relate classes of sounds to muscle groups and their respective innervation.

The final component of the innervation systems is the *autonomic nervous system*. A division of the peripheral nervous system, this system supplies smooth muscles, viscera, and glands. It is sometimes referred to as the visceral, afferent, or vegetative nervous system. It is composed of the sympathetic and parasympathetic divisions, which help to maintain a constant internal body environment or prepare the body for impending danger and for more localized reactions. By definition the autonomic system is a motor system and functions subconsciously, that is, below the level of the cortex. There are also sensory impulses coming into this system (Barr, 1974). This system is closely related to the central and peripheral nervous systems. Lesions of the autonomic nervous system, although not directly affecting the segmental features of articulation, can result in problems of the eye, heart, blood vessels, lung, stomach, intestine, gallbladder, skin, salivary glands, and spleen. The effects of autonomic nervous system involvement on speech may perhaps be in terms of the suprasegmental features: rate, rhythm, inflection, loudness, pitch, stress, duration, juncture, tempo, and voice quality.

One final consideration regarding the innervation systems, and all of the bodily systems for that matter, is *blood supply*. The human body, particularly the central nervous system, requires a rich blood supply in order to maintain a balance of oxygen, glucose, and vitamins necessary for

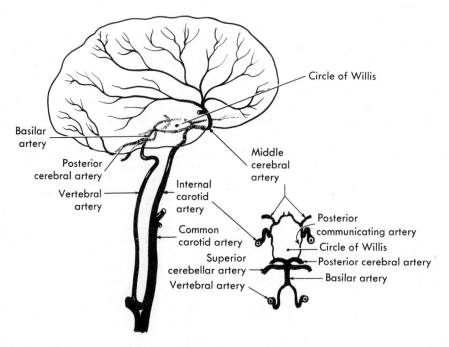

Fig. 2-8. Blood supply to the brain.

metabolism. One sixth of all the blood in the human body goes to the brain. Deprivation of blood supply to the brain for 6 to 8 minutes results in irreversible brain damage.

Blood supply to the brain is derived from the common carotid and vertebral arteries (Fig. 2-8). The common carotid artery divides into the external and internal carotid arteries in the neck, where the internal carotid artery ascends to the cranial cavity through a canal in the base of the skull dividing into the anterior and middle cerebral arteries. The vertebral arteries ascend to the cranial cavity through the foramen magnum (the large hole in the base of the skull) joining to form the basilar artery and then joining into two posterior cerebral arteries. Here the anterior and middle cerebral arteries anastomose (to open, one into another) with the vertebral arteries to form the circle of Willis (a circle of arteries at the base of the brain) (Fig. 2-8). From the circle of Willis the anterior and middle cerebral arteries ascend to supply blood to the front and middle parts of the brain and the two posterior cerebral arteries ascend to provide blood to the back of the brain. Over 60% of all cardiovascular accidents causing brain damage are related to the middle cerebral artery.

To summarize, the common carotid artery conducts the original blood supply to the anterior and middle parts of the brain, and the vertebral arteries conduct the original blood supply to the posterior part of the brain. Venous drainage from the brain, which completes the circulation process, is mainly into dural sinuses within the cranial cavity via jugular veins and returns to the heart (Gardner, 1975).

Summary of the innervation systems

The central, peripheral, and autonomic nervous systems are composed of a complex network of neural structures that function synergistically to mediate speech. It becomes readily apparent that normal functioning of these systems is absolutely essential to normal speech. These innervation systems interrelate with each other and with other bodily functions to effect oral communication. Any problems in their interconnections, degree of timing of motor impulses, or defective sensory feedback to the brain and ear can be detrimental to speech. However, these innervation systems are not solely and totally responsible for oral communication. Several bodily systems, made functional in part by the innervation systems, are also indispensable to normal speech.

ANATOMY AND PHYSIOLOGY OF BODILY SYSTEMS

There are between nine and eleven interrelated systems in the body, depending on the reference used (Gray, 1959; Zemlin, 1968), that participate in mediating speech. Obviously some systems are more closely involved than others in the development and production of speech. Nevertheless integration of all the systems of the human body is essential for normal speech to occur. The systems are:

Skeletal: Bones and related cartilages
Articular: Joints, ligaments, and other connective tissue
Muscular: Intrinsic and extrinsic muscles
Digestive: Digestive tract and related digestive glands
Vascular: Heart, blood vessels, and lymphatic systems
Nervous: Brain, spinal cord, cranial and peripheral nerves, ganglia, and sense organs
Respiratory: Air passageways, larynx, and lungs
Urinary: Kidneys and urinary passages
Reproductive: Organs of reproduction
Endocrine: Ductless glands
Integumentary: Skin, nails, and hair

The skeletal, articular, and muscular systems provide the structures of the speech mechanism. The vascular, nervous, respiratory, and muscular systems provide the functional aspects of the speech mechanism. In essence these seven systems constitute the anatomy and physiology necessary for producing speech. The remaining four systems assist with the emotional, prosodic, pragmatic, and other nonverbal aspects of speech.

Traditionally in speech science these eleven bodily systems have been condensed into four primary but overlapping systemic processes involved in oral communication. They include respiration, phonation, resonation, and articulation (Kaplan, 1960; Lillywhite and Bradley, 1969). Actually these processes are mainly a combination of what was previously listed as muscular, digestive, nervous, and respiratory systems. A brief discussion of these four processes will conclude the anatomy and physiology of the speech mechanism.

Respiration

The system of respiration is made up of the lungs, bronchi, abdomen, trachea, thorax, larynx, and air passageways of the pharynx, nose, and sometimes mouth. It is this system that provides the body with oxygen, carries away carbon dioxide, and provides the major source of energy for speech. Closely related to inhalation and exhalation is the diaphragm, innervated by the phrenic nerve, the thoracic cavity, which houses these structures, and the medulla oblongata, which controls respiration at the subconscious level.

During inhalation a person takes air in either through the nose or mouth. The air passes through the pharynx and larynx into the trachea, which splits (bifurcates) into the left and right bronchi and finally into the respective and comparatively unfilled left and right lungs. For this usually subconscious process to occur, there must be less air pressure inside the respiratory system than there is outside the body. This imbalance between external and internal air pressure is created by enlarging the thoracic cavity. This is accomplished by lifting the rib cage, primarily by the intercostal muscles, and by lowering the diaphragm, after exhaling the carbon dioxide from the lungs (Zemlin, 1968). A complex neuromuscular network is involved in inhalation.

Exhalation is achieved by a natural compression of the thoracic cavity because of the untorquing and elastic recoil of the rib cage, the relaxing and pushing upward of the diaphragm, and the greater internal air pressure caused by the air-filled lungs after inhalation. These activities result in greater air pressure internally than externally, permitting exhalation of the used air. This passing air between the vocal folds helps to set them into vibration and carries the vibrations through the vocal tract for speech purposes. A number of muscles play an integral part in both inhalation and exhalation (Judson and Weaver, 1965).

The respiratory cycles are controlled by the medulla oblongata as long as they occur subconsciously. Conscious or forced respiration involves the cortex. The number of respiratory cycles per minute varies with age, physical activity, and emotions. Adults typically average between 14 and 17 respiratory cycles per minute during quiet breathing. Respiratory cycles in children are considerably faster—up to 1 per second in the very young child. Males tend to have slightly slower respiratory cycles than fe-

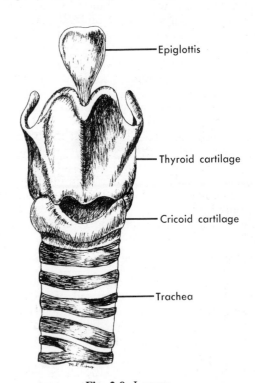

Fig. 2-9. Larynx.

- Epiglottis
- Thyroid cartilage
- Cricoid cartilage
- Trachea

males. The ratio of inhalation to exhalation is different during breathing for life-sustaining breathing than for speech. Exhalation takes approximately as long as inhalation during breathing for life-sustaining purposes, whereas during speech exhalation can take up to ten times as long as inhalation. For speech purposes, inhalation is also deeper and more rapid, and exhalation is more forced and controlled. In effect the demands for conversational speech are far more complex than for nonspeech respiration.

Situated at the top of the trachea is the larynx (Fig. 2-9). Biologically the larynx is the protective valve for the lower respiratory system. By closing or adducting, the vocal folds of the larynx prevent foreign matter from being aspirated into the trachea and lungs. More recently in the phylogenetic development of human beings, the larynx has been converted into a vibrator or vibration source for producing sounds (all vowels and voiced consonants) for articulation, with the energy source being respiration, specifically exhalation.

Phonation

Phonation, an overlaid function of the larynx, is the process of producing sound by the vocal folds of the larynx and is the acoustic source of all oral communication except unvoiced consonants. As mentioned previously, the laryngeal mechanism consists of cartilages, ligaments, membranes, muscles, joints, and part of cranial nerve X. This sound-producing mechanism includes the lower respiratory, laryngeal, and upper airway, which must function in concert (Fig. 2-9). The larynx is made up of a number of intrinsic and extrinsic muscles surrounding its cartilaginous framework. A number of excellent sources are available that explain the anatomy and physiology of the larynx (Palmer, 1972; Crafts, 1966; Gray, 1959; Negus, 1949). The mechanism also includes (1) physical properties such as vocal cord mass, (2) mechanical restraints such as one structure restraining the movement of another, (3) aerodynamic influ-

ences such as subglottic air pressures and flows, and (4) gravity such as it is affected by posture (Minifie, Hixon, and Williams, 1973).

Phonation also involves the sucking-together action of the vocal folds as the breath stream passes between them (Bernoulli effect), subglottic air pressure, elasticity, compliance, and vibratory capability of the muscular edges of the vocal folds (thyroarytenoid and vocal muscles), and innervation by cranial nerve X. Phonatory theories that explain the process of phonation are the myoelastic-aerodynamic theory (Müller, 1843) and the neurochronaxic theory (Husson, 1950).

The sound quality at the level of the vocal folds is best described as a buzzing sound rather than the differentiated vocal qualities that are perceived during articulation. This monotonic buzz is altered by the resonators of the speech mechanism, which modify the quality of the laryngeal buzz, but not the frequency. Voice registers are terms used to describe resonance such as chest and head. As with a number of aspects of the speech mechanism, not all is known about voice production.

Resonation

Resonation, the capacity of a resonator to vibrate optimally and change position, is the process of modifying the voiced breath stream. The resonating or vocal tract cavities (nasopharynx, oropharynx, and laryngopharynx; oral cavity; nasal cavity; and possibly the sinuses of the head), along with positional changes of the articulators, velum, epiglottis, and pharyngeal walls, bring about the changes in voice from what is produced at the level of the vocal folds to what is perceived by the listener. These cavities modify the buzzing laryngeal sound produced by the vocal folds into perceptibly different voice qualities. These resonators act as variable acoustic filters that let proportionately more acoustic energy pass at different frequencies as the speaker changes the shape of the vocal tract (Lieberman, 1977). However, no other frequencies are emitted from the mouth than those that appear at the glottis.

Resonation can also be adverse because of unfavorable coupling with another cavity. For example, if the nasal cavity is coupled too closely with the oral or pharyngeal cavities, hypernasality and nasal sound emission may result. Resonation is intricately involved with articulation since nearly all of the resonating cavities function in molding, shaping, and in other ways modifying the airstream coming from the larynx to produce articulated phonemes. Conversely disordered resonation often results in misarticulations, such as the distorted articulation that nearly always accompanies hypernasality (see Chapter 4 for more detailed discussion of this). In fact resonation and articulation are so interdependent that they are sometimes referred to as a single hyphenated process—"articulation-resonance" (Darley, 1964; Perkins, 1977).

Articulation

This process of pronouncing approximately fifty phonemes and at least half again as many phonetic combinations in contextual speech involves the use of fifteen or so movable and immovable articulators (Table 1) of the speech mechanism (Fig. 2-10) and innervation of these structures by cranial nerves V, VII, IX, X, XI, and XII. Rather than divide the speech structures into vocal tract cavities (oral, pharyngeal, nasal, and laryngeal) and articulators, we will consider all of the structures as articulators, since

Table 1. Articulators

Movable	Immovable
Cheeks	Alveolar ridge
Fauces	Hard palate
Hyoid bone	Nose
Larynx	Teeth
Lips	Sinuses
Lower jaw	
Pharynx	
Soft palate	
Uvula	
Tongue	

they are all part of the articulation system. In actuality these speech structures constitute a large part of the vegetative system; that is, these structures and muscles used in speech also have basic biologic functions of mastication (chewing) and deglutition (swallowing). A brief discussion of each articulator follows.

Movable articulators

Although not directly involved in articulation, the *cheeks* provide added stability to the sides of the oral cavity, mainly by the buccinator muscle, and contribute to the cosmetic aspects of facial expression in speech. To a minimal degree the cheeks contribute to resonation. In persons who have undergone a laryngectomy, the cheeks may play a major role if buccal speech is taught. Innervation is by cranial nerves V and VII (trigeminal and facial).

The *fauces,* or pillars of fauces as they are sometimes called, are curtains of muscle and mucosa partially separating the oral cavity from the pharyngeal cavity. The muscles of the fauces interconnect with muscles of the soft palate, pharynx, and tongue and are located on either side of the oral cavity at the back of the mouth. They function primarily in resonation but probably also influence the articulation of back vowels and velar consonants through velopharyngeal movement and control. Their lateral movement during phonation may be an indication of the amount of lateral movement of the pharyngeal walls (Darley and Spriestersbach, 1978), which is very important in achieving velopharyngeal closure. Located between the anterior and posterior fauces on each side are the tonsils. Sensory and motor innervation is provided by cranial nerve IX (glossopharyngeal).

The U-shaped *hyoid bone*, located just below the mandible, does not articulate with any other bone. Suspended by a number of muscles attached to it from above and below, this bone facilitates articulation by forward and upward movement for production of front-of-mouth sounds and upward and backward movement for production of back-of-mouth sounds. Movement of the hyoid bone is the result of contraction and relaxation of various muscles.

Although not an articulator per se, the *larynx* as a vocal tract cavity and sound generator is directly involved in the production of every voiced phoneme. In a pathologic sense it has been used as an articulator by completely obstructing the breath stream, as in stuttering and spastic dysphonia, or by partially obstructing the breath stream, as in laryngeal paresis. Abnormal presence of glottal stops among some speakers with repaired cleft palate and normal production of /h/ are other examples of the larynx functioning as an articulator. Certain dialects use the larynx as an articulator of normal glottal stops. Sensory and motor innervation is by cranial nerve X.

The *lips* are made up mainly of the orbicularis oris muscle and a composite of other muscles of the mid and lower face including the incisive, compressor, caninus, risorius, quadratus labii, zygomaticus, triangularis, platysma, and mentalis muscles. The lips are primarily responsible for the production of /p/, /b/, and /m/, are partially responsible for /f/, /v/, and other consonants and vowels requiring varying degrees of lip movements, that is, lip-rounding, lip-protrusion, lip-retraction, and are responsible for cosmetic aspects of facial expression. Because of their mobility, involvement of the lips has to be quite extreme before articulation is affected, such as in lip paralysis or severe scarring from trauma or surgical repair. Innervation of the lips is by cranial nerves V and VII.

The *lower jaw* or mandible is a facilitator of articulation and resonance. As the only movable bony articulator, excluding the hy-

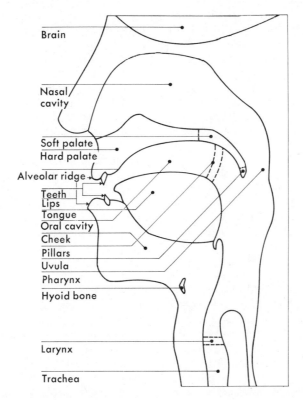

Brain

Nasal cavity

Soft palate

Hard palate

Alveolar ridge

Teeth

Lips

Tongue

Oral cavity

Cheek

Pillars

Uvula

Pharynx

Hyoid bone

Larynx

Trachea

Fig. 2-10. Speech mechanism. (From Weiss, C.: Weiss Comprehensive Articulation Test, Hingham, Mass., 1978, Teaching Resources Corp. Reproduced by permission of the publisher. All rights reserved.)

oid bone, the mandible can increase or decrease the size of the oral cavity and can facilitate tongue elevation by narrowing the vertical dimension of the mouth. However, jaw movement to assist tongue movement declines as the place of articulation moves back in the mouth (Kent and Moll, 1972). By altering the size and shape of the oral cavity, the mandible also plays a role in resonation. Although lateral movements of the mandible are also possible and necessary for mastication and deglutition, these movements, mediated by the pterygoid muscles, are not necessary for articulation. The masseter, temporalis, and pterygoid muscles are responsible for mandibular movements. Innervation is provided by cranial nerve V.

An important movable vocal tract cavity in the production of sounds is the *pharynx*. This tubelike structure is surrounded by muscles and can be divided into the hypopharynx, oropharynx, and nasopharynx or epipharynx. The epipharynx is the narrowest part of the pharynx and also the site of velopharyngeal closure. The pharynx functions in modifying resonance and in assisting the production of speech sounds. This structure serves as a variably sized resonating cavity and as an articulator for closing off the nasal cavity, with the help of the soft palate, for all but the three nasal phonemes—/m/, /n/, and /ŋ/. Velopharyngeal closure is sphincteric (circular) in nature. If the pharynx is incapable of such sphincteric closure, then speech will probably be characterized by nasal air flow on pressure consonants and hypernasality on vowels. Interestingly children have greater intraoral breath pressures than adults for production of pressure consonants (Bernthal and Beukelman, 1978). In both cases articulation is affected because the oral-nasal air flow balance is disturbed. Muscles that provide the functional capability for the pharynx include the superior, medial, and inferior constrictors, salpingopharyngeus, palatopharyngeus, and stylopharyngeus. The adenoids situated in the nasopharynx may also contribute to velopharyngeal closure in children. Sensory and motor innervation is provided by cranial nerves IX, X, and XI.

The *soft palate* or velum begins at the end of the hard palate and extends backward to the pharynx terminating at the tip of the uvula. It completes the back portion of the roof of the mouth (or floor of the nasal cavity) and is the only movable structure in the roof of the mouth. It is the site of contact for back-of-mouth phonemes—/k/, /g/, and /ŋ/—and adds the final component for adequate velopharyngeal closure necessary for all phonemes except the three nasal sounds. It contains the following muscles: levator veli palatini, tensor veli palatini, palatoglossus, palatopharyngeus, and uvulae. Damage to the soft palate or nerves that innervate it can be devastating to the production of any oral speech (see Chapter 4). Innervation is provided by cranial nerves V, IX, X, and XI.

Generally considered part of the soft palate, the *uvula* is not important to velopharyngeal closure or articulation, except perhaps in producing a "uvular trill." It has been implicated in snoring. Innervation is by cranial nerve XI.

The most important and most mobile articulator is the *tongue*. It fills a large part of the oral cavity and is the primary modifier of oral cavity configurations. Attached only on one end, it is involved in the production of the phonemes and in resonation. The basic biologic functions of the tongue are tasting, chewing, and swallowing. The tongue may be divided into tip, blade, dorsum, body, and root. It has two distinct functional parts, the anterior two thirds and the posterior one third (Fig. 2-11). It may also be divided into body and root.

The tongue consists of four intrinsic muscles (superior and inferior longitudinal, transverse, and vertical), which change the shape of the tongue and are more important to consonant production, and four extrinsic muscles (genioglossus, hyoglossus, chondroglossus, and styloglossus), which move the tongue within the oral cavity and are important to vowel production. The longitudinal muscles shorten the tongue; the transverse and vertical muscles narrow and lower the tongue mass; the hyoglossus and

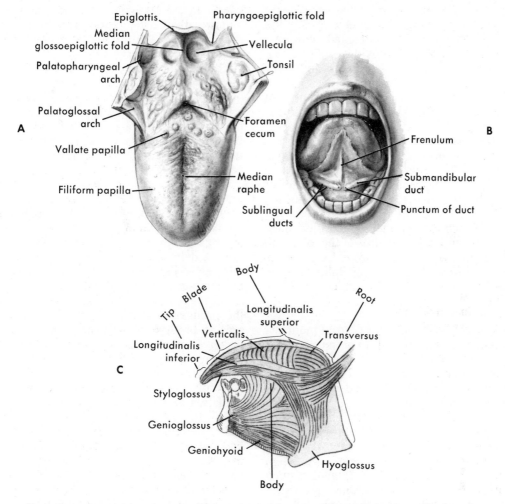

Fig. 2-11. A and **B,** Anterior two-thirds and posterior one-third of the tongue. The frenulum is shown in B. **C,** Intrinsic and extrinsic muscles of the tongue and its divisions.

chondroglossus muscles lower the back of the tongue and aid in retracting it; and the styloglossus muscle raises the tongue tip, retracts the tongue, and lateralizes it. These intrinsic and extrinsic muscles function in concert to produce speech. However, if the speaker talks too fast, some tongue positions are omitted, causing speech to become less distinct.

Perkell (1969) observed that the tongue tip is more active in consonant articulation, whereas the body of the tongue is active in articulating both consonants and vowels. Thus he suggests that the speech production mechanism is composed of two neuromuscular systems with different behavioral characteristics that respond in general to different feedback. This observation, coupled with the observed differences in velocity, complexity, precision of movement, and anatomy, suggests that different types of muscles are generally responsible for consonant production than for vowel production.

A restricting factor in tongue mobility can be the frenulum (frenum), a slip of connective tissue attached to the anterior undersurface of the tongue. If the frenulum is attached too far forward or too near the tip of the tongue, tongue-tie or ankylosis of the tongue is the result. Attached appropriately, the frenulum provides control and stability of the tongue for speech and vegetative purposes.

Since the tongue is the most important articulator, its malfunction as in paralysis, injury, or atrophy can result in severe articulation disorders. Cranial nerve XII is primarily responsible for lingual functioning in speech. This nerve provides proprioceptive or kinesthetic feedback from the anterior two thirds of the tongue to the brain and motor supply to this portion of the tongue. Cranial nerve V provides tactile feedback from the anterior two thirds of the tongue to the brain, and cranial nerve IX provides both sensory and motor capabilities to the posterior one third of the tongue.

Immovable articulators

Located behind the upper front teeth is a rough, bony surface (rugae) of the maxillary dental arch known as the *alveolar ridge*. It is this immovable structure that is either directly or indirectly involved in the front-of-mouth phonemes such as /t/, /d/, /n/, /l/, /s/, /z/, /ʃ/, /ʒ/, /tʃ/, and /dʒ/. These sounds are produced by the tongue tip contacting part or most of the alveolar ridge. The alveolar ridge is a common place of articulation and the preferred place of lingual contact during rest and during swallowing. Structural deviations, resulting from clefts or other damage to the alveolar ridge, can cause articulation problems with the phonemes mentioned above. Innervation of its mucosa is provided by cranial nerve V.

Located immediately behind the alveolar ridge is the *hard palate*. The hard palate, or roof of mouth, separates the nasal cavity from the oral cavity and includes the maxillary teeth. It extends from the alveolar ridge to the soft palate. It is lined with mucosa and serves as a passageway for the oral breath stream. The hard palate and the tongue are directly involved in the production of /r/ and /j/. The hard palate can be narrow, wide, high, or low. Any of these

conditions, if excessive or if cleft, may adversely affect articulation. Innervation of the mucosa of the hard palate is also provided by cranial nerve V.

The *nose* or nasal cavity provides the air passageway for production of /m/, /n/, and /ŋ/. It also serves as one of the resonating cavities for speech. Divided by a septum, the nasal passageways on either side must be unobstructed for normal articulation-resonance. Innervation of the mucosa of the nose is provided by cranial nerve V.

Contributing to the cosmetic as well as the articulatory aspects of speech are the *teeth*. The teeth may be deciduous (baby) or permanent, depending on the age of the person. The number and alignment of teeth vary widely among persons. The average number of deciduous teeth is twenty, and the average number of permanent teeth is about thirty-two. The teeth are important in the production of /f/, /v/, /θ/, and /ð/ and help to produce the friction quality of the fricative sounds because of the breath stream passing over the cutting edges of the incisor teeth. As with the lips, the teeth are not indispensable to essentially normal articulation in many persons because of their ability to compensate for dental malocclusions and other dental deviations (Bankson and Byrne, 1962). Other persons, however, may not be able to compensate adequately so that their articulation can be adversely affected by severe dental abnormalities. Innervation of the teeth is provided by cranial nerve V.

Although the paranasal *sinuses* are sometimes thought to be related to resonation, research has not substantiated this claim (Curry, 1940). Nevertheless, upper respiratory infections sometimes appear to alter the resonatory quality of speakers.

Excluded from the list of articulators is the ear. Since it is not an articulator per se, it was purposely omitted from Table 1. Because it is so important to speech acquisition, development, production, and perception, some mention of the auditory system appears warranted.

The *auditory mechanism* consists of the

outer ear, middle ear, inner ear, cranial nerve VIII, and auditory cortex within the temporal lobe. This mechanism has a number of parts that function together in perceiving sound. Some of the parts include the eardrum, ossicular chain of three tiny bones in the middle ear, and the cochlea, where the vibrations are transformed into electrical energy, accomplished by the shearing action of the moving hair cells therein. This neural response travels up cranial nerve VIII to the appropriate receptive area in the temporal lobe. The sense of balance is also mediated by the semicircular canals located in the inner ear.

A speaker perceives himself somewhat differently than does the listener because of differing modes of sound transmission. When speaking, some sound vibrations pass through the bones of the face and skull, as well as the outer ear, resulting in distorted perception on the part of the speaker. The listener, unlike the speaker, perceives the sound vibrations coming through the outer and middle ears, a process that is essentially distortion free. However, this distortion factor in self-perception does not seem to affect how one speaks or learns to speak, at least in most persons.

Most persons would agree that speech is learned or stimulated, to a great extent, through the sense of hearing, assuming, of course, the absence of hearing loss or auditory perceptual problems. Maintenance of normal speech may be related more to tactile and kinesthetic feedback. The hearing mechanism then is important to self-monitoring of speech, which involves auditory recognition and discrimination of distinctive and other features of speech. As such, it has an integral role in oral communication and could logically be considered an indirect articulator.

CONCLUDING REMARKS

In this chapter we have outlined the anatomy and physiology of the speech mechanism without specific reference to speech science, since most students using this text will have had courses in speech science. In this concluding section some general ideas about speech science such as acoustics and perception will be discussed because of their importance to articulation.

Acoustics of speech is defined as sound and wave qualities and characteristics that underlie the processes of speech production and speech perception. It has been described as the link between speech production and speech perception (Minifie, Hixon, and Williams, 1973). The three parameters controlling the acoustics of vowel production are vocal tract length, position of the tongue, and configuration of the lips. The latter two parameters are closely related to the acoustics of consonant production. Acoustics also involves wave motion parameters such as displacement, velocity, energy, acceleration, pressure, power, and intensity.

The acoustic aspect of speech science helps us to classify vowels and consonants as well as the special factors and features involved in speech perception. Denes and Pinson (1973) have indicated that most of the data on the acoustics of speech concern intensity levels of speech and their spectra, yet the acoustic energy of speech is very small. In fact our vocal folds utilize only a fraction of the energy from the breath stream, about one twentieth of 1%. This energy is dispersed in all directions and varies greatly within and between speakers. Thus it is not surprising that the intensity of telephone conversations varies over a range of about 100 to 1 (from 75 to 55 dB). Even someone who speaks at a normal conversational level has approximately a 700 to 1 range of intensities between the weakest and strongest speech sounds. Intensity variations from quiet to normal to loud speech range from 45 to 85 dB. Different productions of the same sound vary, as do productions of the same sound in different contexts even though the differences may be imperceptible.

Speech energy is generated roughly from 50 to 10,000 Hz with the greatest energy between 100 and 600 Hz. Vowels are the strongest sounds, generating the most energy. That is partly why they convey more "meaning" or intelligibility (understandability) than most consonants. The strongest vowel is /ɔ/ as in "bought," and the weakest vowel is /i/ as in "be." The strongest consonant is /r/ as in "red," which is 200 times as intense as the weakest consonant /θ/ as in "think." This might provide a reason why /r/ is easier to perceive than /θ/.

The spectrum of speech, which is concerned with the frequency and intensity of each harmonic of the speech wave, is important to intelligibility. It enables us to perceive sounds as being recognizably different. The most important features of the vowel spectrum are frequencies and amplitudes of the different formants. Analysis of these resonances and peaks has shown that speech is a continuously varying process and the acoustic characteristics of speech vary with time (Denes and Pinson, 1973). These aspects of speech science certainly help us to appreciate the dynamics of speech.

The chain of events that results in oral communication has been succinctly described by Denes and Pinson (1973):

The movements of the vocal organs generate a speech sound wave that travels through the air between speaker and listener. Pressure changes at the ear activate the listener's hearing mechanism and produce nerve impulses that travel along the acoustic nerve to the listener's brain. In the listener's brain a considerable amount of nerve activity is already taking place, and this activity is modified by the nerve impulses arriving from the ear. This modification of brain activity, in ways we do not fully understand, brings about recognition of the speaker's message.*

They add that in a speaker-listener situation there really are two listeners, not one, since the speaker is also engaged in self-listening while speaking.

To transmit a thought orally, the speaker begins by selecting appropriate words and

*Excerpt from *The Speech Chain: The Physics and Biology of Spoken Language* by Peter B. Denes and Elliot N. Pinson. Copyright © 1963 by Bell Telephone Laboratories, Incorporated. Reprinted by permission of Doubleday & Company, Inc.

sentences (linguistic level). Thus oral communication begins with the occurrence of neural and muscular activity (physiologic level) and is terminated by the speaker with the generation and transmission of a sound wave (physical or acoustic level). This process is reversed by the listener. How the message is interpreted by the listener depends on a number of factors, including type of phonology, vocabulary, syntax, prosodic features, and pragmatics used. Perkell (1969) describes speech events as a set of phonetic features characterized by the articulatory correlates of pressure, airflow, sound, motions and positions of vocal tract organs, and electrical activity of the musculature. There obviously are many alternative ways of looking at the sound patterns of language (Ingram, 1976) and of how they are perceived.

As we suggested earlier, differences in velocity, complexity, and precision of tongue movement suggest that different muscles are responsible for consonant and vowel productions. Vowels are produced by the larger, slower extrinsic muscles of the tongue, muscles that control general tongue position. Consonant articulation additionally requires the more precise, complex, and faster functions of the smaller, intrinsic tongue muscles. Hence the speech mechanism, insofar as the tongue is concerned, appears to be composed of two neuromuscular systems (extrinsic and intrinsic neuromuscular systems of the tongue) responding to different feedback (Perkell, 1969).

Closely related to the acoustics of speech is *speech perception*. Several theories of speech perception have been postulated, one of which is the motor theory of speech perception. According to this theory, the listener perceives speech by matching the incoming signal against an internally generated signal. However, this theory does not necessarily imply that the same neural mechanisms that control speech production also control speech perception; it also does not seem to explain all the facts of speech perception. There appear to be innately determined neural property detectors that respond to specific acoustic signals (Lieberman, 1977). Some listeners respond to bursts in speech, whereas others respond to formant transitions. Moreover, some theories are more plausible for consonants than for vowels, such as the traditional articulation-based phonetic theory. Lindau, Jacobson, and Ladefoged (1972) concluded that tongue contours for several vowels are nearly identical. These slight differences in tongue contour cannot be the factors that differentiate these vowels and certain other sounds. The acoustic differences that differentiate these sounds must be the functional result of the total supralaryngeal tract area.

Regardless of the perceptual theory advocated or refuted, some common factors related to speech perception are present. First the dominant hemisphere of the brain, usually the left, is more involved in speech perception than in nonspeech perception. This is substantiated by the fact that there are greater electrical potentials recorded in the left hemisphere during perception of speech signals. Second, although discrimination and identification of speech are quite different, both are integrally involved in the perceptual aspects of oral communication. Third the phonetic features are differentially perceived (Jakobson, Fant, and Halle, 1963; Chomsky and Halle, 1968). That is, the distinctive features of the cardinal vowels (see Chapter 3) are more readily distinguishable than the features of some of the intermediate vowels. Fourth prosodic features such as breath group and cadence pattern, coarticulation, and the duration and intensity of speech sounds also affect their perception. Fifth the nature of some vowels are much more likely to be auditory than articulatory (Lindau, Jacobson, and Ladefoged, 1972), because normal adult speakers actually make use of different articulatory maneuvers to effect similar phonetic contrasts. Likewise consonant stops are variably produced by having a range from an airtight intraoral seal to a somewhat open intraoral configuration, and the presence of nasal airflow may be perceptible or imperceptible. Even though we cannot precisely separate a consonant from a vowel in context, we can hear both components. Finally, if sounds are transmitted and put together at a rate of twenty to thirty segments per second, and the fastest rate at which we can identify sounds is approximately seven to nine segments per second, how is speech perceived? Speech sounds would have to be compressed into an indivisible composite so that they are perceived, produced, and perhaps programmed on a nonsegmental basis, perhaps in syllable units. Also important to speech perception are speech context, our expectations of what will be spoken, knowledge and familiarity of the communication to which we are listening, and characteristics relating to speaker identity.

As with the acoustics and perception of speech, the *production of speech* is likewise complex and not entirely understood. Much more research has to be done before we can fully explain how the characteristics of the produced sounds depend on vocal tract configurations. Speech production includes the generation of variably noisy sounds within the vocal tract and the selective modification of these sounds by resonance characteristics of the vocal tract (Minifie, Hixon, and Williams, 1973). These sounds may or may not have one sound source. An example of a sound having more than one sound source is /z/. Sounds may or may not be voiced and have varying times of voice onset.

Much more could be said about such parameters as coarticulation, pressure control, respiratory programming for speech, functioning of the muscle spindle system, physiology of the subglottal, laryngeal, and supralaryngeal vocal tract, and timing factors, to mention but a few. However, additional information on these subjects can be found in the references cited at the end of this chapter.

SUMMARY

Respiration, phonation, resonation, and articulation constitute the primary processes involved in speech production. These processes, along with the functions of the innervation systems, must interact and interrelate in a synergistic manner for normal speech to occur. Although speech production and perception place greater demands on some of these processes than on others, all systems must be basically intact in order for speech to develop and be used intelligibly. Respiration, if adequate for sustaining life, usually will provide an adequate energy source for setting the vocal folds into vibration and for transmitting their vibrations. Normal phonation requires normal functioning of the vocal folds, which includes normal laryngeal structures, innervation, and aerodynamic function. Resonance relies on selective filtering or modification of the vocal tract cavities. These cavity configurations, along with the tonus (normal state of continuous slight tension of the muscles) of their walls modifies the laryngeal buzz into usually acceptable voice quality. Articulation, the last major process, includes the modification of the vocal tract by partially or completely interrupting the flow of breath to produce the distinctively different sounds in our language. These four processes work together with the innervation systems to mediate speech and, therefore, can be considered the anatomy and physiology of the speech mechanism.

STUDY SUGGESTIONS

1. In what way is articulation an "overlaid" function? How may this relate to articulation disorders?
2. Explore the meaning and implications of the statement that "Articulation is a relatively late development in the history of human development."
3. Relate the need for an understanding of anatomy and physiology of speech to diagnosis and treatment of disordered articulation.
4. If a lesion involving cranial nerve XII has been medically established, how might a knowledge of the functions of that nerve aid the speech-language diagnostician to anticipate certain kinds of articulation disorders? Cranial nerve IX? Others?
5. Explain why some clinical experts prefer to link articulation and resonance together

as one hyphenated label for both processes.
6. How do the nervous systems function in the production and perception of speech?
7. What are some of the activities important to speech that occur in each hemisphere of the brain?

REFERENCES

Abbs, J.: The influence of the gamma motor system on jaw movements during speech, Ph.D. thesis, University of Wisconsin, 1971.

Ajuriaguerra, J.: Speech disorders in childhood. In Carterette, E., editor: Brain function, Berkeley, Calif., 1966, University of California Press.

Bankson, N., and Byrne, M.: The relationship between missing teeth and selected consonant sounds, J. Speech Hear. Disord. 27:341-348, 1962.

Barr, M.: The human nervous system, ed. 2, Hagerstown, Md., 1974, Harper & Row, Publishers.

Bernthal, J., and Beukelman, D.: Intraoral air pressure generated during the production of /p/ and /b/ by children, youths, and adults, J. Speech Hear. Disord. 21:361-371, 1978.

Berry, M.: Language disorders of children: the basis and diagnoses, New York, 1969, Appleton-Century-Crofts.

Carpenter, M.: Human neuroanatomy, Baltimore, 1978, The Williams & Wilkins Co.

Chomsky, N., and Halle, M.: The sound pattern of English, New York, 1968, Harper & Row, Publishers.

Chusid, J., and McDonald, J.: Correlative neuroanatomy and functional neurology, Los Altos, Calif., 1967, Lange Medical Publications.

Coppoletta, J., and Wolbach, S.: Body length and organ weights of infants and children, Am. J. Pathol. 9:55-70, 1933.

Crafts, R.: A textbook of human anatomy, New York, 1966, The Ronald Press.

Curry, R.: The mechanism of the human voice, New York, 1940, Longmans Green and Co., Inc.

Darley, F.: Diagnosis and appraisal of communication disorders, Englewood Cliffs, N.J., 1964, Prentice-Hall, Inc.

Darley, F., and Spriestersbach, D.: Diagnostic methods in speech pathology, ed. 2, New York, 1978, Harper & Row, Publishers.

Darley, F., Aronson, A., and Brown, J.: Motor speech disorders, Philadelphia, 1975, W. B. Saunders Co.

Denes, P., and Pinson, E.: The speech chain, Bell Telephone Laboratories, Indianapolis, Ind., 1973.

Eccles, J.: The neurophysiological basis of mind, London, 1953, Oxford Press.

Egolf, D., and Chester, S.: Nonverbal communication and the disorders of speech and language, ASHA 15:511-518, 1973.

Espir, M., and Rose, C.: The basic neurology of speech, Philadelphia, 1970, F. A. Davis Co.

Gardner, E.: Fundamentals of neurology, ed. 6, Philadelphia, 1975, W. B. Saunders Co.

Gray, H.: Anatomy of the human body, Philadelphia, 1959, Lea & Febiger.

Husson, R.: Etude des phénomènes physiologiques et acoustique fondamentale de la voix chantie, Thesis presented in Paris, 1950.

Ingram, D.: Phonological disability in children, London, 1976, Edward Arnold.

Jakobson, R., Fant, G., and Halle, M.: Preliminaries to speech analysis, Cambridge, Mass., 1963, The M.I.T. Press.

Johnson, W., Darley, F., and Spriestersbach, D.: Diagnostic methods in speech pathology, New York, 1963, Harper & Row, Publishers.

Judson, L., and Weaver, A.: Voice science, ed. 2, New York, 1965, Appleton-Century-Crofts.

Kaplan, H.: Anatomy and physiology of speech, New York, 1960, McGraw-Hill Book Co.

Kaplan, H.: Anatomy and physiology of speech, ed. 2, New York, 1971, McGraw-Hill Book Co.

Kent, R., and Moll, K.: Cinefluorographic analyses of selected lingual consonants, J. Speech Hear. Disord. **15:**453-473, 1972.

Lieberman, P.: Speech physiology and acoustic phonetics, New York, 1977, Macmillan Publishing Co., Inc.

Lillywhite, H.: General concepts of communication, J. Pediatr. **62:**5-10, 1963.

Lillywhite, H., and Bradley, D.: Communication problems in mental retardation: diagnosis and management, New York, 1969, Harper & Row, Publishers.

Lindau, M., Jacobson, L., and Ladefoged, P.: The feature advanced tongue root, UCLA Phonetics Laboratory, Working Papers in Phonetics **22:**76-94, 1972.

McDonald, E., and Chance, B.: Cerebral palsy, Englewood Cliffs, N.J., 1964, Prentice-Hall, Inc.

Minifie, F., Hixon, T., and Williams, F., editors: Normal aspects of speech, hearing, and language, Englewood Cliffs, N.J., 1973, Prentice-Hall, Inc.

Müller, J.: Von Stimme und sprache. In Hülscher, J.: Handbuch der Physiologie des Menschen für Vorlesunge, Coblenz, Germany, 1843, vol. 2.

Negus, V.: The comparative anatomy and physiology of the larynx, New York, 1949, Grune & Stratton, Inc.

Noback, C.: The human nervous system, New York, 1967, McGraw-Hill Book Co.

Paff, G.: Anatomy of the head and neck, Philadelphia, 1973, W. B. Saunders Co.

Palmer, J.: Anatomy for speech and hearing, ed. 2, New York, 1972, Harper & Row, Publishers.

Penfield, W., and Rasmussen, T.: The cerebral cortex of man: a clinical study of localization of function, New York, 1950, Macmillan Publishing Co., Inc.

Penfield, W., and Roberts, L.: Speech and brain mechanisms, Princeton, N.J., 1959, Princeton University Press.

Perkell, J.: Physiology of speech production: results and implications of a quantitative cineradiographic study, Cambridge, Mass., 1969, The M.I.T. Press.

Perkins, W. H.: Speech pathology: an applied behav-ioral science, ed. 2, St. Louis, 1977, The C. V. Mosby Co.

Sperry, R.: Neurology and the mind-brain problem. In Isaacson, R., editor: Basic readings in neuropsychology, New York, 1964, Harper & Row, Publishers.

Van Riper, C., and Irwin, J.: Voice and articulation, Englewood Cliffs, N.J., 1958, Prentice-Hall, Inc.

West, R., and Ansberry, M.: The rehabilitation of speech, ed. 4, New York, 1968, Harper & Row, Publishers.

Zemlin, W.: Speech and hearing science, Englewood Cliffs, N.J., 1968, Prentice-Hall, Inc.

GLOSSARY

adducting Parts of the body pulling toward each other, such as the vocal folds moving toward approximation at the midline.

afferent Nerves that conduct sensory impulses inward toward the spinal cord or brain.

agnosia Inability to recognize or understand incoming stimuli (afferent) to the brain by one or more of the sensory modalities, such as vision, audition, and taction.

anarthria Inability to articulate because of neuromuscular involvement of the articulators.

anastomose To open one into the other, such as one artery opening into another.

aphasia Loss of ability to comprehend verbal symbols or to speak as a result of central nervous system damage or deterioration.

aphonia Inability to produce voice; lack of voice or phonation.

arrhythmic Absence of normal rhythm of speech.

ataxia Irregularity or lack of muscular coordination that usually interferes with articulation and sometimes body balance.

bifurcate Divide into two.

bilateral Both sides, two sided.

cerebral peduncle A stalklike bundle of nerves connecting various parts of the cerebrum.

choreiform Involuntary irregular movements.

coccygeal Pertaining to the coccyx or small bone at the end of the spinal column.

cochlear Pertaining to the cochlea or spiral-shaped, auditory portion of the inner ear.

colliculi Small elevations on the midbrain structures of the brain.

convoluted surface A surface of the brain that appears to be coiled or rolled together.

decussation The crossing or intersecting of nerve tracts.

deglutition Swallowing.

diplopia Seeing a single object as double or two.

dorsal Back, behind, or dorsum.

dysarthria Articulation disorder caused by a

neuromuscular involvement of the articulators.

dysphagia Difficulty in swallowing resulting from injury, inflammation, or other problems with the esophagus and vegetative tract.

dysphonia Partial loss of ability to voice or phonate sounds.

effector A nerve end-organ that distributes incoming impulses from the brain to the periphery; from inside toward outside.

eustachian tube Small tube between the middle ear and the upper pharynx serving to equalize air pressure in the middle ear with the outside.

extrinsic muscle Muscle originating outside the structure with which it is involved.

facial anesthesia Lack of feeling or movement of a portion of the face.

flaccidity Pertaining to weak, lax, or flabby muscle tone.

hemianopia, hemianopsia Blindness in one half of the field of vision in one or both eyes.

hemiplegia Paralysis of one side of the body.

homunculus A very small model of a human body used to illustrate sensory representation of body parts on the cortex.

hypotonia Diminished muscle tone or flaccidity.

imprinting Impressions (imprints) of physiologic patterns of bodily activity on the brain and neural pathways.

intrinsic muscle A muscle originating and functioning entirely within the structure with which it is involved, such as an intrinsic muscle of the tongue.

kinesthetic The "muscle sense" by which motion, weight, and position are perceived.

lacrimation The secretion of tears.

lumbar The body region pertaining to the loins, or the part of the back and sides between the ribs and pelvis.

mandibular Pertaining to the lower jaw, or mandible.

mastication The act of chewing.

maxillary Pertaining to the upper jaw, or maxilla.

myoelastic-aerodynamic theory A theory relating the process of phonation to airflow and elasticity of the laryngeal muscles.

neural patterning The imprinting of physiologic patterns of bodily activity on neural pathways.

neurochronaxic theory A theory relating the process of phonation to the excitation and conduction of nerve impulses.

neurophysiology Physiology of the nervous system.

nystagmus Involuntary, rapid movements of the eyeball in any of several directions.

ontogenetic Pertaining to the developmental history of the organism.

ophthalmic Pertaining to the eye.

overlaid function Structures and processes of the body that perform functions secondary to their main purposes, such as the tongue being used for speech even though its primary functions are taste, mastication, and deglutition.

paresis Slight or incomplete paralysis.

phylogenetic Pertaining to the biologic history of a race.

phylogenetic neophyte A latecomer in the biologic history of the race.

proprioception Body information concerning movements and body position provided by sensory nerve terminals chiefly within muscles, tendons, joints, and the labyrinth. This term is sometimes used interchangeably with kinesthesis.

ptosis Usually used to refer to drooping of the upper eyelid, but may refer to prolapse of a body part.

receptor A sensory nerve ending that responds to various kinds of stimuli, such as touch and taste.

rigidity Stiffness and inflexibility, usually of the limbs, as with hemiplegia or other forms of spasticity.

sacral Pertaining to or situated near the sacrum, which is a part of the lower spinal column.

servosystem A sensory feedback system, such as cranial nerve XII, which provides kinesthetic feedback from the tongue allowing monitoring of tongue function in articulation.

spasticity A form of cerebral palsy characterized by hypertonicity of the muscles making movements stiff and awkward.

sphincteric Pertaining to a ringlike muscle or group of muscles that narrows a natural orifice, such as the pharynx in velopharyngeal closure.

strabismus Abnormal deviations of the eye that the individual cannot control.

synergistic Pertaining to correlated action or cooperation on the parts of two or more structures to achieve a unified function.

tinnitus Noises or ringing in the ear, which may be associated with Meniere's disease.

tympanic Referring to the membrane (eardrum) between the outer and middle ear.

unilateral One side; single-sided function or activity.

vegetative Basic, involuntary biologic functions of the organism.

velopharyngeal closure Closure of the nasal port

by synergistic action of the velum and the upper pharynx to direct the airstream into the oral cavity.

ventral Pertaining to the belly; toward the belly. It may also refer to anterior or front as opposed to dorsal or back.

vermis The narrow connecting mass of fibers between the two cerebral hemispheres.

vertigo A sensation of seeming to revolve in space or having things revolve around the individual. This term is sometimes erroneously used as a synonym for dizziness.

vestibular Pertaining to the vestibule, or the oval cavity of the inner ear, forming the approach to the cochlea.

visceral Pertaining to the cavities and organs of the abdomen, thorax, and pelvis.

CHAPTER THREE

Acquisition and development of speech

"A child, when it begins to speak, learns what it is that it knows."
WHEELOCK

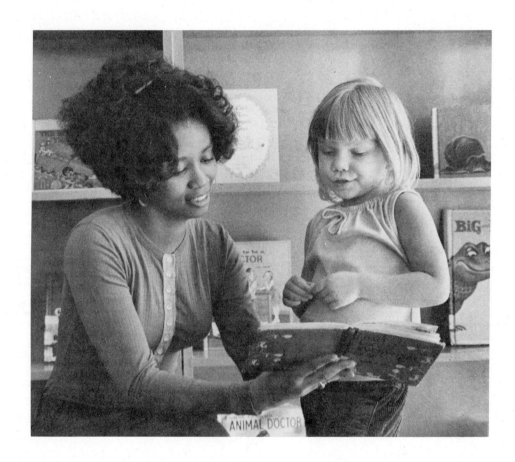

The answers to three questions are critical to an understanding of speech: (1) What is speech? (2) How did speech originally occur in human beings? (3) How does speech develop in the child? The first question may be answered in several ways: as the phonologic component of an established oral communication system; as a series of individual phonemes intricately blended and sequenced to form words; as a vehicle for conveying language; as a part of resonance and language; as a composite of arbitrary symbols produced by structures and muscles not originally intended for communication; and as vocal tract movements or adjustments, air turbulence, constriction, or interruption of the breath stream (Perkins, 1977). In this book we will refer to speech, articulation, and phonology interchangeably as the production and perception of speech sounds in meaningful units and their rules mediated by the bodily systems and the structures referred to as the articulators.

Because the speech structures are simultaneously responsible for speech and resonance characteristics and because resonator adjustments are an unavoidable consequence of speech movements, Darley (1964) considered speech and resonance as being inseparable aspects of oral communication. Speech may also be viewed as a learned behavior, social phenomenon, novel response, oral gesture, and a means of establishing interpersonal relations, maintaining emotional homeostasis, and manipulating human behavior (Simon, 1957). Speech is unique because of its late ontogeny, because it is exclusive to human beings and different from other forms of human behavior, and because it utilizes a symbol system.

Answers as to how speech evolved and developed are not as easily formulated. Attempts to explain the origin of speech and language have been recorded almost since the beginning of written symbolization (Lillywhite, 1963). Like all theoretic discussions of important topics, the range has been wide and sometimes very near the boundaries of imagination. Nevertheless, theories appear mutually inclusive, overlapping, and similar; they may vary in gestalt, emphasis, purpose, and etiologic philosophy. Some theories seem to explain only a part of communication; others ignore language (as opposed to speech) as a means of human intercourse. And some are based on the assumption that up to the emergence of oral communication, human beings had remained silent, which is highly improbable from a physiologic or psychologic point of view (Jespersen, 1922). Humans would not have had an oral communication system already perfected on the first occasion of its use. It is only by use that a system such as oral communication can be developed and refined. Nevertheless, inherent in most theories is some developmental order and ideas for remediating articulation disorders, not to mention attempts at simply satisfying curiosities of how oral communication might have evolved, even though we may never know how communication was acquired and developed. A brief review of theories follows.

BEHAVIORAL THEORIES OF ACQUISITION

Theories on phonologic acquisition and development can be divided into two major categories: (1) behavioral theories and (2) psycholinguistic theories. Philosophically these two categories are not mutually exclusive. They tend to signify differences in the time the theories originated and their respective emphases. These categories also differ in that behavioral theories, generally defined, seem to explain phonologic acquisition better, whereas psycholinguistic theories appear to provide better insights into phonologic development.

Included in this rather broad behavioral category is a range of theories from Divine Origin to vocal play. Aside from the Divine Origin theory, generally these theories suggest the acquisition of speech as a need for social intercourse, facilitation of group living, and pleasure in oral expressions that are appropriately reinforced. These behavioral theories may not be as specific as some of the more recent theories on phonologic development, and they are not particularly concerned with order of acquisition and development.

Divine Origin theory

Among the earliest theories is the Divine Origin or religious theory. This theory suggests that speech occurred as a miraculous, divine phenomenon, along with the creation of the first man, Adam. The ability or capacity for oral communication was an integral attribute of divinely created human beings according to this theory. Proponents of this theory may query, "How else could such a complex behavior have evolved?" However, almost every other recorded theory has considered the probability of external circumstances creating a need for communication.

Learning theory

A major and quite inclusive theory of speech acquisition and development presupposes learning. Advocates of this theory state that since speech is a learned behavior, it is acquired through practice, training, and experience. If learning can be defined as a change in behavior and perception as a consequence of experience not dependent on, but sometimes related to, maturation, then the learning theory may provide a valid explanation, in part, of how speech developed.

Inherent in this theory is the need to communicate. This theory also necessitates the occurrence of imitating, practicing, experiencing, conditioning, and reinforcing behavior. Implicit in learning is some form of teaching, often indirect and unconscious. Speech could not have initially been learned without the process of teaching, regardless of how crude teaching may have been, according to this theory. The teaching may have been no more than the simple unconscious repitition of sounds for the listener (learner) to hear, which may describe how much of speech is "taught" today. The fact that speech has been taught quite directly

and successfully by speech-language pathologists for decades and by parents more indirectly for centuries makes this theory plausible.

Unfortunately learning connotes different things to different people. It has been defined in several different ways, perhaps reflecting the myriad types of learning—short term, long term, verbal, nonverbal, concrete, and abstract. Hilgard (1943) mentioned ten different theories on how learning occurs, most of which have since been modified. Suffice to say that the extent and manner in which learning contributed to the evolution of speech may never be known. It is a major philosophy from which other theories have evolved and a widely accepted theory in regard to the acquisition and development of communication in modern times and the remediation of all types of communication disorders.

Social need theory

Also called the social pressure theory, this theory was developed by Smith (1792). It states that primitive human beings (*Java* or *Pithecanthropus erectus*), when confronted by the necessity for making wants known, would utter certain sounds to designate familiar objects. Repetition of these utterances eventually resulted in the consistent use of "words." Proponents of this theory indicate that speech evolved out of social necessity, which is closely related to many aspects of speech acquisition and development in the modern child.

Effect theory

The effect theory, also referred to as the association theory, is similar to the social need theory. This theory suggests that responses are learned or imprinted because of their effect or need to be learned. But why did these verbal responses, that is, speech, need to be learned? The answers may well be because they were reinforcing. McGeoch (1943) stated that reinforcing stimuli are reinforcing because they satisfy some internal or external need. The social need theory explains the external need for communication. But what is the internal need? A logical explanation is offered by Hull (1943). He theorized that needs arise from inside and outside the body and that because the body is continually striving to satisfy needs (such as the need for self-expression), in order to maintain equilibrium or homeostasis, responses occur. The successful maintenance of systemic and environmental equilibrium increases the possibility of those responses recurring, hence the continual development and use of oral communication.

Contiguity theory

The contiguity or field theory is a more contemporary derivation of original learning theories. This theory stresses the importance of motivation and reinforcement. To most behavioral scientists, motivation and reinforcement not only are important in learning, but they also achieve behavioral changes because they cause responses to occur. One could assume that *Pithecanthropus erectus,* who existed about 1 million years ago, probably was motivated to talk, if not also reinforced for doing so.

Unlike the effect theory, the contiguity theory considers motivation to talk and not the effect of talking as being responsible for the evolution of communication. Speech developed because it was elicited through motivation and reinforcement and not because of the need to communicate. In considering this theory, one might ask if reinforcement is necessary for learning to occur. Does learning occur as a result of immediate or delayed reinforcement? Could reinforcement interfere with learning? What are the similarities among the contiguity theory, classical conditioning, and operant philosophies?

Innate theory

Sapir (1921) stated that speech is an acquired, "cultural" function. However, for speech to be learned, the rudiments of an innate communication system must be present waiting to become stimulated or activated. Lieberman (1977) and Stampe (1969) have supported the innate theory. These proponents say that human beings are born with the element of a communication system but that if the system is not appropriately activated or if the system is congenitally defective, normal communication may not occur. Thus this theory requires the addition of activating stimuli ("teaching") in order to explain the development of speech.

Onomatopoetic theory

This theory, sometimes referred to as the echoic or bow-wow theory, suggests that speech developed out of human beings' imitation of the sounds around them, such as animal noises, the murmur of a brook, and the crash of a tree. Primitive words were imitations of these sounds. Human beings imitated the barking of dogs and thereby developed a word that meant dog or bark (Jespersen, 1922). Müller (1840), however, stated that it is absurd to think that humans would imitate inferiors when he wrote, "The Onomatopoetic Theory goes very smoothly as long as it deals with cackling hens and quacking ducks; but around that poultry yard there is a high wall, and we soon find that it is behind that wall that language really begins." We are inclined to agree with Müller that this theory would not appear to explain fully the origin and development of communication, although the role of imitation, as in babbling, may be very important for later "deferred imitations" (the ability to retain a speech model for imitation at a future time) (Piaget, 1962).

Interjectional theory

A modification of the onomatopoetic theory is the interjectional, pooh-pooh, or work theory. This theory states that human beings not only imitated the sounds around them but that these sounds were modified by such vocalizations as cries of pain, anger, and pleasure accompanied frequently by gestures. These "interjections" were modified to take on a meaning beyond the original emotional states that produced them. Whitney (1868) suggested that human beings used their voices to give "signs" to their ideas (sign theory). Voice was the preferred modality because it appeared to be the most convenient mechanism to use. Jespersen (1922) stated that when contempt, disgust, surprise, pain, astonishment, and other intense sensations or feelings are accompanied by a tendency to exhale air from the mouth or nose, this produced sounds like "pooh or pish." He added that interjections are the negation of language. They occur when one cannot or will not speak. Besides, interjections often contain phonemes not used in language, that is, nonvoiced vowels, inspiratory sounds, and clicks. An accidental interjection may have been the primordium of communication development, but not much more.

Phonetic type theory

This theory, also called the theory of roots or nativistic theory, is based on the proposition that everything that is struck "rings" and that each substance has its own peculiar "ring." Müller (1840) thought that human beings had their own peculiar "ring" and that within humans were "roots" or typical sounds (phonemes). Under sufficient stimulation these typical sounds were "rung" from the human organism, such as the ring of a bell produced by striking it. It was only natural that this was called the ding dong theory by those not overly impressed with its significance.

Noire (1891) elaborated the idea of "roots" with the explanation that whenever a person extended a forcible emission of breath the vocal folds were made to vibrate and phonated sounds resulted. These sounds came to be recognized as having some peculiar "phonetic type," consistency, and symbolic meaning. In spite of Noire's support, however, Müller later abandoned this theory.

Gesture theory

Also called the oral gesture theory, this theory indicates that primitive communication consisted originally of gesture and pantomime but that there must have been vocalizations too. Wundt (1897) assumed that humans eventually discovered the utility of vocal communication over gesture and thus vocalization developed as a more meaningful method of transferring ideas. Piaget (1962) contended that as human beings developed tools that required the use of hands, there was a greater need for oral gesture. This oral gesture (vocalization) eventually came to have consistency and meaning. Modern communication continues to incorporate a considerable number of gestures.

Vocal play theory

This theory proposed by Jespersen (1922) maintains that language developed out of the "poetic side of life." His delightful contention was that primitive human beings must have indulged in more or less extended periods of dancing and lovemaking. Out of the exultation of these activities and perhaps primitive chanting or song, language was born in the courting days of mankind. Interestingly this explanation relates rather closely to the belief in the necessity for a child to experience considerable pleasure from vocalizing (babbling) before developing a language adequate for communication. Some of the prosodic features of communication may also have evolved from vocal play.

Yo-heave-ho theory

This theory, also called the work theory, postulates that vocalization occurred originally during work. Under any strong muscular effort it is a relief to the system to let breath come out strongly and repeatedly, causing the vocal folds to vibrate in different ways, thus producing sound. When primitive acts such as group work were performed in common, they would naturally be accompanied with some sounds that were eventually associated with the idea of the act performed and became a name for that act. The first words that may have occurred accidentally were associated with "heave" or "haul," thus "yo-heave-ho."

Novel response theory

An interesting concept regarding the development of communication is that it occurred because oral communication was considered a novel (original or different) response. Such an accidental form of behavior could have been considered a novel act that was encouraged and rewarded. Vocalizations by infants (vocal play) are still rewarded as novel behavior and often are encouraged and rewarded.

Social control theory

DeLaguna (1927) accepted the existence of vocal expressions in primitive human beings. She attempted to find a motive for the transition from these primitive, concrete expressions to the complex languages that we now know. She thought that language must have developed out of the necessity for group cooperation for purposes of survival. As humans found it necessary to band together to defend themselves, to gather food, and to make tools, it was necessary to be able to command, describe, and predict by means of complex verbal symbols. Note the similarity between this theory of development of language and its development in the modern child. In both cases oral communication develops as a means to control, in a systematic way, the behavior of others toward oneself (Lillywhite, 1963).

PSYCHOLINGUISTIC THEORIES OF DEVELOPMENT

Of more recent origin are the psycholinguistic theories of phonologic development related more to speech acquisition in the child than how it may have developed in the human race. At least three major theories have attempted to explain the development of speech. They are the (1) structural, (2) natural, and (3) prosodic theories (Ferguson and Garnica, 1975).

Structural theory

Structural theory contends that phonologic development occurs through the establishment of predictable series of sound contrasts (Jakobson, 1968; Chomsky and Halle, 1968). This process of learning contrasts rather than individual sounds has set the stage for rather new areas of research. Structuralists advocate an orderly sequenced, innately generated phonologic process rather than acquisition as a modification of the adult phonologic processes. They think that acquisition and development of distinctive features is a universal process, one that is fixed in its order of acquisition, but not necessarily in its rate of acquisition.

Natural theory

Natural theory emphasizes the presence of an innate set of hierarchically structured orderly processes that simplify adult words (Stampe, 1969; Smith, 1973). This theory focuses on the adult word, which the child is constantly attempting to produce by a process of simplification, rather than the child having a phonologic system of his own. The importance of generating internal phonologic rules (Ingram, 1976; McNeill, 1970), also referred to as generative phonology, stresses rule behavior orientation necessary to transform adult speech to child speech.

Prosodic theory

Prosodic theory (Waterson, 1971) suggests that phonologic development is achieved through the process of perceiving prosodic features of speech rather than specific speech sounds. Thus the child acquires speech by perceiving crucial prosodic cues in adult speech and then tries to duplicate these prosodic features. It is conceivable that the young child perceives and acquires these suprasegmental features before acquiring features of speech sounds.

Much of modern linguistic theory suggests that children creatively construct their language in accordance with innate and intrinsic capacities (Slobin, 1973) and that they have a communication system of their own and not one that is a direct copy of the adult systems. Psycholinguists (Lenneberg and Lenneberg, 1975) further postulate the existence of complex, genetically programmed perceptual and cognitive mechanisms that develop neither through reinforcement nor by imitation. Precisely how rules and contrastive features of oral communication are learned remains to be answered.

Additional theories, not only on the original development of speech but also on the present learning of speech, or parts thereof, exist, such as the autism theory, inventory theory, emergence theory, motor theory, and cultural acquisition theory. Since these theories are not exclusive of the theories already discussed, no additional mention will be made.

In response to the initial question of how oral communication came about, a precise, definitive answer is obviously not possible. An indefinite, eclectic theoretic answer must prevail for now. It seems plausible that the initial acquisition of oral communication, possibly like much of the oral communication development in any child, has occurred as the combined result of any or all of the aspects proposed in the various theories: need, learning, reinforcement, gesture, novelty, control, work, play, imitation, innate potential, divine assistance, and perhaps also accident. With the presently renewed interest in child phonology (Ferguson and Farwell, 1975; Ingram, 1976; Moskowitz, 1970; Smith, 1973; and Stampe, 1969), answers to the existing unknowns of speech development, and even speech acquisition, may eventually be found.

PHONOLOGIC SYSTEM

There has been little research to determine the general stages of phonologic development (Ingram, 1976). Therefore, few definitive statements can be made concerning how and when speech develops in the child. The following discussion will begin with a review of the phonetics of speech and conclude with the stages of phonologic development (phonemics of speech). Both processes must be considered in the total management of persons with defective articulation.

There are approximately fifty sounds in General American English that comprise our phonetic system. However, the number will vary from regional dialect to regional dialect, from phonetician to phonetician, from discipline to discipline, from classification system to classification system, and, in some cases, from speaker to speaker. These sounds, or speech segments, are traditionally indicated by symbols of the International Phonetic Alphabet (IPA), although other symbol systems have been used (Gleason, 1961).

Phonemes, simply described by Carrell (1968) as "The building blocks out of which meaningful or grammatically functional forms are composed" are the differentially used sounds in oral language. McDonald (1964) further states that a phoneme is not an entity, but rather a class, group, or family of similar sounds or allophones that are phonetically similar and show characteristic patterns of distribution. These allophones, which are subtle, systematic, acceptable variations in pronunciation of a phoneme, typically vary so little acoustically that they remain part of the phoneme family, such as an aspirated /k/ still being an acceptable allophone of the phoneme /k/. Allophones are noncontrastive or nondistinctive; they do not change the meaning of a word. Irwin (1972) gives good illustrations of how sounds vary even though meaning does not change (that is, aspirated /p/ in "pin" and nonaspirated /p/ in "spin"). If there is a change in meaning because of how the sound is produced, then the feature of that production is contrastive or distinctive. No change in meaning indicates a noncontrastive or nondistinctive feature, as in the examples just cited. If the allophones of a particular phoneme were to vary considerably, they would probably no longer be acceptable variations of that phoneme but would most likely become allophones of another phoneme. Technically speaking, no two sounds or pronunciations are exactly alike, although they may seem to be because our auditory discriminative abilities are not sensitive enough to perceive the subtle allophonic differences.

A phoneme is a family of phonetically similar sounds. Phonemes contrast with one another in order to differentiate the meaning of spoken words (Tiffany and Carrell, 1977). Thus a phoneme, or phonemic unit, is semantically distinctive. It denotes "meaning," which is the key word in this explanation. Contrasting pairs or minimal pairs are good examples of how one sound can change the meaning of otherwise similar words, such as "pat" and "bat." Phonetics, then, may be described as the study of the science of speech sounds without regard to meaning, and phonemics is the study of the science of speech sounds with regard to meaning (Stetson, 1951). Phonetics may also be considered the motoric aspect of articulation, whereas phonemics is the linguistic aspect of articulation, which further complicates the problem of trying to discuss articulation as a process separate from language.

Phonemes are used to represent all possible phonetic productions, acceptable or unacceptable, by every possible speaker of every possible phoneme. They are the smallest perceptible unit of nonmeaningful oral language. This is not to be confused with the term "morpheme," which is the irreducible unit of meaningful speech (Winitz, 1969). Similarly allophones refer to all possible acceptable variations in the production of a phoneme. Phones represent sounds that may or may not be produced correctly, such as variations of the lateral /s/. Misarticulated phones are called malphones. As Tiffany and Carrell (1977) point out, the use of the word "phoneme" to indicate a misarticulated sound is semantically incorrect; a misarticulation should be referred to as a misarticulated phone or malphone rather than a misarticulated phoneme.

The following basic considerations are important to the discussion of our phonetic system (Judson and Weaver, 1965): (1) speech sounds are produced by structures that are part of the vegetative system; (2) speech sounds are perceived by the auditory mechanism; (3) speech sounds are symbol units; (4) speech sounds are learned; (5) speech sounds are influenced by forces that work to produce variation, such as duration, rate, and stress; and (6) speech sounds are influenced by forces that work to prevent variation such as auditory, tactile, and kinesthetic feedback. These considerations coupled with the fact that articulation consists of (1) fixed, (2) guided, and (3) ballistic movements lay the foundation for analyzing and describing phonemes, allophones, and phones (McDonald, 1964). However, caution should be used in generalizing from isolated speech samples such as phonemes, syllables, and isolated words to contextual speech. Also, speech movements really cannot be described as specific events or as containing exact articulator placements for individual sounds. Concepts such as overlapping movements (p. 69) (Shohara, 1964), assimilation (p. 68) (Stetson, 1951), abutting consonants (p. 68) (McDonald, 1964), coarticulation (p. 68) (Winitz, 1969), and ellipsis (p. 69) (Tiffany and Carrell, 1977) may not be adequately representative when considered in a context other than connected speech. The fact that articulation is a dynamic and variable function including both segmental (sounds) and nonsegmental (prosodic) features cannot be overlooked. All of these characteristics of speech, along with speech perception by the listener as well as by the speaker, must be considered in the development and use of speech.

The contributions of descriptive linguistics, psychology, anthropology, sociology, phonetics, psycholinguistics, and, of course, speech-language pathology toward understanding the contemporary concepts of articulation are immeasurable. To most lay people, an understanding of speech acquisition and development is unimportant; its use, however, is considered very important. In this section we will examine the production of speech sounds according to their anatomic, physiologic, perceptual, and acoustic correlates. We will consider the speech sounds: sounds that are the essence of oral communication and that are the primary medium by which the more than 3000 oral languages of the world are mediated; sounds that are amazingly stable in the presence of a 20% mortality rate for vocabulary every 1000 years (Gleason, 1961); sounds that vary from dialect to dialect and from phonetic context to phonetic context; and sounds that are identified and described according to some of their distinctive features.

Several approaches to analyzing phonology have been employed. They include (1) physiologic, (2) acoustic, (3) perceptual, and (4) other distinctive feature analyses. These approaches typically utilize the human ear in perceptual analysis. Although more objective approaches have been advocated and tried, the human ear still appears to be the most effective and practical approach for the diagnostician (Curtis, 1954; Fairbanks, 1940; Fairbanks and Grubb, 1961; Perkins, 1977). The following phonologic system will be discussed mainly from the standpoint of the physiology and perception of each sound: (1) fourteen vowels, (2) eleven diphthongs, and (3) twenty-five consonants.

Vowels

As with all phonemic classes, vowels defy exact definition. They are an integral part of nearly all syllables and have characteristic vocal tract configurations. Phoneticians use four to fourteen distinct vowels to represent General American Dialect (Jones, 1932; Tiffany and Carrell, 1977; Wise, 1957). Wise (1957) lists eight basic vowel positions, four at the corners of the vowel diagram (cardinal vowels) and four interspersed between the cardinal vowels. It should be remembered that "General American Dialect" is the term used to encompass the dialect in English speech that supposedly is used by most Americans, primarily living in "Middle America" and on the West Coast. It does not include "Southern American Dialect," "Eastern American Dialect" (which is somewhat akin to "British Dialect"), "stage diction," and the hundreds of minor dialects throughout the country, such as "Brooklynese" and "Bostonese." The International Phonetic Alphabet is commonly used to symbolize the different sounds in our language, and it is reasonably adequate to record and describe the sounds of all of the dialects related to English. Interestingly the International Phonetic Alphabet is not international. It was developed in France, based on the Latin alphabet.

Description of vowels as well as consonants can employ the system of distinctive features. Jakobson, Fant, and Halle (1952) list a number of features recognized or judged on an either-or (binary) basis. However, their features, although quite widely accepted, are not without controversy. There still is disagreement concerning the best set of distinctive features that should be used, if any. A system was developed by Chomsky and Halle (1968) that is somewhat more widely accepted, although more applicable to language than to articulation. These features will merely be listed here and compared with a more traditional description. For explanation of distinctive feature terminology, the reader is referred to the original source.

Distinctive features
  I. Major class features
     A. Syllabic and nonsyllabic
     B. Sonorant and obstruent
  II. Cavity features
     A. Coronal and noncoronal
     B. Anterior and nonanterior
     C. High and nonhigh
     D. Low and nonlow
     E. Back and nonback
     F. Front and nonfront
     G. Rounded and nonrounded
     H. Distributed and nondistributed
  III. Secondary aperture features
     A. Nasal and nonnasal
     B. Lateral and nonlateral
  IV. Manner of articulation features
     A. Stop and nonstop
     B. Tense and lax
  V. Source and features
     A. Voiced and nonvoiced
     B. Strident and nonstrident

These sixteen features, although somewhat foreign to traditional descriptions, will be employed, in part, in describing the pho-

Table 2. A comparison of traditional and distinctive feature descriptions of the vowel /i/*

Feature	Traditional description	Distinctive feature description
Major class features	Vowel	Syllabic, sonorant
Cavity feature	Front, high, nonrounded	Coronal, anterior, high, nonback, front, nonrounded, distributed
Secondary aperture features	Closed velopharyngeal mechanism	Nonnasal, nonlateral
Manner of articulation features	Since all vowels are continuants, the first part of this category (stop vs nonstop) would usually be excluded in traditional descriptions Tense	Nonstop, tense
Source and features	Since all vowels are voiced and nonstrident, this category would usually be excluded in traditional descriptions	Voiced, nonstrident

*Whereas distinctive feature descriptions appear to be more thorough, they also seem to be somewhat more redundant.

netic system. A more traditional distinctive feature system is included in Appendix G. A comparison of traditional and distinctive feature descriptions of a selected vowel follows (Table 2).

Identification and description of vowels are further complicated by the following:

1. There are no "pure" vowels
2. They are very similar to diphthongs
3. They are the combined result of the coupling of the articulation-resonance system
4. They have both periodic and aperiodic acoustic features
5. Their features vary depending on whether a system of narrow or broad transcription is used
6. Not all of the vowel symbols used in the International Phonetic Alphabet are considered vowels; some are considered allophones of other vowels
7. Some phoneticians regard vowels as sequences of phonemes
8. Vowels, as well as the other phonetic classes, contain considerable arbitrariness, which is necessary in order to maintain uniformity
9. There is no "preferred" standard of pronunciation in this country
10. Articulation varies continually, depending on such nonsegmental features as stress, rate, and duration
11. There is a lack of agreement as to which features make phonemes distinctive
12. They are influenced by coarticulation

For purposes of review, we shall describe vowels in regard to: (1) horizontal tongue placement in the oral cavity, (2) vertical tongue placement in the oral cavity, (3) degree of lip-rounding, (4) presence or absence of tension of the speech mechanism musculature, (5) vertical position of the lower jaw, and (6) duration of phonation. Fig. 3-1 illustrates approximate tongue positions for all vowels except the nonstressed /r/ (Bloodstein, 1979). The features of voicing and continuant-noncontinuant need not be included because all vowels are voiced and continuant. Thus vowels may be described as having maximum vocal tract constriction toward the front, middle, or back of the mouth; with the tongue assuming positions of varying height—high, mid or low; with lip positions ranging from neutral to rounded, to retracted; with the speech muscles assuming varying degrees of tenseness and laxness; and with the lower jaw ranging from near approximation (neutral position) with the upper jaw to moderately lowered.

Fourteen vowels are included, and their

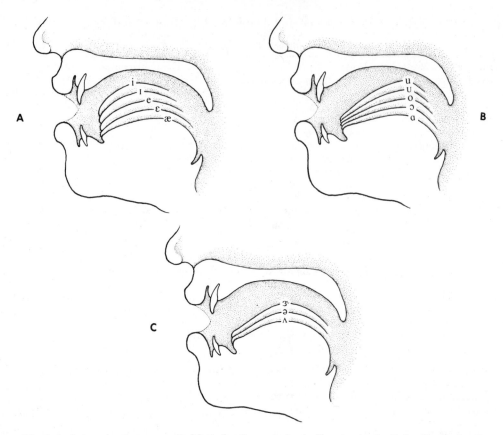

Fig. 3-1. Approximate tongue positions for the vowels. **A,** Front vowels; **B,** back vowels; **C,** central vowels. (From Oliver Bloodstein: *Speech Pathology: An Introduction.* Copyright © 1979 by Houghton Mifflin Company. Used by permission.)

distinctive features are summarized in Appendix G. Cardinal vowels will not be referred to specifically because the vowels do not represent equal degrees of acoustic and physiologic separation, or basic vowel positions, and therefore are not truly cardinal. A brief discussion of each vowel (vocoid or vocalic phoneme) follows.

Front vowels /i/, /ɪ/, /e/, /ɛ/, and /æ/

/i/ as in "heat" is the highest tongue positioned (a relative expression denoting vocal tract [oral cavity] constriction rather than precise tongue placement) front vowel. It is tense, long, and produced with considerable tongue–hard palate constriction. The lips are nonrounded and perhaps slightly retracted, varying with context, duration, rate, and stress of the speech in which it appears. The jaws are nearly in approximation. This vowel is perceived as a very high frequency vowel that may be diphthongized.

/ɪ/ as in "hit," the next highest tongue positioned front vowel, is produced with the lips a little more lax than for /i/. The lips are nonrounded and slightly parted. It is a short sound produced with constriction between the tongue and front part of the hard palate. The jaw is lowered slightly. Acoustically this is also a high frequency vowel. As with all vowels and diphthongs, this frequently occurring stressed vowel may vary physiologically and acoustically depending on context, rate, stress, and duration. Perceptual discrimination between /ə/ and /ɪ/ is sometimes difficult and confusing for children, persons with hearing loss or poor sound discrimination, and persons with foreign dialect.

/e/ as in "wait" is made with mid-high tongue position and somewhat parted and nonrounded lips. It is a tense, long front vowel that has less tongue–hard palate constriction and lower jaw position than /ɪ/. One of the most important features of this vowel is its diphthongal quality, such as /eɪ/. When articulated more as a diphthong than a vowel, the diphthong symbol should be used.

/ɛ/ as in "bet" is another of the more frequent sounds in spoken English language. Tongue position is slightly lower than for /e/. The lips are parted a little more but are nonrounded. The jaw is lowered somewhat more than for the preceding sound. This sound is considered a lax, short, low, front vowel. It causes frequent difficulty for persons with a foreign dialect who are learning to speak English.

/æ/ as in "bat" is produced with the bulk of the tongue in the lowest position of all the front vowels. The lips are parted considerably, and the jaw is lower than for the other front vowels. This sound is generally thought to be tense, long, and low with no lip-rounding or lip-retraction. Its frequency of occurrence is about average among all the vowels.

Central vowels /ʌ/, /ə/, /ɝ/, and /ɚ/

As indicated in Fig. 3-1, the central vowels are produced with the highest part of the tongue and the major vocal tract constriction occurring near the middle of the mouth, hence the name central vowel or midvowel. Even though the number of central vowels may vary according to phoneticians (Fairbanks, 1940; Gleason, 1961), we have elected to include four.

/ʌ/ as in "cup" has also been described as a back vowel (Heffner, 1952). It is lax, short, and typically considered the stressed counterpart of the neutral schwa /ə/ vowel;

that is, it appears in the stressed syllables in words. Maximum tongue–hard palate constriction is near the middle of the oral cavity, both vertically and horizontally. The lips are nonrounded, and the jaw is lowered a little for this sound. Although some phoneticians consider this vowel the highest central vowel, we prefer to consider /ɝ/ and /ɚ/ the highest.

/ə/ as in "about" has been the subject of disagreement among phoneticians because its features are not readily distinctive. This symbol is used to represent the nonstressed counterpart of /ʌ/, occurring in nonstressed syllables in words. It is lax, short, and of similar tongue height as its stressed counterpart. The lips are nonrounded and parted somewhat, and the jaw is lowered slightly.

/ɝ/ as in "heard" is a tense, long stressed vowel. Vertical tongue position is mid to midhigh, depending on the speaker and the speech context. The lips are slightly rounded and parted, and the jaw is lowered less than for /ə/. It is the symbol used in stressed syllables. It should not be confused with consonant glide /r/.

/ɚ/ as in "better" is the nonstressed counterpart of /ɝ/. It is slightly more lax than /ɝ/ and is produced with primary constriction of the vocal tract in the middle of the mouth, both horizontally and vertically. The lips, although slightly rounded, are in a little more neutral position than for /ɝ/, and the jaw is depressed slightly. This symbol is usually used in the nonstressed syllable in words. It is produced almost identically as its stressed counterpart. Whether or not the most appropriate or most common tongue position for articulating this sound and its stressed counterpart is retroflexed or bunched is still an issue in debate (Delattre and Freeman, 1968). One point is certain; these two members of the /r/ family are the most difficult vowels to produce and, as such, are not learned until around 6½ years of age. Because of their frequency of occurrence, their misarticulation can cause a very conspicuous articulation deviation. Misarticulation is also very difficult to correct in some persons.

Back vowels /u/, /ʊ/, /o/, /ɔ/, and /a/

The last group of vowels, five in all, are those produced toward the back of the oral cavity, logically called the back vowels. They are generally produced by retracting the body of the tongue, which causes maximum linguapalatal constriction of the vocal tract toward the back of the mouth.

/u/ as in "boot" is produced with the primary tongue-palate constriction high toward the back of the mouth. The lips are rounded and narrowly parted, and the jaw is lowered slightly. It is a high, tense, long vowel that may be diphthongized as in /ju/.

/ʊ/ as in "book" is produced with the tongue somewhat lower than for /u/, although it is still a high vowel. It is lax, short, and made with the lips mildly rounded. The jaw is lowered slightly. This sound is the shortest of the back vowels.

/o/ as in "boat" is a tense, long vowel with moderately rounded lips. Vertical position of the tongue is near the middle. The jaw is lowered slightly more than for /ʊ/. This vowel may be diphthongized as in /ou/ in some stressed positions and, as such, should be symbolized as a diphthong.

/ɔ/ as in "bought" is a low, lax, long back vowel that includes mild lip-rounding in most speakers. The jaw is lower than for the preceding back vowels. It can be diphthongized as in /ɔɪ/.

/a/ as in "cot" is the lowest back vowel. The tongue is on the floor of the mouth. The jaw is moderately lowered, and the lips are widely parted and nonrounded. It is a lax, long vowel that can be diphthongized as in /aɪ/, /aʊ/, and /aɚ/.

Diphthongs /aɪ/, /aʊ/, /ɔɪ/, /eɪ/, /ou/, /ju/, /ɪɚ/, /ɛɚ/, /aɚ/, /ɔɚ/, and /ʊɚ/

Features of eleven diphthongs are included in the following discussion, realizing that two, /eɪ/ and /ou/, are not regarded as true, distinctive diphthongs by some phoneticians. However, since many persons tend to diphthongize /e/ and /o/ in stressed syllables, /eɪ/ and /ou/ will be treated as separate diphthongs (Fig. 3-2).

By definition a diphthong is "a continually changing blend of one vowel sound into

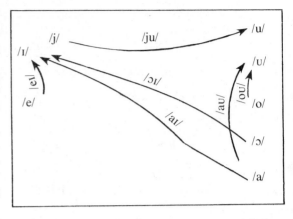

Fig. 3-2. Schema of rising diphthongs and /ju/.

another, occurring within the same syllable" (Leutenegger, 1963). Some phoneticians consider a diphthong as a blending of two sound elements (digraph), whereas others regard it as a spreading of only one given vowel sound, as an on- or off-glide (moving toward or away from a glide consonant), or as having a prominent shift of resonance (Tiffany and Carrell, 1977). Physiologically there is a shifting of articulator positions either upward or toward the middle of the oral cavity, and phonetically they are symbolized by approximations of two-vowel phonemes.

If vowels can be described as having resonance, then diphthongs can be described as having resonance shifts or changes as the result of a shift or adjustment of the vocal tract. All diphthongs are continuants and are of similar duration—relatively long. Two distinct vocal tract constrictions occur for each diphthong. The reader is cautioned that future studies and publications may include other systems of classification and different terminology. Nevertheless, one should always be more concerned with the sound features than with terminology. A brief discussion of the rising and centering diphthongs follows.

Rising diphthongs /aɪ/, /aʊ/, /ɔɪ/, /eɪ/, /ou/, and /ju/ (Fig. 3-8)

/aɪ/ as in "pie" is an approximate combination of /a/ and /ɪ/; it is approximate because no diphthong is an exact replication of any two vowels. The tongue glides smoothly and quickly from a low, neutral position to a high, front position, and the jaw moves from a moderately lowered position to a slightly more raised position producing a resonance change. Vocal tract constriction occurs at two different places. The lips are nonrounded. Because the tongue rises from one position to another, this diphthong and all of the other diphthongs that are produced by raising the tongue for the second part of the sound are called rising diphthongs.

/aʊ/ as in "cow" is described as resembling a combination of /a/ and /ʊ/ and producing a rather subtle resonance change, especially in some persons and in some contexts. The tongue shifts from a low, back position to a high, back position. The lips move from a neutral position to a moderately rounded position, while the jaw moves from a wide open position to a nearly approximated position with the upper jaw.

/ɔɪ/ as in "toy" is a resonance change caused by articulator and vowel tract constriction shifts from the midback vowel /ɔ/ to the high front vowel /ɪ/. The lips change from a mildly rounded position back to a neutral position. The tongue moves upward and forward, and the jaw likewise moves upward for this rising diphthong.

/oʊ/ as in "owes" is considered a diphthong when it is stressed so that a resonance shift is perceived. The tongue moves from a midback position to a highback position, and the lips move from a mildly rounded position to a slightly more rounded position. The lower jaw moves to a more nearly approximated position with the upper jaw as it goes from /o/ to /ʊ/. Vocal tract constriction increases as the tongue is elevated.

/eɪ/ as in "sail" also has a subtle resonance change as the speech mechanism makes its adjustment from /e/ to /ɪ/. The tongue again rises from the first part of the sound to the second part, but the lips retain a neutral position throughout. The jaw moves upward, contributing to the resonance change.

/ju/ as in "use" is the off-glide diphthong. It is not truly a rising diphthong because the tongue moves from a high, front position to a high, back position. The lips move from a neutral or slightly retracted position to a mildly rounded position. The jaw maintains a relatively stationary position.

Centering diphthongs /ɪɚ/, /ɛɚ/, /aɚ/, /ɔɚ/, and /ʊɚ/ (Fig. 3-3)

/ɪɚ/ as in "cheer" is the first of the centering diphthongs to be discussed. In centering diphthongs the terminal position of the tongue is toward the center of the oral cavity. The tongue moves from a rather high, front position for /ɪ/ toward the center of the mouth for the central vowel /ɚ/. The final resonance of this and the remaining centering diphthongs is accomplished either with the tip of the tongue or by bunching the body of the tongue. The lips move from a neutral position to a mildly rounded position, although this varies among speakers. The jaw is essentially stable.

/ɛɚ/ as in "pear" is produced by combining the midfront vowel /ɛ/ with the central vowel /ɚ/, or a close approximation thereof. The tongue moves from the midfront of the mouth toward the center of the mouth. The lips move from a neutral position to a mildly rounded position, while the lower jaw moves toward an approximation with the upper jaw.

/aɚ/ as in "car" combines the low, back vowel /a/ with the midcentral vowel /ɚ/. The tongue moves from the back of the mouth upward and forward toward the center of the mouth. The lips again move from a neutral position to a mildly rounded position. The jaw moves from an open position toward approximation with the upper jaw. The jaw and tongue move further for this sound than for any of the other rising diphthongs.

/ɔɚ/ as in "for" combines the relatively low, back vowel /ɔ/ with the central vowel /ɚ/. The tongue moves from a rather low, back position in the oral cavity toward the middle of the mouth. The lips move from a mildly rounded position to a less rounded position. The jaw moves from a slightly

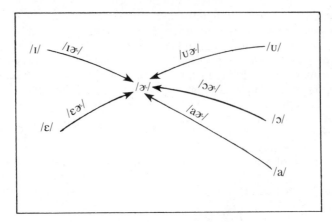

Fig. 3-3. Schema of centering diphthongs.

lowered position to near approximation with the upper jaw.

/ʊɚ/ as in "poor" is featured as a combination of the high, back vowel /ʊ/ with the central vowel /ɚ/. The tongue moves from a high, back position toward the middle of the mouth. The lips move from a moderately rounded position to a mildly rounded position. The jaw tends to move from a mildly open position toward a slightly more open position.

Consonants

The consonants, also called nonvocoids or nonsyllabics with some exceptions, are of more concern to the diagnostician and clinician of articulation disorders than are the vowels and diphthongs. This is because more children and adults have difficulty with consonants than with vowels, with the sole exception of the stressed and nonstressed /r/ sounds. Because of this, more attention will be given to the physiologic and acoustic properties of the consonants.

Twenty-five consonants will be discussed in terms of (1) place of articulation (where the sound is made), (2) manner of articulation (how the sound is made), (3) laryngeal activity (vibration of vocal folds or none), (4) degree of vocal tract constriction (amount of interruption of breath stream), and (5) tension of speech musculature (whether muscles are relatively tense or lax). Other distinctive features that could be applied are listed on p. 277 and in Appendix L. Table 3 provides a comparison of traditional and distinctive feature descriptions of the consonant /p/.

Consonants are nonsyllabic sounds or changes in resonance caused by varying the degree of vocal tract constriction that produces the syllabic pulses of speech. They can also be described as sounds produced by occluding (stops and affricates), diverting (nasals), obstructing (fricatives), and gliding articulator movements (glides) of the outgoing breath stream (Nemoy and Davis, 1954). An understanding of how each phoneme is made and how each one sounds is important in becoming a competent diagnostician and clinician of articulation disorders.

The following phonetic categories will be used for the consonant sounds: (1) stops, (2) fricatives, (3) nasals, (4) lateral, and (5) glides. These categories are displayed in terms of place and manner of articulation (Table 4) and are illustrated in regard to oral cavity configurations in Fig. 3-4. The primary feature of stops is obstruction of the breath stream by completely occluding the vocal tract, building up of air pressure behind the point of obstruction, and sudden release of air pressure, causing an explosive sound. Fricatives feature a constricted, but not completely obstructed, breath stream

Table 3. A comparison of traditional and distinctive feature descriptions of the consonant /p/

Feature	Traditional description	Distinctive feature description
Major class features	Stop, consonant	Nonsyllabic, obstruent
Cavity feature	Bilabial	Noncoronal, anterior, nonhigh, nonlow, front, nonback, distributed, nonrounded
Secondary aperture features	Closed velopharyngeal mechanism	Nonnasal, nonlateral
Manner of articulation features	Stop	Stop, tense
Source and features	Nonvoiced	Nonvoiced, nonstrident

Table 4. A common traditional description of consonants according to place and manner of articulation

Consonant	Stop	Fricative	Nasal	Lateral	Glides
Bilabial	p, b		m		w (hw)
Labiodental		f, v			
Linguadental		θ, ð			
Lingua-alveolar	t, d	s, z	n	l	
Linguapalatal	tʃ, dʒ	ʃ, ʒ			j, r
Linguavelar	k, g		ŋ		
Glottal		h			

and considerable intraoral breath pressure resulting in a friction, or hissing sound. The only exception is /h/, which has minimal vocal tract constriction. Nasals feature an occluded oral tract and an open nasal tract resulting in nasal airflow and resonance. The lateral /l/ is the result of air flowing past either side of the elevated tongue tip. Glides feature movement rather than exact placement or position in producing the important acoustic characteristics. These sounds are produced as the result of the gliding movements of the articulators.

Stops /p/, /b/, /t/, /d/, /tʃ/, /dʒ/, /k/, and /g/

Stops are also called plosives, stop plosives, and unreleased stops.

/p/ as in "pal" is categorized as a front, bilabial (both lips) stop that requires complete obstruction of the nonvoiced (surd) outgoing breath stream and muscular tension, primarily of the lips, which are closed, while the velopharyngeal port is also closed

enabling the breath stream to be trapped and built up inside the mouth without escaping through the nose before the lips are parted quickly causing an explosive (plosive) sound. Depending on the phonetic context, this and other stops may be produced with aspiration (audible airflow) or without aspiration (inaudible airflow). Tiffany and Carrell (1977) state that the plosive sounds are a combination of the airstream turbulence at both the glottis and the alveolar contact. Regardless of the type of aspiration, four stages of articulator movements are present in their production: (1) closure of the velopharyngeal port (implosion stage), (2) articulator movements leading to vocal tract occlusion (implosion stage), (3) brief occlusion of the vocal tract (hold stage), and (4) a sudden release of the impounded breath stream (explosion stage). For /p/, the jaw is slightly lowered and the tongue is in the neutral position if this sound is produced in isolation. In contextual

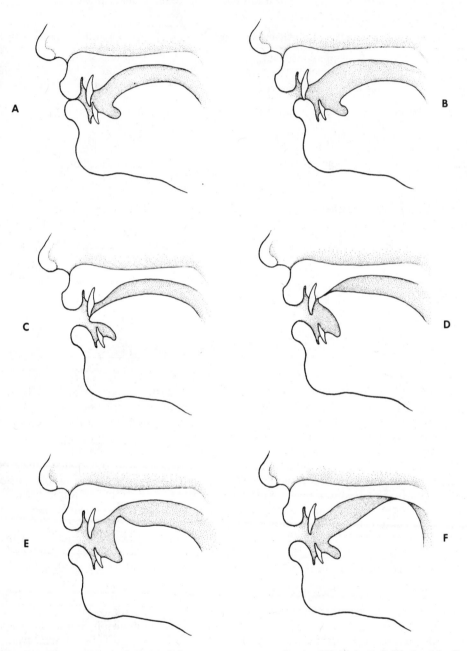

Fig. 3-4. Place of articulation of the consonant sounds. **A,** Bilabial; **B,** labiodental; **C,** linguadental; **D,** lingua-alveolar; **E,** linguapalatal; and **F,** linguavelar. (From Oliver Bloodstein: *Speech Pathology: An Introduction,* p. 70. Copyright © 1979 by Houghton Mifflin Company. Used by permission.)

speech the positions of the tongue and jaw are influenced by preceding and following sounds. All stops are noncontinuants; that is, they cannot be prolonged indefinitely as can fricatives, for example. For a more in-depth discussion of the physiology of this and subsequent consonant sounds, including the muscles involved, the reader is referred to Van Riper (1978) and Irwin (1972).

/b/ as in "bat" is the voiced cognate or homophone of /p/. It is produced similarly except the larynx is in vibration (voiced or sonant) and the muscles of the speech mechanism are more lax. This sound is produced with less aspiration than its cognate.

/t/ as in "to" is a midfront lingua-alveolar (tongue–upper midfront alveolar ridge behind the front teeth) aspirated sound that has no laryngeal activity. It requires complete obstruction of the breath stream and muscular tension, primarily of the tongue. It is the most frequently occurring consonant sound in spoken English (Table 5). As with most of the consonants, the velopharyngeal port is closed in varying degrees. This sound is made by momentarily holding the tip and blade of the tongue against the alveolar ridge with the lateral margins of the tongue contacting the contiguous teeth or alveolar ridge or both in order to impound completely the breath stream. The breath pressure is thus built up inside the mouth and suddenly released by quickly pulling the tongue tip and blade away from the alveolar ridge, producing an explosive sound. The lips are in a neutral, slightly parted position, and the jaw usually is lowered a little as the sound is produced.

/d/ as in "do" is the voiced cognate of /t/. It is made the same way except it requires vibration of the vocal folds and more lax speech musculature. It also has less aspiration, depending on the phonetic context, than its nonvoiced counterpart. This is quite typical for all nonvoiced stops.

/tʃ/ as in "chew" is a stop but is also called an affricate. It has been described as a blending of the nonvoiced lingua-alveolar plosive /t/ and the nonvoiced palatal (tongue–hard palate) or lingua-alveolar as-

Table 5. Frequency of occurrence of all phonemes

Number	Phoneme	Percentage of occurrence
	Consonant	
1	t	6.60
2	n	6.12
3	s	5.04
4	d	4.68
5	r	4.65
6	l	3.78
7	k	3.09
8	z	2.88
9	w*	2.88
10	m	2.60
11	ð	2.37
12	h	2.34
13	b	1.74
14	v	1.74
15	p	1.68
16	g	1.62
17	f	1.50
18	ŋ	1.25
19	j	1.02
20	ʃ	0.88
21	tʃ	0.77
22	θ	0.66
23	dʒ	0.62
24	ʒ	0.04
	Vowel	
1	ə	6.4
2	ɪ	5.4
3	i	4.0
4	a	3.5
5	æ	3.1
6	ɛ	2.5
7	ɔ	2.5
8	ɝ	2.42
9	ɚ	2.23
10	u	2.0
11	e	1.8
12	ʊ	1.5
13	ʌ	1.4
14	o	0.7
		100

*/hw/ has been combined with /w/.

pirated consonant /ʃ/ that requires no laryngeal activity. Its production includes complete obstruction or constriction of the breath stream and tension of the speech musculature, mainly the tongue. The velopharyngeal mechanism is closed, and the lips are mildly rounded. During its production the jaw is lowered slightly. This sound is made by obstructing the breath stream with the tongue tip and blade at the alveolar ridge similar to the production of /t/, except that the tongue is spread more widely. The margins of the tongue are in contact with the contiguous teeth and gums. The tongue is released by retracting and grooving it into the position of /ʃ/ rather than lowering it suddenly as in /t/, resulting in a combination of explosion and friction noise.

/dʒ/ as in "just" and "angel" is the voiced cognate of /tʃ/ and is made similarly except that the vocal folds are vibrating, the speech musculature is lax, and it has less aspiration. This sound may be described as a blending of /d/ and /ʒ/.

/k/ as in "cat" or "kite" is a back, nonvoiced linguavelar (tongue–soft palate) consonant that requires complete, momentary constriction of the vocal tract. It includes muscular tension and, of course, considerable aspiration. This sound is made with the back of the tongue sealing off the breath stream by contacting the soft palate. These movements are preceded by closing of the velopharyngeal mechanism, which enables a buildup of air pressure behind this point of obstruction. The back of the tongue is then suddenly lowered to permit the rushing of air through the mouth and the accompanying explosive sound. The tip of the tongue and lips are in a relatively neutral position, whereas the jaw is quite stationary. As Tiffany and Carrell (1977) point out, the sound heard may be a combination of (1) rapid explosion, (2) turbulent noise of air passing through the oral cavity, and (3) the release of air through the glottis.

/g/ as in "go" is the voiced cognate of /k/ and is made similarly except that the vocal folds are in vibration, the speech musculature is lax, and there is less aspiration.

Fricatives /f/, /v/, /θ/, /ð/, /h/, /s/, /z/, /ʃ/, and /ʒ/

Fricatives are also called oral continuants. Fricatives are phonemes having a distinct "friction" or "hissing" sound caused by the airstream passing through a narrow opening. All the sounds listed are fricatives because of their "friction" quality, and the last four are also called sibilants because of their "hissing" quality. All of them are continuants.

/f/ as in "fun" is a front, labiodental (lipteeth) nonvoiced fricative. The speech musculature is tense, and the degree of breath stream constriction is considerable. The tongue is in a neutral position, the velopharyngeal mechanism is closed, and the jaw is slightly lowered. This sound is typically articulated with aspiration. It is made by closing the velopharyngeal port, lowering the jaw slightly, raising the lower lip and drawing it backward against the cutting edges of the upper front teeth, and forcing air through this constricted vocal tract in the front of the mouth. The tongue is not involved in the articulation of this fricative. This sound is sometimes difficult to discriminate from /θ/ and /s/ because of their similar high frequency and low intensity components.

/v/ as in "very" is the voiced cognate of /f/. It differs in production in that it requires laryngeal activity and less aspiration and tension. Since these homophones are readily visable, they have certain advantages in remediation if they are faulty.

/θ/ as in "thin" is a front, linguadental (tongue-teeth), nonvoiced, aspirated fricative that has lax speech musculature and moderate obstruction of the breath stream. The jaw is lowered slightly, the lips are in a neutral position, and the velopharyngeal mechanism is closed. This sound is made by closing the velopharyngeal port, dropping the jaw slightly, lightly placing the flattened tip of the tongue near or on the cutting edges of the upper front teeth, and forcing the breath stream through the space between the tongue and teeth. Some persons tend to interdentalize the tongue (protrude it between the teeth) when articulating this sound.

/ð/ as in "this" is the voiced cognate of /θ/. Its features differ only in voicing, less aspiration, and more lax musculature.

/h/ as in "high" is the last of the "friction-sounding" fricatives. It is a back nonvoiced glottal (larynx) sound having only limited, if any, airflow constriction and relatively lax musculature. The articulators are relatively inactive, except for the necessary postures for the sound to follow in contextual speech. The jaw is lowered, and the velopharyngeal port is closed, at least to some degree. It is made by lowering the jaw slightly, closing the velopharyngeal mechanism, and forcing nonvoiced air through the glottis until it produces an audible friction noise. Because it is so influenced (assimilation) by sounds that immediately follow it in speech, its features are difficult to specify. It usually is coarticulated with the vowel that it follows. It has no cognate.

/s/ as in "say" and "cent" is the first of the four sibilants to be discussed. It is described as a midfront, nonvoiced, aspirated lingua-alveolar (tongue–alveolar ridge behind the upper, front teeth) sibilant having tense speech musculature and considerable vocal tract constriction. It is produced by closing the velopharyngeal port, placing the tongue blade and tip behind the upper front teeth (although some persons make it with the tip down) near the alveolar ridge with the lateral margins contacting the contiguous teeth or gums or both. The tongue blade assumes a narrow groove at the midline necessary for producing a "hissing" sound. The lips are retracted somewhat, and the lower jaw is almost in approximation with the upper jaw. The sound that is perceived is the result of the breath stream being forced through the narrow lingua-alveolar orifice and the cutting edges of the upper front teeth. Tiffany and Carrell (1977) list seven factors that can affect the quality and cause variability of this high-frequency, weak-intensity sound: (1) air pressure, (2) airflow rate, (3) constriction of airflow, (4) configuration of constriction, (5) anatomic nature of structures in contact with airflow, (6) presence of air cavity in front of air turbulence, and (7) resonance frequency of that air cavity. Any deviations in these seven factors can cause acoustic differences. Because this consonant is vulnerable to so many possible deviations and occurs so frequently in spoken English, it is a problem frequently encountered by the speech-language pathologist.

/z/ as in "zoo" and "is" is the voiced cognate of /s/. Its features differ in voicing, less aspiration, and lax musculature.

/ʃ/ as in "shoe" and "sugar" is a midfront nonvoiced linguapalatal (tongue–hard palate) aspirated sibilant. The degree of breath stream obstruction is considerable, although not as much as for /s/, and the speech muscles are tense. It is produced by closing the velopharyngeal port and elevating the flattened tip, blade, and body of the tongue so that the blade nearly touches the alveolar ridge. The sides of the tongue contact the contiguous teeth and gums of the hard palate, and the tongue is broadly grooved in such a way that the breath stream must pass centrally down the tongue and out of the mouth, rather than past the lateral margins of the tongue as in /l/. The tongue is grooved somewhat broader than for /s/, resembling placement for /tʃ/. The jaw is lowered slightly, and the lips are mildly rounded. This sound is the loudest of the sibilants and fricatives.

/ʒ/ as in "treasure" and "azure" is the voiced cognate of /ʃ/. It is produced similarly to its cognate except for voicing, less aspiration, and more lax speech musculature.

Nasals /m/, /n/, and /ŋ/

Nasals are also called semivowels. These three consonants have in common the prominent features of resonance or vowel-like quality, complete oral tract constriction, and nasal airflow. They also are frequently assimilated with vowels that are in juxtaposition. /m/ and /n/ are sometimes syllabic, that is, produced as separate syllables. /n/ is the second most frequently occurring consonant in spoken English.

/m/ as in "me" is featured as a front, bilabial (both lips) voiced nasal. Constriction of airflow is complete, and the speech muscles are quite lax. This sound is made by occluding the lips, having the velopharyngeal port open, and emitting the vocalized breath stream through the nose. The tongue remains in a neutral position, and the jaw is lowered slightly. This continuant sound has no cognate. However, if one were to produce it by occluding the nose, the result would be an approximation of /b/.

/n/ as in "no" is a midfront, lingua-alveolar (tongue–upper front gum ridge) voiced nasal. The degree of airflow constriction is complete, and the speech muscles are rather lax. This sound is made by placing the tongue tip and blade on the alveolar ridge with the lateral margins of the tongue contacting the contiguous teeth and the gums providing complete obstruction of oral airflow. The velopharyngeal mechanism is open, the jaw is lowered slightly, and the lips are in a neutral position. The vocalized breath stream passes through the nasal cavity. It has no cognate, but if the nose were occluded, the produced sound would resemble /d/.

/ŋ/ as in "sing" is categorized as a back, voiced lingua-alveolar (tongue–soft palate) nasal. The vocal tract is completely constricted, and the speech muscles are somewhat tense. It is produced by elevating the posterior part of the tongue body against the soft palate and emitting the breath stream through the nose. The jaw is lowered slightly, and the lips are in a neutral position. It has no cognate. A sound resembling /g/ is made when producing /ŋ/ with the nose occluded.

Lateral /l/

/l/ is sometimes referred to as a semivowel, liquid, or glide. /l/ as in "life" is the only lateral in the English language. It is similar in quality to both the nasal and glide sounds. It is classified as a midfront, voiced lingua-alveolar (tongue–upper front alveolar ridge) consonant requiring little breath stream constriction and muscular tension.

It is produced by closing the velopharyngeal port and elevating and holding the tongue tip lightly against the alveolar ridge with its lateral margins not in contact with the contiguous structures. The breath stream passes on either side of the elevated tongue tip to produce this lateral sound. The jaw is lowered slightly, and the lips are in a neutral position. This continuant does not have a cognate but is produced in the final position of a word or syllable as a dark /l/. It can also function solely as an entire syllable, and as such is indicated by /l̩/.

Glides /j/, /r/, /w/, and /hw/

Glides are sometimes called semivowels. The label for these sounds was derived from their manner of production. The acoustic properties are the result of the articulator movements toward or away from the target position, rather than the position itself. It is the movement pattern that distinguishes these phonemes.

/j/ as in "yes" is classified as a midfront, voiced linguapalatal (tongue–hard palate) glide requiring little breath stream constriction and muscular tension. It is produced as the tongue tip and blade move or shift to the position of the following vowel while the vocalized breath stream passes over the elevated tongue. The jaw also shifts to a lower position, depending on the following sound in contextual speech, contributing to the perceptible change in resonance, similar to that of diphthongs. The lips are in a neutral position, and the velopharyngeal mechanism is closed. The first part of this sound, in isolation, resembles /i/. This glide does not have a cognate.

/r/ as in "read" is a middle, voiced linguapalatal (tongue–hard palate) continuant consonant. It is part of the /r/ family. This sound requires some breath stream constriction and muscular tension. It is produced by a gliding movement of the articulators, primarily the elevated tongue tip and blade, while the velopharyngeal port is closed. It can also be produced by assuming a rather stable tongue posture, either retroflexed or centrally bunched. It is made similarly to /ɝ/ and /ɚ/. The lips tend to be mildly rounded, and the jaw is lowered slightly. These postures will vary according to the following sound to be produced and with the speaker. This consonant is one of the frequently misarticulated sounds in the English language and one of the most difficult to correct. It has no cognate.

/w/ as in "we" is classified as a front, voiced bilabial (both lips) glide requiring limited breath stream obstruction and speech muscle tension. It is made by closing the velopharyngeal mechanism, rounding the lips moderately, and emitting the vocalized breath stream between the rounded lips. The jaw is lowered slightly, but the tongue is in a neutral position, or preparing for the sound to follow. The diphthong-like resonance change occurs as a result of the movement of the lips and jaw.

/hw/ as in "when" is rapidly becoming extinct in spoken English. It can be considered a cognate of /w/ varying mainly in aspiration, tension, and voicing. Because it is aspirated so seldomly, it has been deleted in the articulation battery of the Weiss Comprehensive Articulation Test (W-CAT) (Appendix G). The nonaspirated /w/ appears largely to have replaced it in conversational speech.

STAGES OF PHONOLOGIC DEVELOPMENT

Even though no stages, besides those mentioned by Ingram (1976), have been proposed, phonologic development must be considered in the overall management of articulation disorders. We certainly have some ideas about when vowels, diphthongs, consonants, and consonant clusters are acquired (Weiss and Lillywhite, 1976), but we do not know exactly how phonemic development compares with cognitive development, learning of meaningful phonemic rules, and when phonologic development really begins and ends. Knowing when these landmark behaviors occur provides the clinician with some information in deciding if articulation is delayed or disordered and perhaps where and when to begin treatment.

How some of the normative data were derived, through diary studies, large sample studies, or linguistic studies, may account for some of the differences reported (Morehead and Morehead, 1976). Where normative differences exist between reported studies, they may relate to methodology (Olmsted, 1971; Prather, Hedrick, and Kern, 1975; Poole, 1934; Templin, 1957; Wellman and associates, 1931). For example, there may have been differences in how the target sounds were elicited. They may have been elicited spontaneously or imitatively. The mastery criterion also varied among studies; some researchers considered a sound mastered when 75% of the children produced it correctly, whereas others required 100% correct for mastery. Whether or not the sounds were produced in isolation, in isolated words, or in contextual speech would introduce another variable. When the data were obtained is another consideration. Since speech sound acquisition has shown a steady increase in development, that is, the motoric aspects of sounds are learned earlier now than in the 1930s or 1940s, this historical fact could explain differences among studies. Notwithstanding, all vowels ("r" excluded) and most consonants are acquired by 4 years of age, and the speech sounds are acquired quite orderly and systematically (Templin, 1957; Olmsted, 1971).

One caution is offered in regard to normative data. Norms are a mythical average. No individual child should be expected to be "on target" in phonologic development at every age interval; individual differences are always present. Norms can be informative and helpful as a guide, but not as a yardstick. Norms can be of assistance in determining the need for referral, prevention, intervention, and a way of measuring progress, if used appropriately.

Most of the existing normative data on acquisition of sounds may be inappropriate because the mastery criterion regarding acquisition was too high (Sander, 1972). Some data were based on 90% of the children correctly articulating the phonemes. Perhaps we should follow the concept of customary speech (age at which more than one half of the children correctly produce the sound) rather than the concept of speech mastery (age at which 75% to 90% of the children correctly produce the sound). Changing the criterion would lower the age of sound acquisition. As a rule of thumb, the diagnostician is encouraged to lower most of the normative age levels by at least 6 months for each phoneme.

Phonologic development appears to be an inseparable part of cognitive development. As such, phonology has a complex system of morphophonemic (sound changes that result from joining one morpheme with another) rules, for example, rules that pertain to vowel shifts such as the vowel change that occurs when the child goes from the word "explain" to the word "explanatory." To learn such a vowel shift rule, the child must be able to compare pairs of words such as these and determine that the words share a particular morpheme. Then the child must be able to isolate the sound change that occurs and establish a rule to explain the change. Explanation of these functions resides in the cognitive abilities of the child (Ingram, 1976), suggesting that phonologic development and cognitive development are inseparable.

Does phonologic development begin with the first words (around 1 year of age) and end around 6 or 7 years of age? Is it really true that the most rapid sound development occurs between 2 and 4 years of age? Must phonologic development be considered in relation to the other aspects of child development? How important are the prelinguistic vocalizations to later phonologic development? These are only a few of the questions that continue to be discussed and studied by phoneticians and psycholinguists. Since definite answers await further research, many of the following comments must be regarded as tentative.

Before proceeding with a more traditional discussion of phonemic development, we would like to review Piaget's stages of cognitive development and the phonologic stages that correspond to each (Ingram, 1976) (Table 6). The corresponding linguistic stages will not be discussed.

Stage one (sensorimotor period, birth to 18 months of age) occurs when the child develops systems of movements and perception. The phonologic stages that correspond with Piaget's cognitive stage one are (1) prelinguistic vocalization and perception (from birth to 1 year of age) and (2) phonology of the first fifty words (1 to 1½ years of age). During the prelinguistic vocalization and perception stage the child explores objects and learns about their properties and functions, develops preverbal vocalizations (babbling) and perceptual skills, and begins the processes of simplifying speech use. The child communicates through crying and gestures (reflexive vocalizations), which may not be as important to speech development as the nonreflexive vocalizations (vocal play). Imitative abilities are also increased and perhaps improved during this time to be used later in deferred imitations. Perceptual and discriminative abilities may be present as early as 1 month of age (Morse, 1974).

Phonology of the first fifty words shows the child acquiring the ability of representing reality through the use of linguistic symbols, even though much of the oral communication is holophrastic in nature (one word representing a complete thought). New sounds are added and advanced forms (better pronunciations of some sounds now than as the child gets older) (Moskowitz, 1970), and voiced for nonvoiced consonant substitutions before vowels occasionally are present. This period, which lasts about 6 months, ends with a marked increase in vocabulary and the first two-word utterances. Nelson (1973) indicated a rapid growth in vocabulary after the first fifty words are acquired.

Jakobson (1968) suggested that there is a universal order of acquisition as follows:

1. The first syllables are CV (consonant-vowel) or CVCV reduplicated
2. The first consonants are labial, most commonly /p/ or /m/

Table 6. Piaget's cognitive stages of development with approximate ages, and the grammatical and phonological stages that correspond to each

Piaget's stages	Linguistic stages	Phonological stages
SENSORIMOTOR PERIOD (0;0-1;6)		
Development of systems of movements and perception. Child achieves notion of object permanence.	1. Prelinguistic communication through gestures and crying. 2. Holophrastic stage. Use of one-word utterances.	1. Prelinguistic vocalization and perception (birth to 1;0). 2. Phonology of the first 50 words (1;0-1;6).
PERIOD OF CONCRETE OPERATIONS (1;6-12;0)		
Preconcept subperiod (1;6-4;0) The onset of symbolic representation. Child can now refer to past and future, although most activity is in the here and now. Predominance of symbolic play.	3. Telegraphic stage. Child begins to use words in combinations. These increase to point between 3 and 4 when most sentences become close to well-formed, simple sentences.	3. Phonology of single morphemes. Child begins to expand inventory of speech sounds. Phonological processes that result in incorrect productions predominate until around age 4 when most words of simple morphological structure are correctly spoken.
Intuitional subperiod (4;0-7;0) Child relies on immediate perception to solve various tasks. Begins to develop the concept of reversibility. Child begins to be involved in social games.	4. Early complex sentences. Child begins to use complements on verbs and some relative clauses. These early complex structures, however, appear to be the result of juxtaposition.	4. Completion of the phonetic inventory. The child acquires production of troublesome sounds by age 7. Good production of simple words. Beginning of use of longer words.
Concrete operations subperiod (7;0-12;0) Child learns the notion of reversibility. Can solve tasks dealing with conservation of mass, weight, and volume.	5. Complex sentences. Child acquires the transformational rules that embed one sentence into another. Coordination of sentences decreases, v. the increase in complex sentences.	5. Morphophonemic development. Child learns more elaborate derivational structure of the language; acquires morphophonemic rules of language.
PERIOD OF FORMAL OPERATIONS (12;0-16;0)		
Child learns the ability to use abstract thought. Can solve problems through reflection.	6. Linguistic intuitions. Child can now reflect upon grammaticality of his speech and arrive at linguistic intuitions.	6. Spelling. Child masters ability to spell.

From Ingram, D.: Phonological disability in children, London, 1976, Edward Arnold.

3. These consonants are followed by /t/ and later /k/
4. The first vowel is /a/ followed by /i/ or /u/
5. A homorganic fricative is acquired only if the stop has been acquired

Ferguson and Garnica (1975) add that /h/ and /w/ are also among the first consonants to be acquired. With regard to syllable structure, CV is common, but VC is also present.

Cognitive stage two, the period of concrete operations (1½ to 4 years of age), includes the onset of symbolic representation, symbolic play, and the concepts of past and future. The phonologic stage that corresponds to this cognitive stage is the occurrence of single morphemes. The inventory of speech sounds is increased, and misarticulations of most words nearly disappear by age 4 years.

In the third cognitive stage (intuitional subperiod—4 to 7 years of age), the child relies on immediate perception to solve various tasks. The child also begins to develop the concept of reversibility and begins to become involved in social games. The corresponding phonologic stage is the completion of the phonetic inventory. The child learns the production of all troublesome sounds by age 7 years and shows good production of most simple words and some longer, more difficult words.

Piaget's fourth cognitive stage is referred to as the concrete operations subperiod (7 to 12 years of age). During this period the child learns the concept of reversibility and learns to solve tasks dealing with conservation of mass, weight, and volume. Phonologic development continues as the child acquires morphophonemic rules and more elaborate derivational structure of the language. The child learns how to spell and read, vowel shifts, and contrastive stress for differentiating compound words from noun phrases such as "blackboard" from "black board." Morphophonemic alterations are learned such as changes between "electric" and "electricity" where the final /k/ in "electric" becomes /s/ in "electricity" (Ingram, 1976). Thus phonologic acquisition is not complete by age 7 years as has been traditionally thought. It continues until 12 years of age and perhaps even longer if mastery of spelling is considered. However, sound production of the approximately fifty sounds in the English language is usually mastered by 7 years of age.

The last cognitive stage is the period of formal operations (12 to 16 years). During this time the child learns the ability to use abstract thought and to solve problems through reflection. The phonologic counterpart is mastery of spelling ability.

In summary a general sequence of some phonologic landmarks can be specified; however, an exact timetable cannot be indicated (Ervin-Tripp, 1966): (1) vowel-consonant discrimination is acquired first; (2) stop-continuant discrimination is acquired early; (3) the development of stops and nasals precedes the development of fricatives, affricates, and semivowels; (4) labial sound development precedes dental, alveolar, and velar sound development, in that order; (5) place of articulation precedes acquiring of voicing features; (6) high and low features of vowel development precede acquisition of front-back features; (7) single consonants precede consonant clusters in development; (8) consonants are acquired first in the initial position of words; and (9) syllabic patterns develop as follows: CV, CVC, and CVCV, where C represents consonants and V represents vowels.

Conversely many aspects of phonologic development cannot be delineated specifically. For example, reductions of consonant clusters occur at various development ages. Likewise, suprasegmental features of speech begin to develop early; however, we do not know precisely when this development begins or stops, if ever. Perception and discrimination develop gradually and relate to overall maturation. Furthermore, when phonologic universalities exist, their existence may relate to neurophysiologic factors of the speech mechanism and correlate with motoric development. One point appears certain; different phonologic processes are used by different children, and these processes seem to involve learning of features as well as learning of individual sounds through the interaction of perception and production. Also, abnormal speech development generally parallels normal speech development, except that it lags behind (Compton, 1975).

In a more traditional sense we can say that vowels are acquired before consonants, followed by nasals, glides, stops, fricatives, and affricates. The infant is first heard to vocalize some front and back vowels and by 2 months of age is producing all front vowels. The consonants /h/, /w/, and /k/ as well as some nondistinguishable sounds also appear by this age. By 6 or 7 months of age the child's repertoire has increased to fourteen vowels as well as occasional consonants (Table 7). However, these sounds are not mastered at this age; they are merely babbled. Somewhere between 6 months and 2½ years of age the vowels, some diphthongs, and a few consonants are learned, totaling at least twenty-seven phonemes. Acquisition is not an all-or-nothing event; individual sounds are not acquired suddenly but rather gradually over time with extended periods during which the sounds are produced correctly and incorrectly. Ferguson and Farwell (1975) indicate that the acquisition of specific patterns and sounds may be greatly influenced by the words in which they occur. Furthermore, the acquisition of a new part of a word, such as a prefix, may distort the production of another part of that same word, such as the suffix (Edwards and Garnica, 1973). Words may first be acquired outside the child's phonologic system only to become part of that system later.

The sequence of vowel development generally begins with those made toward the front of the mouth followed by those made toward the back of the mouth and proceeds to those made toward the middle of the mouth. Two of the four middle or central vowels, the stressed and nonstressed /r/ sounds, are not acquired until around 6 or 6½ years of age. Frequency of vowel occurrence, based on studies by Black and Irwin (1969) and Barker and England (1962) of speakers of General American Dialect is listed in Table 5. The consonants /p/, /b/, and /m/ are also learned between 2 and 3 years of age. After the first year, consonant acquisition exceeds vowel acquisition. Also sex differences in regard to rate of sound development slightly favor females.

Next in the developmental hierarchy are the five or six rising diphthongs, which are typically learned by 3½ years of age. One reason they are learned a little later than most of the vowels is that they require a smoothly coordinated blending of two different articulator positions. The five centering diphthongs develop considerably later because they all include the /r/ vowels as part of the sound.

Few deletions of final consonants are present after age 3 years. Deletions of unstressed syllables occur up to 4 years of age. When deletions by reduction of clusters occur, they show predictable patterns, as do deletions of marked members of a cluster. Greenlee (1974) gave the following example of how a child reduced or simplified the consonant cluster in the word "play." The following predictable patterns were observed:

Stage 1: Deletion of entire cluster /ey/ [eɪ]
Stage 2: Reduction of cluster to one member /pey/ [peɪ]
Stage 3: Use of cluster with substitution for one of the members /pwey/ [pweɪ]
Stage 4: Correct articulation /play/ [pleɪ]

Following the development of rising diphthongs are the nasals /n/ and /ŋ/ and the glides /w/ and /h/. These sounds are usually learned before 4 years of age. /hw/ is deleted from discussion because it is practically extinct among speakers of English. For those persons who still use it, /hw/ should appear around 4 years of age.

By age 4½ years /t/, /d/, /k/, and /g/ are learned. Their production requires a somewhat higher level of neuromuscular integrity than those sounds previously mentioned. By age 5 years /f/, /v/, and /j/ are learned, followed by /θ/, /ð/, and /l/ by age 5½ years.

Between 6½ and 7 years of age the remaining sounds are learned. These include /r/, /ɝ/, /ɚ/, /s/, /z/, /ʃ/, /ʒ/, /tʃ/, and /dʒ/, all centering diphthongs, and all of the consonant blends or clusters. Thus somewhere between the beginning and the end of the first grade, virtually all children have mastered the approximately fifty sounds in our language. Exceptions, of course, include children with physical, psychologic, neuro-

Table 7. Sequential characteristics of phonologic development

Age*	Behavior
Birth	Crying
1 week	92% of front vowels present—/i/, /ɪ/, /e/, /ɛ/, /æ/
	7% of middle vowels present—/ɝ/, /ɚ/, /ʌ/, /ə/
	No back vowels present—/u/, /ʊ/, /o/, /ɔ/, /a/
1 month	Reflexive vocalization (undifferentiated vocalizations)
	One half of the vowels and a few consonants present—/æ/, /ɛ/, /ʌ/, /ɪ/, /e/, /u/, /l/, /h/, /k/, /g/, /m/, /n/
2 months	Vocal play and babbling (differentiated vocalizations)
	Perceptual development begins
	Behaviors up to and including this level are derivative of chewing, suckling, and swallowing movements
	Vowel distribution—front vowels, 73%; middle vowels, 25%; back vowels, 2%
	Consonants present—/m/, /b/, /g/, /p/, /j/, /w/, /l/, /r/
	Occasional diphthongs are heard
3 months	Sounds added—/ə/, /j/, /ŋ/
	Increased vocal play and babbling
4 months	Sounds added—/t/, /v/, /z/, /θ/, /ɔ/, /o/
	Vowel distribution—front vowels, 60%; middle vowels, 26%; back vowels, 14%
5 months	Syllable repetition
	Sixty-three variations of sounds present
6 months	Lalling begins
	Imitation of sounds
	Vowel distribution—front vowels, 62%; middle vowels, 24%; back vowels, 14%
7 months	Syllables and diphthongs continue to develop
8 months	Marked gain in back vowels and front consonants
	Babbling peaks
9 months	Echolalia appears
	Continued imitation of sounds
	Jargon (jabber)
	More back vowels, central vowels, and consonants appear
10 months	Invention of words
	Continued imitation of sounds and words

*It should be noted that whereas many vowels and consonants are used by the infant in the first weeks or months of life, they are not actually "learned" or used consistently and meaningfully, not usually for the purpose of communication, but are random vocalizations and babbling. These sounds are gradually refined (learned) and assume semantic significance. It is interesting that a number of consonants, which are relatively late to be "learned," such as /l/, /r/, /t/, /v/, /z/, and /θ/, are used very early by the infant but often do not reappear until the child is ready to learn them and use them for purposeful communication.

logic, and unfavorable environmental problems. It should also be pointed out that sounds that a child made correctly at an earlier age may subsequently be made incorrectly, such as an interdental lisp that may develop when the front deciduous (baby) teeth fall out.

Another consideration regarding the sequence of phonetic development is intelligibility (understandability) of articulation.

A true measure of articulation proficiency is how a child uses the sounds in contextual speech. The sounds may be articulated correctly in isolation or in isolated words, but not in conversation. This point will be stressed more when diagnostic methods are discussed.

There appears to be a residual diathesis or unknown variable operating in regard to intelligibility. When comparing a child's ar-

Table 7. Sequential characteristics of phonologic development—cont'd

Age	Behavior
11 months	First true word may appear
12 months	Vowel distribution—front vowels, 62%; middle vowels, 16%; back vowels, 22%
	Consonants begin to develop faster than vowels
	Diphthongs continue to develop
	Word simplification begins
	Reduplication occurs
16-24 months	Intelligibility is 25%
	Deletion of unstressed syllables
	Word combinations begin to develop
	Use of holophrastic words
	Diphthongs continue to develop
	Better production of some sounds now than later
24-30 months	90% of all vowels and diphthongs are learned
	Mean length of utterance—three and one half words
	Articulation is intelligible 60% of the time
	Front consonants continue to develop
30-36 months	All vowels are learned except /ɝ/ and /ɚ/
	All rising diphthongs—/aɪ/, /aʊ/, /oʊ/, /eɪ/—are learned except /ju/
	Consonants /p/, /b/, /m/, /w/ are learned
	Articulation is intelligible 75% of the time
	Mean length of utterance—five words
36-54 months	Centering diphthongs develop /iɚ/, /ɛɚ/, /aɚ/, /ɔɚ/, /uɚ/
	Some stops are substituted for fricatives
	Consonants /n/, /ŋ/, /j/, /t/, /d/, /k/, /g/ are learned
	Mean length of utterance—six words
54-66 months	Consonants /f/, /v/, /j/, /θ/, /ð/, /l/ are learned
66-78 months	Consonants /r/, /s/, /z/, /tʃ/, /dʒ/, /ʃ/, /ʒ/ are learned
	The remaining middle vowels /ɝ/ and /ɚ/ are learned as well as all centering diphthongs
84 months	All consonant clusters are learned, and articulation is completely normal; morphophonemic rules continue developing to age 12 years

ticulation with the developmental norms of speech sounds, one may find articulation on target, yet the speech may be very difficult to understand, suggesting that factors other than developmental schedule of speech sounds influence the intelligibility, such as rate, stress, inflection, and loudness of speech. Articulation development should be compared with norms not only on the basis of test results but also on the basis of correctness as determined during contextual speech. Table 7 is provided as a guide to the approximate times when a child learns the different sounds in context. If speech is characterized by more misarticulations in contextual speech than on a single-word articulation test, then those discrepant sounds were not mastered in all contexts.

When determining abnormal or atypical speech development, several aspects must be considered: (1) Is the child's speech sound development behind the normal time schedule? (2) Does the speech deviate from the norms in terms of omissions, substitutions, and distortions? (3) Does the child use an insufficient number of sounds? (4) What other factors might be related to the speech problem? (Berry and Eisenson, 1956). Delayed or disordered speech then can be a matter of manner, quality, and quantity of performance.

Although Table 7 outlines some of the landmarks of speech development, it does not stress the dramatic perceptual and pre-linguistic changes that occur during the first year of life. Wood (1964) stated that observing an infant during this early period of life is like watching a time-lapse motion picture of flowers unfolding before one's very eyes, it is so rapid and beautiful. The landmarks also do not emphasize the non-segmental or prosodic features of articulation that are so important.

Setting specific timetables for the non-phonetic features of speech, as well as for the phonetic features, would indeed be a formidable task, but one that should eventually be done. We do know that most children, at very young ages, learn to smile, pout, frown, and use other body language quite appropriately. We also know that they begin to show awareness of their environment long before 1 year of age by withdrawing from strangers, grasping for small pieces of wearing apparel, such as a button, and exploring objects by placing them inside the mouth, but we do not know exactly when these behaviors begin and when they end. We are not certain if speech perception is considerably ahead of speech production or vice versa (Smith, 1973) and if speech perception facilitates speech learning or if speech production improves speech perception (Shvachkin, 1973; Salus and Salus, 1974). There certainly seems to be some interaction between speech perception and speech production. During this first year of life, when many facets of the child are developing simultaneously, the speech mechanism is also developing and is being tried and tested by the infant.

In learning speech the child is not passive but is continually acting upon the environment and restructuring it in many ways. This active role of organization, assimilation, and accommodation eventually results in the child having his own phonologic system. Moreover, the child does not learn just any adult word, but perhaps those words that are comparatively simple in structure. Each child seems to have a preference for certain words, for certain sounds, and for certain prosodic features of speech. Indeed the child is a selective listener.

SUMMARY

Three basic questions were raised in this chapter: (1) What is speech? (2) How did speech originally occur in human beings? and (3) How does speech develop in the child? Of these three questions, perhaps only the first one can be answered with any degree of certainty or understanding, and even this question is not easily or universally answered. How speech was originally acquired remains an enigma, as does much of phonologic theory and development. Nevertheless, it would appear that speech development begins at birth and probably is seldom mastered even during a lifetime (Van Riper, 1978), because it is such a complex and intriguing process. With the preceding review of the phonologic system, theories on speech acquisition and development, and the sequence of phonemic development in mind, the reader is ready to explore the types and causes of defective articulation.

STUDY SUGGESTIONS

1. Relate the pertinent aspects of various theories of how speech-language developed in the human race to the development of speech-language in a child.
2. Try to develop a rationale for the claim of some linguists that the human child is born with an innate capacity for the development of speech-language.
3. Relate and compare imitation, motivation, reinforcement, and learning theory to the development of articulation in the child.
4. Show how a knowledge of the distinctive features of the most used phonemes can be used in diagnosis and treatment of articulation disorders.
5. Relate the development of phonemes and morphemes to the development of syntax, grammar, and semantic content in speech-language.
6. Relate the factors in the preceding study suggestion to developmental sequence of speech-language and age level of the child.

REFERENCES

Barker, J., and England, G.: A numerical measure of articulation: further developments, J. Speech Hear. Disord. **1:**23-27, 1962.

Berry, M., and Eisenson, J.: Speech disorders: principles and practices of therapy, New York, 1956, Appleton-Century-Crofts.

Black, J., and Irwin, R.: Voice and diction, applied phonation and phonology, Columbus, Ohio, 1969, Charles E. Merrill Publishing Co.

Bloodstein, O: Speech pathology: an introduction, Boston, 1979, Houghton Mifflin Co.

Carrell, J.: Disorders of articulation, Englewood Cliffs, N.J., 1968, Prentice-Hall, Inc.

Chomsky, N., and Halle, M.: The sound pattern of English, New York, 1968, Harper & Row, Publishers.

Compton, A.: Generative studies of children's phonological disorders: a strategy of therapy. In Singh, S., editor: Measurements in hearing, speech and language, Baltimore, 1975, University Park Press.

Curtis, J.: Systematic research in experimental phonetics. 3. The case for dynamic analysis in acoustic phonetics, J. Speech Hear. Disord. **19:**147-157, 1954.

Darley, F.: Diagnosis and appraisal of communication disorders, Englewood Cliffs, N.J., 1964, Prentice-Hall, Inc.

DeLaguna, G.: Speech: its function and development, New Haven, 1927, Yale University Press.

Delattre, P., and Freeman, D.: A dialect study of American r's by x-ray motion pictures, Linguistics **44:**29-68, 1968.

Edwards, M., and Garnica, O.: Patterns of variation in the repetition of utterances by young children, unpublished paper, Stanford University, 1973.

Ervin-Tripp, S.: Language development in review of child development research. In Hoffman, M., and Hoffman, L., editors: Ann Arbor, Mich., 1966, University of Michigan Press.

Fairbanks, G.: Voice and articulation drillbook, New York, 1940, Harper & Row, Publishers.

Fairbanks, G., and Grubb, P.: A psychophysical investigation of vowel formants, J. Speech Hear. Disord. **4:**203-219, 1961.

Ferguson, C., and Farwell, C.: Words and sounds in early language acquisition: English initial consonants in the first 50 words, Language **51:**1-61, 1975.

Ferguson, C., and Garnica, D.: Theories of phonological development. In Lenneberg, E., and Lenneberg, E., editors: Foundations of language development, New York, 1975, Academic Press, Inc.

Gleason, H.: An introduction to descriptive linguistics, New York, 1961, Holt, Rinehart and Winston, Inc.

Greenlee, M.: Interacting processes in the child's acquisition of stop-liquid clusters, PRCLD **7:**85-100, 1974.

Heffner, R.: General phonetics, Madison, Wis., 1952, University of Wisconsin Press.

Hilgard, E.: Theories of learning, ed. 2, New York, 1943, Appleton-Century-Crofts.

Hull, C.: The principles of behavior, New York, 1943, Appleton-Century-Crofts.

Ingram, D.: Phonological disability in children, London, 1976, Edward Arnold.

Irwin, J.: Disorders of articulation, Indianapolis, 1972, The Bobbs-Merrill Co., Inc.

Jakobson, R.: Child language, aphasia, and phonological universals, The Hague, 1968, Mouton.

Jakobson, R., Fant, G., and Halle, M.: Preliminaries to speech analysis, Cambridge, Mass., 1952, The M.I.T. Press.

Jespersen, O.: Language: its nature, development and origin, London, 1922, George Allen & Unwin, LTD.

Jones, D.: An outline of English phonetics, New York, 1932, E. P. Dutton & Co., Inc.

Judson, L., and Weaver, A.: Voice science, ed. 2, New York, 1965, Appleton-Century-Crofts.

Kernahan, D., and Stark, R.: A new classification for cleft lip and cleft palate, Plast. Reconstr. Surg. **22:**435, 1958.

Lenneberg, E., and Lenneberg, E., editors: Foundations of language development, New York, 1975, Academic Press, Inc.

Leutenegger, R.: The sounds of American English: an introduction to phonetics, Chicago, 1963, Scott, Foresman and Co.

Lieberman, P.: Speech physiology and acoustic phonetics, New York, 1977, Macmillan Publishing Co., Inc.

Lillywhite, H.: General concepts of communication, J. Pediatr. **62:**5-10, 1963.

McDonald, E.: Articulation testing and treatment: a sensory-motor approach, Pittsburgh, 1964, Stanwix House, Inc.

McGeoch, J.: The psychology of human learning, New York, 1943, Longman, Inc.

McNeill, D.: The acquisition of language: the study of developmental psycholinguistics, New York, 1970, Harper & Row, Publishers.

Metraux, R.: Speech profiles of the preschool child 18-54 months, J. Speech Hear. Disord. **15:**37-53, 1950.

Morehead, D., and Morehead, A., editors: Normal and deficient child language, Baltimore, 1976, University Park Press.

Morse, P.: Infant speech perception: a preliminary model and review of literature. In Schiefelbusch and Lloyd, 19-53, 1974.

Moskowitz, A.: The two-year-old stage in the acquisition of English phonology, Language **46:**426-441, 1970.

Müller, M.: The science of language, New York, 1840, Longman, Inc.

Nelson, K.: Structure and strategy in learning to talk, Monogr. Soc. Res. Child Dev. **38:**1-2, 1973.

Nemoy, E., and Davis, S.: The correction of defective consonant sounds, Magnolia, Mass., 1954, Expression Co., Publishers.

Noire, L. In Müller, M.: The science of language, New York, 1891, Longman, Inc.

Noll, J.: Articulatory assessment in speech and

the dentalfacial complex, ASHA **2:**283-296, 1970.

Olmsted, D.: Out of the mouth of babes, The Hague, 1971, Mouton.

Perkins, W.: Speech pathology: an applied behavioral science, ed. 2, St. Louis, 1977, The C. V. Mosby Co.

Piaget, J.: Play, dreams, and imitation in childhood, New York, 1962, W. W. Norton and Co., Inc.

Poole, I.: Genetic development of articulation of consonant sounds in speech, Elementary English Review **11:**159-161, 1934.

Prather, E., Hedrick, D., and Kern, C.: Articulation development in children aged two to four years, J. Speech Hear. Disord. **40:**179-191, 1975.

Salus, P., and Salus, M.: Developmental neurophysiology and phonological acquisition order, Language **50:**151-160, 1974.

Sander, E.: When are speech sounds learned? J. Speech Hear. Disord. **37:**55-63, 1972.

Sapir, E.: Language, an introduction to the study of speech, New York, 1921, Harcourt Brace Jovanovich, Inc.

Shohara, H.: Significance of overlapping movements in speech. In McDonald, E.: Articulation testing and treatment: a sensory-motor approach, Pittsburgh, 1964, Stanwix House, Inc.

Shvachkin, N.: The development of phonemic speech perception in early childhood. In Ferguson, C., and Slobin, D., editors: Studies of child language development, New York, 1973, Holt, Rinehart and Winston, Inc., pp. 91-127.

Simon, C.: The development of speech. In Travis, L.: Handbook of speech pathology, New York, 1957, Appleton-Century-Crofts.

Slobin, D.: Cognitive prerequisites for the development of grammar. In Ferguson, C., and Slobin, D., editors: Studies in child language development, New York, 1973, Holt, Rinehart and Winston, Inc.

Smith, A.: A dissertation on the origin of language. In The theory of moral sentiments, ed. 7, London, 1792.

Smith, N.: The acquisition of phonology: a case study, New York, 1973, Cambridge University Press.

Stampe, D.: The acquisition of phonetic representation, PCLS, Fifth Regional Meeting, 1969.

Stetson, R.: Motor phonetics, ed. 2, Amsterdam, 1951, North-Holland Publishing Co.

Templin, M.: Certain language skills in children: their development and interrelationships, Minneapolis, 1957, University of Minnesota Press.

Tiffany, W., and Carrell, J.: Phonetics, theory and application, ed. 2, New York, 1977, McGraw-Hill Book Co.

Van Riper, C.: Speech correction: principles and methods, ed. 6, Englewood Cliffs, N.J., 1978, Prentice-Hall, Inc.

Waterson, N.: Child phonology: a prosodic view, J. Linguistics **7:**170-221, 1971.

Weiss, C.: Weiss Comprehensive Articulation Test, Boston, 1978, Teaching Resources.

Weiss, C. E., and Lillywhite, H. S.: Communication disorders: a handbook for prevention and early intervention, St. Louis, 1976, The C. V. Mosby Co.

Wellman, B., and associates: Speech sounds of young children, University of Iowa Studies in Child Welfare **5:**2, 1931.

Whitney, W.: Language and the study of languages, New York, 1868, Charles Scribner's Sons.

Winitz, H.: Articulatory acquisition and behavior, New York, 1969, Appleton-Century-Crofts.

Wise, C.: Applied phonetics, Englewood Cliffs, N.J., 1957, Prentice-Hall, Inc.

Wood, N.: Delayed speech and language development, Englewood Cliffs, N.J., 1964, Prentice-Hall, Inc.

Wundt, W.: Outlines of psychology, Leipzig, 1897, W. Engleman.

GLOSSARY

abutting consonants A consonant that is closely next to or abutting another consonant.

air turbulence Air passing through the oral cavity but being affected by the oral structure in such a manner that a "noisy" movement or sound is created.

allophone Subdivision of a phoneme; unit of sound making up or belonging to a particular phoneme.

alveolar contact Contact of the tongue, usually tip or blade, with the alveolar ridge.

assimilation The influence of one spoken sound on another as articulators change movements from one to another.

ballistic movement Force and direction—trajectory—of articulatory movements.

bilabial Refers to function of both lips in producing a sound, such as /b/.

coarticulation Overlapping articulatory movements that occur when two contiguous sounds are produced in speaking.

cognate A sound that is much like another, varying mainly in that one is voiced and the other is unvoiced, such as /s/ and /z/.

consonant A speech sound produced by modification of the voiced or unvoiced breath stream.

constriction Narrowing of an opening or passageway.

continuant A speech sound that can be "continued" for a period of time through either the oral or nasal passageway, such as /s/ as compared to /p/.

diathesis Congenital predisposition toward certain diseases or conditions.

diphthong A speech sound produced by smoothly adjusting the articulators within the same syllable to bring two vowels together to form one sound unit, such as bringing /a/ and /ɪ/ together to form /aɪ/ as in "high."

distinctive features Observable articulatory features that differentiate the production of phones and phonemes.

distortion Phones and phonemes are produced but are faulty or "distorted" as opposed to being omitted or substituted.

ellipsis Omitted but understood and unconsciously supplied elements of a sound.

fricative A sound having a "friction" quality caused by forcing the breath stream between two constricted articulators.

General American Dialect English speech supposedly used by most Americans, especially those living in "Middle America" and the western states.

glide A sound produced by movement of articulators causing the breath stream to flow or "glide" rather than being stopped or constricted.

glottal Pertaining to the glottis, the opening between the vocal folds.

holophrastic Expressing an entire phrase or sentence in one word.

homeostasis State of equilibrium of the body.

interdental lisp Distortion of sibilant sounds by placing the tongue between the front teeth.

juxtaposition Next to each other or side by side.

labial Pertaining to the lips.

lateral To the side of the body or articulator, such as the breath stream passing over the side of the tongue as in a lateral lisp. Lateral also refers to the /l/ because the breath stream passes on either side of the elevated tongue in its production. May also refer to lateral pharyngeal walls, lateral movement, etc.

lingual Pertaining to the tongue.

liquid Sometimes used to describe the lateral phonemes or the glides.

malphone Misarticulated phone or sound.

nasal Pertaining to the nose or nasal passages. It may also refer to sounds produced by the breath stream passing through the nose.

obstructing Partially occluding the airstream causing friction or friction sounds

occluding Stopping the breath stream as in the production of plosive and affricative sounds.

omissions Leaving out phones, phonemes, or syllables during speech.

orifice Opening.

overlapping movements Articulator movements for one sound overlapping with those movements of a contiguous sound.

phone A speech sound. The only aspect of spoken language that can be observed and measured; perhaps the basic unit of language.

phoneme Sound or units of sound; a family of allophones or phonetic units.

phonemics Study of the science of speech sounds with regard to meaning.

phonetics Study of the science of speech sounds without regard to meaning.

plosive A phone produced by stopping and suddenly releasing the breath stream by the articulators.

prosody Stress, inflection, rhythm, and melody of speech.

rate A nonsegmental characteristic that influences spoken phones; the speed of talking.

segmental features Features of a speech sound and how it is produced.

sibilant A phoneme characterized by a "hissing" quality as the breath stream is forced between articulators.

stop The occluding of oral or nasal passages causing the breath stream to stop momentarily; a category of consonant sounds.

substitution A phone or phoneme used incorrectly as a substitute for another.

syllabic Having the features of a syllable; a vowel or, more commonly, a vowel plus a consonant.

vocoid Sound that is "voiced."

voiced sound Sound that results from vibration of the vocal cords.

voiceless sound A phone or phoneme in which no sound is produced by vocal cord vibration. Also called unvoiced sound.

CHAPTER FOUR

Types and causal patterns
of articulation disorders

"That is not good language that all understand not."
PROVERBS

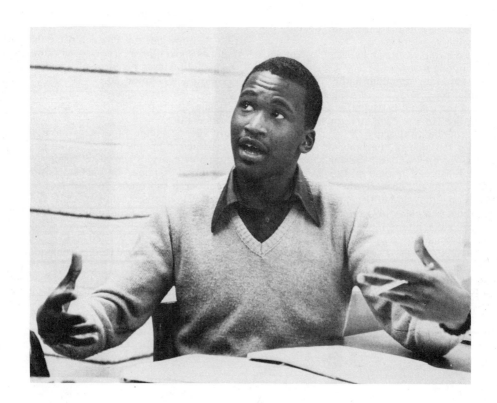

Articulation disorders have been defined by Powers (1971) as the "faulty placement, timing, direction, speed or integration of articulation movements resulting in absent or incorrect speech sounds," or what some would consider phonetic errors. Using a somewhat different viewpoint, Winitz (1969) described defective articulation as the "incorrect learning of the phoneme system of the language," that is, the person uses a system, or a part thereof, that is deviant from the phonetic system of the community in which the language has been learned; this is also referred to as phonemic errors. As pointed out in Chapter 3, misarticulations occur normally during the early stages of speech development. Thus, when some articulation errors occur at certain age levels, the child is not considered to have an articulation disorder. Rather, use of such articulation patterns is characteristic of normal phonologic acquisition.

This information leads one to ask, "When do misarticulations constitute a disorder?" As Johnson and associates (1967) stated, "It is not easy to decide whether or not a given primary child should be regarded as having impaired articulation." At least one study has shown that acquisition of phonemes, that is, spontaneous correction of misarticulations without articulation treatment, sometimes continues until the fifth grade (Bralley and Stoudt, 1977). Roe and Milisen (1942) found that articulation continues to develop until the fourth grade. Nevertheless, it is generally agreed that by the second grade or by 7 years of age most children have acquired normal articulation as judged by adult standards. If misarticulations are regularly present after this age or if sound development is behind the expected norms, articulation is considered to be deviant. Probably the most critical variable in determining if articulation is defective is to compare the child's articulation with normative data (see Chapter 3) relative to the age at which specific phonemes are acquired. If the child's errors are atypical for the age level, it is regarded as an articulation delay or disorder. Additional factors to be considered are the number of errors, consistency of errors, types of errors (described below), conspicuousness of errors (either auditory or visual), ease of imitating correct production of misarticulated sounds, whether the errors interfere with speech intelligibility (understandability), and how the individual and others view the speech problem (Johnson and associates, 1967; Skinner and Shelton, 1978). One important variable mentioned previously is intelligibility or understandability, which, according to Powers (1971), is related to the number of misarticulated sounds, the particular sounds that are misarticulated, and the frequency with which misarticulated sounds occur. We add a fourth factor: type of misarticulation. Obviously the more unintelligible the speech, the greater the severity of the problem and the greater the need for articulation treatment.

Leonard (1973) has taken a somewhat different viewpoint for determining what is deviant articulation, although it is consistent with the preceding statements. He differentiates between use of an immature phonologic system and a deviant system (delay vs disorder). In the former instance the individual is following a normal sequence of development, but at a slower rate, whereas in the latter instance the person is using an abnormal developmental pattern. It is Leonard's contention that persons with a deviant pattern should be given priority for articulation management over those who are merely using an immature pattern of articulation. However, for purposes of efficiency we will use the terms interchangeably in this book, realizing that the diagnostician should try to differentiate between an articulation delay and an articulation disorder. In any case it is obviously important to understand and know what characterizes abnormal articulation as discussed in this chapter.

TYPES OF ARTICULATION DISORDERS
Terminology

A myriad of terms have been used to describe articulation disorders. Three widely used terms generally refer to etiologic bases of the disorder. *Dyslalia* has been defined by Wood (1971) as "defective articulation due to faulty learning or to abnormality of the external speech organs and not to lesions of the central (or peripheral) nervous system"; it is also called a nonorganic or "functional" articulation disorder. In contrast, *dysarthria* (p. 35) refers to a "disturbance in the execution of motor patterns for speech, due to paralysis, weakness, or discoordination of the speech musculature" (Canter, 1967); it is also called an organic articulation disorder. Both voluntary and involuntary movements are consistently impaired (Skinner and Shelton, 1978). According to Wood (1971), dysarthria results from impairment of the central nervous system; however, Byrne and Shervanian (1977) state that dysarthria results from impairment of either the central nervous system or the peripheral nervous system. Canter (1967) has attempted to clarify this confusion by indicating that dysarthria originally referred to central nervous system impairment but is now used as involvement of any level of the neuromuscular system. Part of the confusion relates to the fact that there are a number of different types of dysarthria. *Apraxia* or *dyspraxia* (a lesser degree of apraxia) is an articulation disorder caused by impairment of the central nervous system; specifically it is thought to result from damage to Broca's area (left hemisphere of the frontal lobe) of the cerebral cortex (Skinner and Shelton, 1978). Apraxia has been defined by Rosenbek and associates (1974) as the "impaired ability to accomplish the volitional production of speech sounds and sound sequences." The dyspraxic person can produce muscular movements involved in articulation production but may not do so when using these movements in meaningful phonemes or when sequencing the movements to produce words. Dysarthria and dyspraxia are discussed in greater detail on pp. 210 and 213.

Other terms are also used to describe the symptomatology of the articulation deviancy. At one time *infantile perseveration* was a frequently used term that Powers (1971) has described as the persistence of early speech characteristics beyond the age when correct speech sounds should have been acquired; that is, the earlier natural patterns of talking are retained too long. Infantile speech and "baby talk" have also been used in reference to the same symptoms; however, these terms are seldom used today. The most common articulation errors in this category occur with /r/, the sibilants, other fricatives, selective plosives such as /t/, /d/, /k/, and /g/, the affricates, and /l/ (Carrell, 1968).

Some terms are used to indicate articulation errors of certain phonemes. For example, *sigmatism* or lisping refers to errors of sibilant sounds, for example, /s/ and /z/, and *rhotacism* indicates errors of the /r/ family. *Lalling* has been used to indicate misarticulations of /l/ and /r/ and possibly other tongue-tip consonants. Whereas useful in some contexts, the terms sigmatism, rhotacism, and lalling are not widely used by speech-language pathologists since they usually are understood only by other speech-language pathologists and no one else.

Cluttering, described by Weiss (1964), may be described as rapid, jerky, indistinct, poorly phrased, disfluent speech. It has been described as a disorder in speaking rate having a range of possible organic and nonorganic etiologies. Cluttering has also been described as orally inaccurate speech, or speech that is slurred, as in some persons with cerebral palsy.

One other term that is used to describe distortions of speech is *dentalization*. This term refers to errors caused by placing the tongue too far forward so that it erroneously contacts the front teeth. Similar to problems of dentalization are problems caused by substituting front-of-mouth sounds for back-of-mouth sounds, called *fronting* errors. The reverse of this pattern of substitutions is called *backing* errors, such as /l/ made with the dorsum of the tongue against the soft palate rather than with the tongue tip against the alveolar ridge.

Classification systems

Probably the most traditional system for classifying articulation errors describes the nature of misarticulations, that is, how particular phonemes or morphemes are misarticulated. The types of errors include: (1) omission, (2) substitution, (3) distortion, and (4) addition. An individual with articulation deviancies may have one or a combination of these types of errors. For example, the same person may substitute /θ/ for /s/, /ð/ for /z/, omit /l/ in blends or clusters, and distort /r/.

An *omission* is an articulation error in which a phoneme is not produced at a place where one should occur, for example, /kæ/ for /kæt/ in the word "cat" and /teɪ/ for /steɪ/ in the word "stay." Omissions are most common in the final position of words and occur less frequently in the medial position for most sounds. With the exception of clusters, initial consonants seldom are omitted. An exception is the child with an organic articulation disorder or hearing impairment. The use of omissions decreases with age; they appear more frequently in the speech of younger children. According to Byrne and Shervanian (1977), omissions rarely occur in the speech of children ready for preschool.

A *substitution* is a misarticulation in which a standard or nonstandard phoneme replaces the correct phoneme, for example, /tæt/ for /kæt/ and /θɪt/ for /sɪt/. Substitutions are relatively common and normal in the speech of small children and are the most frequent type of articulation error in school-aged children, although the frequency of occurrence tends to decrease with age. Byrne and Shervanian (1977) report that the most frequent substitutions are those shown in Table 8. Often an earlier-acquired sound is substituted for a later-developing one, as illustrated by the substitution of /w/ for /r/. Substitution errors are usually a change in one distinctive feature, not two or more features. Winitz (1975) indicated that the most frequent substitution involves the distinctive feature of *place,* or where the sound is made; less frequently

Table 8. Most frequent phonemic substitutions

Substitution	Example
/w/ for /r/ and /l/	Red, lamp
/θ/ or /t/ for /s/	Bus
/ð/ or /d/ for /z/	Zebra
/f/ for /θ/	Thumb
/d/ for /ð/ and /g/	This, go
/t/ for /k/	Kitten
/b/ for /v/	Valentine
/s/ or /tʃ/ for /ʃ/	Shoe
/l/ for /j/	Yes

the *manner* of production, or how the sound is made, is incorrect; and the least frequent feature error is *voicing,* which is another system for classifying articulation errors. Carrell (1968) essentially agrees by saying that voiced phonemes are usually substituted for voiced phonemes, fricatives for fricatives, plosives for plosives, etc. In other words the distinctive features of voicing and manner of production are often correct. Substitutions are often inconsistent (Johnson and associates, 1967). They occur least often in the initial position of words and most frequently in the medial and final positions.

A *distortion* is an articulation error in which the standard phoneme is modified so that it is approximated, although incorrect; the approximation is also not acceptable as a different standard sound as in substitution errors and may be considered a malphone. Byrne and Shervanian (1977) further clarify the concept of a distortion by indicating that it is perceived as being either visually or acoustically different but that it still retains the basic characteristics of the target phoneme. Distortions occur more often than omissions in older children and adults and tend to be more consistent in usage than omissions and substitutions (Johnson and associates, 1967). Again an exception would be an organically caused articulation disorder.

An *addition* is a misarticulation in which a phoneme is added, for example, /bəlu/ for /blu/. This type of error occurs quite infrequently and is not always considered an articulation error. In fact the addition of the schwa /ə/ is sometimes used as a remedial technique during the early stages of articulation treatment.

Another classification system was mentioned by Winitz (1969). He dichotomized articulation problems into either *phonetic* or *phonemic* disorders. Phonetic errors are the result of faulty planning and executing of motoric movements for speech sound production. Phonemic errors are the result of using speech sounds incorrectly so that meaning is affected even though the motoric movements can be executed adequately. This system is in need of further delineation before being widely accepted.

Chomsky and Halle (1968) recommended a *distinctive feature* system of classification and description. Their system describes features of phonemes in terms of five major categories: (1) major class, (2) cavity, (3) secondary aperture, (4) manner of articulation, and (5) source. Subcategories of these basic categories are listed in Chapter 3.

A final classification system pertains to misarticulations relevant to the position of sounds within a syllable or word. Two methods have been used: (1) initial-medial-final, and (2) prevocalic, intervocalic, and postvocalic. The first method considers misarticulations as they occur in a word, which can be at the beginning, such as /p/ in "*p*ut," in the middle, such as /l/ in "be*l*ow," or at the end, such as /t/ in "ha*t*." Much criticism has been leveled at this system because contextual speech really does not isolate phonemes in the initial and final positions, with the exception of the first and last sound in an utterance. Virtually all sounds in context are medial. More recently consonant sounds have been described in relation to syllables in which they occur or in vowel contexts. Consonants can be described as occurring before, between, or after a vowel or as starting or ending a syllable in contextual speech. This method underscores the importance of considering misarticulations in contextual speech rather than in isolated words. Both methods are still being used with considerable success in diagnosis and treatment.

A digression seems useful here. Since misarticulations frequently involve the sibilants /s/, /z/, /ʃ/, and /ʒ/, specific terminology is commonly used to describe substitutions and distortions of these phonemes. Speech-language pathologists thus need to be familiar with these terms (Fig. 4-1). *Lingual, frontal, dental,* and *interdental lisps* refer to substitutions and distortions in which the tongue is placed too far forward in the mouth so that it approximates the placement for /θ/ and /ð/. In a *lateral lisp* (unilateral or bilateral) the airstream is directed over one or both sides of the tongue rather than over the central portion of the tongue. *Nasal lisp* involves direction of part or all of the airstream through the nasal cavity rather than through the mouth when producing sibilants. It may resemble a nasal fricative or a nasal "snort" or "snore." *Strident lisp* results in a high-frequency whistle or hissing sound caused by grooving the tongue tip too much or by the breath stream passing between the tongue and a hard surface such as that of dentures or other intraoral appliances. The last type of sibilant error is the *occluded lisp*. This lisp is characterized as having essentially no sibilant quality, so that /s/ and /z/ would be perceived more like a /t/ and /d/ substitution. This misarticulation results from occluding the breath stream in the oral cavity, usually by placing the tongue too far forward or not allowing for a narrow, grooved passageway for the breath stream to pass between the tongue and alveolar ridge. It may resemble a nasal fricative or a nasal "snort" or "snore." A malocclusion such as a closed bite or overbite can cause excessive anterior tongue crowding and a resultant occluded lisp.

Powers (1971) has made some generalizations about the types of errors described previously. Misarticulations seldom occur on vowels and, conversely, are noted most frequently on consonants. This pattern is

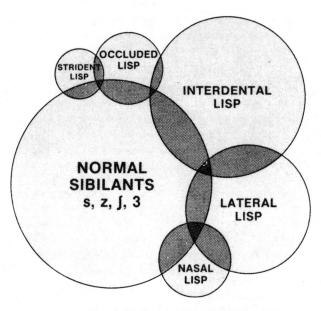

Fig. 4-1. Types of sibilant errors. (From Van Riper, Charles: Speech correction: principles and methods, ed. 6, © 1978. Reprinted by permission of Prentice-Hall, Inc., Englewood Cliffs, New Jersey.)

consistent with the sequence of speech development in that vowels are acquired before consonants. As mentioned before, the most frequently misarticulated sounds are /s/, /z/, /θ/, /ð/, /tʃ/, /dʒ/, /r/, /v/, /ʃ/, /ʒ/, and /l/. These phonemes are the later-appearing ones and thus are presumed to be the more difficult ones to produce, in terms of neuromuscular coordination and precision. Errors occur most frequently on fricatives, often on glides, especially /r/ and the lateral /l/, less often on plosives /t/, /d/, /k/, and /g/, and seldom on nasals. Consonant clusters, such as /spr/ as in "spring," also are frequently misarticulated. Generally the fewest articulation errors are produced in the initial position and more in the medial position, with the most occurring in the final position. There seems to be a progression in articulation development from omissions to substitutions to distortions, with distortions being "closer" to correct articulation. One might say, then, that omissions are more severe errors than substitutions and that substitutions are more severe than distortions, which also follows a progressive dim-

inution in the number of distinctive feature errors. However, severe distortions may make speech less intelligible than either omissions or substitutions because the listener can "fill in" omissions and substitutions more easily.

Severity of articulation disorders varies from mild to severe and from barely perceptible to the trained ear to complete unintelligibility. The number of misarticulated sounds, the consistency of misarticulations, the types of errors, importance of deviant sounds to intelligibility, stimulability of the misarticulated sounds (ability to imitate the sound in error), nonsegmental features (rate, intensity, stress, and rhythm), and the age of the person are some of the factors contributing to the severity level of a particular articulation disorder (Perkins, 1961; Powers, 1971). The prognosis for developing correct articulation and the probable amount of intervention needed for correction of errors are additional factors to be considered in determining severity. For example, if the prognosis is good, the severity level will be less than if the prognosis is poor. Similarly if years of treatment seem necessary for speech improvement, the problem is considered more severe than if the disorder will likely require less time to correct.

CAUSAL PATTERNS OF ARTICULATION ERRORS

Now that systems for classifying articulation disorders have been presented, we need to discuss the causal patterns of misarticulations. As Winitz (1969) has indicated, "When mastery is not achieved by a certain age level, causal interpretations are often made to explain the absence of describable motor responses." Clearly a certain level of neuromuscular development is undoubtedly necessary for learning articulation; however, other factors are also required. Normal articulation development involves both physical characteristics and capacities as well as perceptual and environmental influences. Byrne and Shervanian (1977) explain:

Not all infants are born with the same capacity for mastering a language. In addition, each environment will interact with whatever capabilities the infant brings to it. The varying forces of capacity and environment shape the quality and quantity of language and speech development.

This concept of two influences on articulation development has led to dichotomizing etiology into *organic* and *nonorganic* or "functional" causes. Traditionally the term "functional" has been used as a "wastebasket term" for any articulation disorder for which no cause was apparent or that was assumed not to have a physical cause; as Powers (1971) has stated, they are labeled by default because there is no obvious organic basis. Bloodstein (1979) listed the following attributes associated with nonorganic articulation problems: (1) absence of obvious structural, auditory, neural, or intellectual disorders; (2) delayed onset of talking; (3) tendency toward spontaneous speech improvement; (4) multiple misarticulations; (5) greater involvement of later-

developing sounds; (6) misarticulations that usually consist of substitutions and omissions; and (7) presence of inconsistent misarticulations. We prefer to classify etiologies as organic, nonorganic, or mixed whenever possible. Organic causes are those in which there is a known structural, physiologic, sensory, or neurologic deficit in the vocal tract or related structures. Conversely a nonorganic cause is one in which there are no *obvious* signs of structural, physiologic, sensory, or neurologic deviations. Mixed causes include both organic and nonorganic factors.

When attempting to determine causation, it must be kept in mind that many articulation disorders are not readily classifiable as purely organic or nonorganic, although they will be discussed here as if they were. Additionally there may be multiple etiologic factors involved in a particular case or there may be only one. Thus we agree with Powers (1971), who recommends looking for a *causal pattern* rather than determining *the* cause.

Organic causal patterns

Neuromuscular problems involving the control of the speech mechanism often result in articulation disorders. According to Canter (1967), "When neuromotor mechanisms of speech are impaired, there are rather predictable alterations in the resulting speech pattern according to the level of the lesion," although there is more nearly a one-to-one relationship between the lesion and speech output in adults than is the case for children. These deviancies may occur in the cerebrum such as in the case of dyspraxia. Some impairments involve the central nervous system or the peripheral nervous system, which innervate the speech mechanism as in cerebral palsy, Parkinson disease, paralysis and paresis of the tongue, amyotrophic lateral sclerosis, and Bell palsy. The muscles themselves are involved in myopathies such as muscular dystrophy. Causes of neuromuscular disabilities range across a wide spectrum of impairments: hereditary malformations, prenatal injuries, metabolic and toxic disturbances, tumors, traumas, seizures, infectious diseases, demyelinating diseases, muscular diseases, and vascular impairments (Perkins, 1977). They may occur prenatally, in infancy, during childhood, and during adulthood.

Two major types of neuromuscular problems confronting speech-language pathologists are *dysarthria* and *dyspraxia*. Dysarthria is perhaps more appropriately termed dysarthrias because there are a number of different dysarthric patterns, depending on the site of the lesion (Darley, Aronson, and Brown, 1975). It is a common motor speech problem among persons with cerebral palsy and dysphasia but may result from any damage to the central nervous system. The primary manifestation of this disorder is usually a paresis of the speech musculature, which impairs the motoric ability for both speech and some vegetative functions. Complete impairment of the speech muscles would be called paralysis. Some of the most prominent speech deviations reported among the dysarthrias by Darley, Aronson, and Brown (1975) were hypernasality, imprecise production of consonants, breathiness, monopitch, reduced or excessive stress, monoloudness, variable rate, prolonged intervals, distorted vowels, and harsh vowel quality. These symptoms obviously vary among the types of dysarthria, such as flaccid dysarthria, spastic dysarthria, ataxic dysarthria, and hypokinetic or hyperkinetic dysarthria. Additional information on dysarthria is provided on p. 213.

Dyspraxia, or more correctly called verbal dyspraxia, is also a neuromuscular speech problem; however, the nature of this problem is not one of paralysis or paresis, but rather one of programming the motor cortex and articulators for speech production. Unlike dysarthria, muscle weakness and incoordination are absent and vegetative functions may be essentially normal. Dyspraxia may be present in anyone at any age but is commonly found among post-stroke patients with dysphasia and is characterized by an inability or difficulty in performing speech acts voluntarily. How-ever, both verbal dyspraxia and dysarthria may be present in the same person (LaPointe and Wertz, 1974). More information on verbal dyspraxia is included on p. 91.

Intellectual variables are grossly related to articulation deviancies. Since mental retardation is commonly associated with diffuse neurologic damage, it will be considered an organic disorder. Persons with lower levels of intellectual functioning demonstrate a higher incidence of articulation errors than persons with higher levels of intellectual functioning. Perkins (1977) stated that intelligibility of articulation especially is a prevalent problem among mentally retarded individuals. Intelligence quotients of persons within the normal range do not seem to be related to articulation development.

Mental retardation is defined by the American Association for the Mentally Retarded as:

A group of conditions characterized by inadequate social adjustment, reduced learning capacity, and a slow rate of maturation, present singly or in combination, due to a degree of intellectual functioning below average, and usually present from birth or soon after.

Mentally retarded persons can be functionally classified into three groups:

1. *Educable:* Can develop social and occupational adequacy; capable of unskilled or semi-skilled work. Can achieve academic work to third-, fourth-, or fifth-grade and sometimes sixth-grade level. The intelligence quotient is between 50 and 75.
2. *Trainable:* Can learn self-care and social adjustment. Incapable of academic work. A few are capable of very simple work in a protected work situation. The intelligence quotient is between 25 and 49.
3. *Custodial:* Incapable of self-care. The intelligence quotient is below 25.*

Etiologic factors of mental retardation are summarized in Table 9 (Lillywhite and

---

*From Lillywhite, H., and Bradley, D.: Communication problems in mental retardation, New York, 1969, Harper & Row, Publishers.

Table 9. Simplified medical classification of mental retardation

Category	Description
1	Associated with cerebral infections, both prenatal and postnatal
2	Associated with intoxications such as toxemia of pregnancy, other maternal intoxication, bilirubin, and postimmunization intoxication
3	Associated with conditions caused by trauma or physical agents such as prenatal injury, mechanical injury at birth, asphyxia at birth, or postnatal injury
4	Associated with diseases or conditions resulting from disorders of metabolism, growth, or nutrition; some of these are cerebral lipoidosis, phenylketonuria, galactosemia, disorders of protein metabolism, disorders of carbohydrate metabolism, arachnodactyly, hypothyroidism, and gargoylism
5	Associated with diseases and conditions caused by new growths, including neurofibromatosis, trigeminal angiomatosis, tuberous sclerosis, and intracranial neoplasms
6	Associated with diseases and conditions resulting from prenatal influence resulting in congenital cerebral defects, cranial anomalies, Laurence-Biedl syndrome, and Down syndrome
7	Associated with conditions caused by uncertain cause, with the structural reaction manifest in conditions of brain sclerosis and cerebellar degeneration
8	Resulting from uncertain cause, with the functional reaction alone manifest in the following: cultural-familial mental retardation, psychogenic mental retardation associated with environmental deprivation, psychogenic mental retardation associated with emotional disturbances, and mental retardation associated with psychotic disorders

Bradley, 1969). Mental retardation refers to a lower level of functioning in all areas of development rather than to selected specific areas.

Mentally retarded individuals usually demonstrate deficits in all areas of speech and language development. The incidence of articulation deviancies is high in this population, with over one half of the persons in one study demonstrating articulation disorders (Byrne and Shervanian, 1977). The pattern of articulation development usually is similar to that of normal persons but occurs at a delayed rate. Mentally retarded individuals may never "catch up," depending on the degree of mental retardation. Often problems resulting from neuromuscular deficiencies are present in addition. Types of misarticulations are similar to those of normal persons. Frequency of errors tends to range from fewest to most as follows: nasals, plosives, glides, fricatives, affricates, and sibilants, in that order.

Other physical characteristics such as general physical debility and poor health, frequent illnesses, developmental slowness, glandular deficiencies, endocrine abnormalities, and hereditary or biologic inferiority may contribute to the development of articulation disorders (Powers, 1971). Research has been so sparse in these areas that definite conclusions cannot be made. It has been postulated that such factors may have an indirect effect by restricting the person's activities and thus result in deprivation of speech stimulation and motivation. At this time we do not even know if a causal relationship exists, much less understand the nature of the relationship.

Motor incoordination in the absence of a neuromuscular disorder has been postulated as a possible cause of articulation disorders, but research results have been contradictory and inconclusive (Powers, 1971; Weiss, 1968). Although it generally has been concluded that persons with deviant articulation do not consistently show poor general motor ability, it may be an etiologic factor or part of the causal pattern in selected individuals. Sommers and Kane

(1974) support this statement when they reported that some recent research has shown that fine motor skills involving movement in space may be defective in some children having functional articulation disorders.

Tongue incoordination could be a causative factor in some cases (Johnson and associates, 1967), although this is not easily determined because of the tremendous compensatory abilities of the tongue in some persons. The occurrence of tongue incoordination as an etiologic factor has been supported by studies showing that individuals with articulation disorders perform diadochokinetic tasks more poorly than normal speakers (Weiss, 1968; Dworkin, 1978). Oral diadochokinesis is defined as the rapid repetition of antagonistic speech movements, more appropriately called maximum articulator movement abilities.

Tongue thrust or orofacial muscle imbalance has also been related to speech problems. Tongue thrust swallow includes (1) forward thrusting of the tongue against or between the anterior or lateral teeth, (2) tight lip closure, (3) teeth apart during swallow, and (4) malocclusion. It may be a causative factor, although no conclusions can be made about the relationship between articulation and tongue thrusting (Powers, 1971; Weiss, 1970; Mason and Proffit, 1974). It most commonly is related to the malocclusion of open bite (Bloomer, 1971; Barrett and Hanson , 1978; Weiss, 1970), which may or may not affect articulation. Associated symptomatology of the tongue thrust syndrome includes mouth breathing, upper respiratory problems, tongue-tie, family history of similar problem, slow and messy eater, and history of finger- or thumb-sucking habits (Weiss, 1973). Etiology has been attributed to bottle nursing, delayed maturation, structural deviations, upper respiratory problems, genetic predisposition, psychoemotional factors, and of course neuromuscular incoordination. Barrett and Hanson (1978) reported a higher incidence of articulation problems among persons with tongue thrust, mainly in interdental and lateral lisping and dentalization of lingua-alve-

olar sounds /t/, /n/, and /l/. Fletcher, Casteel, and Bradley (1961) found that frequency of tongue thrust and associated articulation errors decreases with age, although articulation errors decrease at a slower rate among tongue thrusters than among nontongue thrusters. Also tongue thrusting and malocclusion have been reported to be present in normal speakers as well as in speakers with defective speech (Subtelny, Mestre, and Subtelny, 1964). Implicating tongue thrust as being neuromuscularly significant is indeed precarious.

Structural deviations of the face and oral cavity may contribute to the etiology of articulation disorders, although articulation errors do not invariably result from such deviations. As Bloomer (1971) stated, "Orofacial abnormalities may directly affect speech, indirectly affect them, or have no effect." Most structural anomalies are of a developmental nature, even though some result from trauma, surgery, or disease.

Malocclusions (dental and jaw irregularities) may be contributory to misarticulations, although defective articulation is not a necessary consequence of all malocclusions nor is a malocclusion present in all articulation disorders. Dental abnormalities that may affect articulation include *neutroclusion* (anomalies or malalignment of individual teeth and groups of teeth, but excluding malalignment of the dental arches; also called Angle class I malocclusion); *distoclusion* (mandible and mandibular teeth retrusion so that their position relative to the maxillary teeth is posterior; also called Angle class II malocclusion); *mesioclusion* (mandible and mandibular teeth protrusion so that their position relative to the maxillary teeth is anterior; also called Angle class III malocclusion); *open bite* (central and lateral incisors of the maxilla are too far forward in relation to the mandibular incisors), and *closed bite* (maxillary incisors overlap the mandibular incisors more than two thirds the distance of the mandibular teeth). Luchsinger and Arnold (1965) report that malocclusions are more frequently present in lispers; Bernstein (1956) found no higher rate of articulation problems in children with malocclusions. These contradictory findings suggest that more research is needed to relate specific dental deviations to specific types of articulation errors.

Bankson and Byrne (1962) studied the effects of *missing teeth* on articulation in young children. They reported a significant relationship between the absence of teeth and the misarticulations of /f/, /ʃ/, and /z/. Snow (1961) also found a higher percentage of malphones among first grade children with missing teeth. Both studies reported that a number of children with missing teeth had normal speech; therefore, once again the results are inconclusive.

A structural deviation frequently mentioned by laypersons is *tongue-tie* or ankyloglossia. This deviation is the result of a short lingual frenum or frenulum, one that is attached too far forward on the undersurface of the tongue, restricting the range of tongue tip movement. Tongue-tie is seldom a significant factor; however, according to Bloomer (1971):

Indication that the frenum is abnormally restrictive is assumed if the tongue-tip is noticeably indented on protrusion; cannot contact the alveolar arch when the mandible is in normal vertical relationship to the maxilla for speech; if the tip cannot be directed to contact the angles of the mouth; or if the consonants that require linguadental and lingua-alveolar contact cannot be achieved.*

Deviations of the tongue have also been considered from a structural standpoint (Bloomer, 1971; Johnson and associates, 1967). Except for partially or entirely missing tongue (aglossia), correlating lingual deviations with articulation problems has not been fruitful. A tongue that is too large (macroglossia) or too small (microglossia) must be considered in relation to oral cavity size and contour of the hard palate. Decid-

ing the significance of lingual deviations must be an individual matter.

Another oral structure important to articulation is the *soft palate* or velum. Its importance to normal resonance and the production of pressure consonants has been reported extensively (Spriestersbach and Sherman, 1968; Bzoch, 1979; Morley, 1970). Most of the studies have dealt with soft palate physiology, even though structure and function are not easily separated. If the soft palate is too short, does not move far enough, or does not move as quickly or consistently as it should, articulation and resonance usually are disordered because of inadequate velopharyngeal closure. It is not uncommon for a person diagnosed as having congenital palatal inadequacy to have a shorter-than-average velum as part of the problem. Sometimes congenital palatal inadequacy is the diagnosis following removal of the adenoids. Cleft of the soft or hard palate is a major structural anomaly that causes articulation and resonance problems and is discussed further on p. 214.

Historically, different configurations of the *hard palate* have received a fair share of clinical attention concerning their importance to articulation. As with most of the oral cavity structures, a clear determination of cause and effect has eluded researchers, unless the structural deviation is extreme, as in the case of cleft palate or removal of part of the maxilla. Fairbanks and Bebout (1950) found no significant differences in hard palate configurations among superior and inferior adult speakers. Clinical evidence indicates that a low palatal arch may be more detrimental to articulation than an unusually high palatal arch. However, Johnson and associates (1967) mentioned that an unusually high and narrow palate in the presence of an excessively large tongue may be a contributing etiologic factor.

One final structural composite that should be considered is the lymph tissue better known as *tonsils* and *adenoids*. Enlarged or hypertrophied tonsils can obstruct the oral passageway and cause a "drag" on the soft palate, thus forcing the breath stream

---

*From Bloomer, H.: Speech defects associated with dental malocclusions and related abnormalities. In Travis, L., editor: Handbook of speech pathology and audiology, © 1971. Reprinted by permission of Prentice-Hall, Inc., Englewood Cliffs, New Jersey.

through the nose (Blakeley, 1972). Enlarged adenoids can occlude the nasal passageway causing an inadequate amount of air to resonate in the nose. This resulting condition is known as hyponasality or denasality. Conversely, if the adenoids are contributing to velopharyngeal (veloadenoidal) closure because the soft palate may be contacting them in order to achieve closure, then their removal (adenoidectomy) may increase the pharyngeal space to the extent that the soft palate no longer makes contact with the back pharyngeal wall. The resulting condition is hypernasality or excessive nasal resonance and airflow, as well as weak production of the pressure consonants. Neither the tonsils nor the adenoids should be indiscriminately removed and not without regard to their subsequent effect on articulation and resonance. Removing part of the adenoidal tissue rather than all of it is another viable consideration in treatment.

Generally research has not shown palate, tongue, and lip measurements to be related to articulation skills (Fletcher and Meldrum, 1968; McEnery and Gaines, 1941). Nevertheless, according to Bloomer (1971), deformities of mouth opening, such as small mouth opening; facial deformity, such as asymmetric or partially missing facial structures; lingual deformities, such as macroglossia, microglossia, or glossectomy; and nasal deformities, such as a deviated nasal septum or hypertrophied turbinates may contribute to articulation deficits.

Certain *sensory deficits* can cause articulation disorders. There is no question that auditory perceptual problems are significant etiologic factors. *Hearing impairments* account for over 10% of all speech defects and are classified as follows: *deaf* or congenitally deaf, *deafened* or adventitiously deaf, and *hard of hearing*. Deaf refers to severe hearing loss (greater than 85 db in the better ear) occurring prior to the acquisition of speech such that the child is unable to understand and learn speech naturally by hearing. Deafened refers to severe hearing loss after speech was acquired, and hard of hearing refers to auditory abnormality in

which sufficient hearing sensitivity remains to permit oral communication, usually with the assistance of amplification, but may interfere with speech learning if it is present in the infant or young child, or with academic learning if the loss is present at school age.

Hearing impairment is generally categorized into four types, based on the site of the problem. A *conductive loss* is one in which the pathology occurs in the external or middle ear as a result of a "plugged" external ear, perforated eardrum, atypical ossicular chain, middle ear filled with fluid, and otosclerosis. The hearing loss in this type is rarely severe and is usually treatable, but articulation may be affected somewhat if the loss is persistent, especially during infancy and childhood. In a *sensorineural loss* the lesion occurs in the inner ear in the cochlea or in cranial nerve VIII as a result of heredity, toxic effects from drugs, maternal and viral infections, diseases, and injury. If the loss is prominent in the higher frequencies, misarticulations of the nonvoiced fricatives often result. Children who are "deaf" usually have both vowel and consonant misarticulations. For example, they tend not to distinguish between voiced and nonvoiced consonants; to omit, distort, and substitute consonants and sometimes vowels; to nasalize vowels; and to misarticulate diphthongs. A third type of auditory impairment is *central hearing loss,* the cause of which occurs in the auditory processing area of the brain (temporal lobe). This type is not well understood; it may relate more to auditory perception than to auditory acuity. A fourth type is *mixed hearing loss,* in which the individual has a combination of hearing problems.

Hearing loss, depending on the severity, can impair the child's ability to perceive sounds. If these sounds include the speech sounds, then the child does not learn normal articulation. Obviously the type, degree, and age of onset of the hearing loss will affect the type and degree of the articulation problem. Generally more impaired hearing causes more impaired speech (Ling,

1973). If the child has a significant high-frequency loss, then high-frequency sounds—/s/, /f/, /θ/, and /tʃ/—are more likely to be misarticulated.

Inadequate auditory perceptual skills may be a cause of articulation disorders. This kind of deficiency is not to be confused with deficient auditory acuity (hearing loss). One may have normal hearing yet perceive speech sounds in an abnormal manner—out of sequence, reversed, or without recognition. Research on the relationship between articulation deficiency and *speech sound discrimination* is conflicting and inconclusive, but individuals with deviant articulation seem to have inferior speech sound discrimination ability. Winitz (1969) and Powers (1971) agree with this assumption but suggest that this deficiency may be a result rather than a cause of articulation disorders. Whereas some studies (Kronvall and Diehl, 1954) found significant discriminative differences between normal and abnormal speakers, other studies (Prins, 1963) have not found significant differences. Even though it seems logical that if an individual cannot discriminate speech sounds, speech acquisition would be impaired, studies have not consistently supported such logic. Nevertheless it is our contention, based mainly on clinical experience, that a relationship exists between speech discrimination and articulation in many persons and that the studies to date have not been effective in assessing self-discrimination abilities. Studies have merely assessed the child's ability to discriminate speech sounds of other speakers, rather than assessing the child's self-discrimination abilities for the speech sounds that are misarticulated. Furthermore we would caution against discarding speech discrimination training in treatment, for if this is done we may be "throwing the baby out with the bathwater." Difficulties in achieving carry-over may relate directly to lack of adequately developed speech discrimination skills. In the meantime more pertinent research on speech discrimination should be undertaken.

Another auditory perceptual skill that has been investigated is *pitch discrimination*. Studies have shown that normal speakers discriminate varying pitch levels better than persons with disordered articulation (Winitz, 1969). Thus this may be an etiologic factor in some cases. The research on the relationship between articulation and *auditory memory* has also been inconclusive (Winitz, 1969). In some instances poor auditory memory may be a causative factor and should be assessed routinely.

Oral sensation-perception provides the sensory feedback from oral cavity structures to the brain. These sensations are thought to be more important in maintaining articulation than in learning it (Van Riper and Irwin, 1958). However, research in this area, which involves oral stereognosis, tactile threshold sensitivity, tactile discrimination, and two-point discrimination, has not clearly demonstrated a relationship between oral sensation-perception and articulation (McCall, 1969; Weiss and Skalbeck, 1975).

Another consideration on the role of sensory feedback and articulation acquisition deals with *sensory deprivation*. We are not concerned here with studies on short-term deprivation, such as tactile or kinesthetic deprivation caused by anesthesia (Scott and Ringel, 1971; Prosek and House, 1975). Rather we are concerned with longer-term sensory deprivation such as that caused by general deprivation of the child because of environmental isolation, neglect, lack of stimulation, and lack of teaching. For example, what is the effect of prolonged auditory, visual, or tactile-kinesthetic sensory deprivation on a child? More specifically, what are the effects of prolonged sensory deprivation on articulation? Even if sensory deprivation is quite subtle, can it result in future articulation problems? Answers to these questions may eventually provide direction to the habilitation process of some children.

One final factor that may be related to speech acquisition is *visual acuity*. Although little research has been done in this area, there is a higher incidence of articulation errors in blind persons (Powers, 1971). Since formation of one third of the speech sounds is visible, inability to see them could cause a delay in their acquisition.

Nonorganic causal patterns

Environmental and personal factors are important in the development of normal articulation. According to Johnson and associates (1967), no significant organic factor can be found in the majority of articulation cases. It is probably true that the most important single cause of articulation errors is the lack of sufficiently favorable conditions for learning good speech. Environment is highly influential in a child's articulation development. Research has investigated selected environmental variables. It has been shown that there is a higher incidence of articulation disorders among *lower socioeconomic levels* (Powers, 1971). Winitz (1969) reports that there is a low, positive correlation between articulation skills and socioeconomic status. His review of the literature showed that persons from upper socioeconomic levels provide a more favorable linguistic environment in that they model better speech patterns for the child to imitate and may be more reinforcing. They also tend to create more stimulation for speech development and provide a greater amount and better quality of articulation training. Yet Everhart (1953) and Prins (1962) did not find a correlation between frequency of articulation problems and parental occupation. Cultural factors appear to influence articulation development more than socioeconomic factors.

Sibling status has been shown to be an environmental factor related to articulation skills (Perkins, 1977; Powers, 1971; Winitz, 1969). Children without siblings, first-born children (Koch, 1956), and children with greater age spacing between siblings demonstrate better articulation skills. Articulation of twins tends to be inferior to that of singletons. This might reflect differences in the frequency or quality of parental attention or of sibling interaction. In the preceding favorable circumstances the parents spend more time with the child, providing a greater amount of and better quality of speech patterns for imitation, especially during the formative years. In the cases of children from families with more than one child and smaller age spacing between siblings, the children probably spend less time with parents and more time with siblings, possibly resulting in inadequate articulation models. Siblings also may not be as reinforcing. Residing in a home in which a foreign language is spoken may result in articulation deviancy as the result of inadequate articulation models for the language of the community (Carrell, 1968). Although differences exist in regard to sibling status, these differences seem to disappear rapidly after the child begins school.

Two other environmental variables—*sex* and *rural living*—have been investigated. A review of the literature (Perkins, 1977; Templin, 1963; Winitz, 1969) shows that females frequently demonstrate better articulation skills than males; however, the differences are seldom statistically significant. Males are also more frequently identified as having articulation problems than are females. Residing in a rural rather than in an urban area does not seem to affect speech development.

Winitz (1969) wrote, ". . . when obvious physical and mental abnormalities are not present, most if not all, phonetic errors are the result of incorrectly learned phonemic systems." In this light one cause of deviant articulation may be *poor speech models* or inadequate speech models as some children may tend to imitate the articulation patterns heard. These poor models may be provided by busy parents, inarticulate older siblings, or others presenting unfavorable models but who are important to the child. The child may be in an environment in which little speech is used. Consequently speech would seldom be heard, resulting in insufficient stimulation and modeling.

Another environmental or personal factor is *lack of speech stimulation and motivation*. For example, a child's wants may be anticipated or gestures accepted in the place of oral speech so that the child does not need to use speech to communicate needs and wants. This anticipation may be done by parents, siblings, and others. Similarly parents usually are excellent interpreters. They can understand virtually everything the unintelligible child says; thus the child really does not need to speak more intelligibly until associating with other children. In other instances the child may be relatively isolated so that there is seldom a need to speak. In other situations the child may be punished for incorrect articulations or not praised for good speech efforts and consequently choose not to speak. Although scientific data are inconclusive in regard to this area, clinical evidence indicates the importance of stimulation and motivation in speech development.

A third environmental variable is *inadequate or inappropriate reinforcement*. If a child is not reinforced for accurate articulation or is reinforced for inadequate articulation, use of articulation errors may persist. If people in the environment do not attend to or respond to the child's utterances and positively reinforce speech attempts, the child may choose not to speak in later situations. On the other hand Winitz (1969) believes that a parent can be too tolerant of deviant speech and reinforce it; thus the child will not attempt to alter misarticulations. A child is reinforced for such errors by the parent who does not rephrase error-filled sentences and who acknowledges understanding of misarticulated words.

A final consideration concerns *educational achievement*. Several investigators (Winitz, 1969; Ham, 1958) reported significant relationships between reading and spelling problems and articulation problems. Although the correlation may not be as high as Winitz suggests—"a delay in reading is the result of a delay in articulation development"—there does seem to be a relationship. Furthermore this relationship might also include linguistic variables. A child with an articulation problem not uncommonly also has a language problem as well as reading and spelling problems.

Psychologic and emotional factors may also influence articulation development. According to Carrell (1968), infantile speech is often emotionally based, reflecting immaturity, insecurity, or some other psychologic influence. Perkins (1977) reports that dependency and regression are often associated clinically with immature articulation, but there is little research evidence for this. Winitz (1969) concluded from his review of studies that persons with articulation defects have a greater proportion of adjustment and behavioral problems on nonstandardized personality inventories. At variance with Winitz, Powers (1971) found the results of studies on *personality traits* and adjustment to be inconsistent in their findings, with some showing a difference between articulatory-deficient children and normal speakers. In the instances in which there is a personality or psychologic difference, one wonders if this difference is the cause or the result of the articulation disorder. Most probably the relationship works both ways.

After reviewing the literature, Powers (1971) concluded that studies consistently show a relationship between articulation skills and *parental adjustment and attitudes*. Some studies have shown that mothers of articulatory-defective children are more poorly adjusted, have less favorable attitudes toward the child, have higher standards, and are more critical. Such characteristics may result in a "rejecting, overcritical, punitive or emotionally-disturbed atmosphere." Such a situation may result in faulty learning of articulation. However, these findings are not consistently reported (Spriestersbach, 1956).

A child may stop developing articulation abilities or regress to more immature articulation patterns as a result of an *emotional reaction* to an experience that is traumatic for the child. Examples are regression resulting from the birth of a sibling, hospitalization of a parent, or death of an important person in the child's environment. Articulation development may be impeded or stopped if a child undergoes a long period of hospitalization (sometimes a relatively short period of hospitalization can be detrimental), illness, or injury. Other similar situations can also adversely affect the child's articulation.

Anxiety, frustration, and discouragement on the part of others concerning the child's speech are etiologic factors. Such emotional reactions to the person with disordered articulation of either organic or nonorganic etiology may result in the perpetuation of the disorder. Powers (1971) has summarized environmental influences very well:

. . . it is obvious that the amount and kind of speech stimulation in the home is a powerful determinant of the child's articulation and language development. Certain environmental conditions and certain types of interaction between the child and his environment are necessary for the development of mature speech. To develop normal patterns of speech a child must hear normal patterns of speech, must have a need and desire to talk, must experience pleasure in hearing speech and in responding with speech, and must have sufficient variety in his speech, and must be reacted to constructively by others.*

Unknown etiology must be indicated in some cases of articulation disorders. A child is subject to a wide range of hazards, which may be physical, environmental, or emotional. It must also be remembered that a child is more vulnerable to unfavorable factors during the first few years and relatively less after the age of 5 or 6 years. Sometimes the evaluator is not able to determine significant etiologic factors, some of which may have been present at an early age and are no longer apparent, such as early injury, illness, or emotional trauma.

Special causes

Cerebral palsy, according to McDonald and Chance (1964), occurs in 3 of every 1000 births. It has many varied definitions and classifications but is defined by Skinner and Shelton (1978) as follows:

A neuromuscular disability including weakness, paralysis, or incoordination. This disorder, which results from brain damage prior to, during, or shortly after birth, may involve different portions of the body, including the speech mechanism. Varieties of cerebral palsy marked by distinctive motor impairments are *athetosis, spasticity,* and *rigidity.**

Usually *ataxia, tremor,* and *mixed* are included also as other major categories, and there are many subcategories of each type. Cerebral palsy is a nonprogressive disorder that can be caused by genetic factors as well as by prenatal, perinatal, and postnatal disease, infection, or trauma. It is primarily a motor transmission problem that may be associated with sensory input, intellectual disturbances and behavioral disturbances.

One classification system for this condition identifies the site of lesion in the brain (Dickson, 1974). Pyramidal lesions result in spasticity, which is characterized by difficulty in executing movement and lack of inhibitory control over muscles. Extrapyramidal lesions result in athetosis, rigidity, and tremor characterized by failure of voluntary control over muscular activity. More specifically, athetosis is identified by involuntary writhing movements that accompany purposeful or postural movement. Cerebellar lesions result in ataxia and atonia (subcategories of cerebral palsy), in which the individual is unable to synchronize fine movements. It must be remembered that multiple types of cerebral palsy may be found in the same individual. Dickson (1974) reports that 90% of individuals with cerebral palsy are spastic or athetoid.

Cerebral palsy is further categorized by the nature of limb involvement. *Monoplegia* refers to involvement of one arm or leg; *paraplegia*, both lower limbs; *hemiplegia*,

---

*From Powers, M.: Functional disorders of articulation: symptomatology and etiology. In Travis, L., editor: Handbook of speech pathology and audiology, Englewood Cliffs, N.J., 1971, Prentice-Hall, Inc.

*From Skinner, P., and Shelton, R.: Speech, language, and hearing: normal processes and disorders, Reading, Mass., © 1978, Addison-Wesley Publishing Co., Inc. Reprinted with permission.

one side of the body; *triplegia,* three limbs; and *quadriplegia*, four limbs.

A wide range of speech and language deviancies occur in individuals having cerebral palsy with severity levels ranging from normal to severe (Mysak, 1971). Incidence figures for communication problems range from 70% to 86%, and there may be problems in respiratory, auditory, phonatory, articulatory, rhythmic, and linguistic systems, with articulation problems being most frequent. The incidence of articulation disorders is high, varying in severity from near normal to very severe. Mysak (1971) reports that articulation development may be complicated by the following factors:

1. Persistence of infantile oroneuromotor patterns
2. Insufficient velopharyngeal closure resulting in inadequate intraoral breath pressure
3. Accompanying mental retardation or hearing loss

Articulation in cerebral palsy is difficult to characterize, although it might be generally described as follows according to type:

1. The athetoid person usually is able to make speech movements, but movements are not under consistent voluntary control.
2. The spastic person is limited in direction and extent of movement, but voluntary control is usually consistent.
3. The ataxic person has defective feedback and often abnormally slow slurred speech.

However, the articulation of each person with cerebral palsy is unique and must be carefully evaluated, even though common symptomatology is present.

Cleft palate is an orofacial anomaly that occurs in approximately 1 in 770 births (Phair, 1947). Koepp-Baker (1971) characterized cleft palate as a deformity that represents an aberrant embryologic tissue disposition. Kernahan and Stark (1958) identify three categories of cleft palate:

1. Clefts of the primary palate (lip and premaxilla, also called prepalatal clefts)
2. Clefts of the secondary palate (posterior to the incisive foramen including both hard and soft palates, also called palatal clefts)
3. Clefts of the primary and secondary palates (includes lip and palates, also called palatal clefts)

Most clefts are "open"; however, occasionally submucous or occult clefts occur in which the bones of the hard palate have failed to unite and the muscles of the soft palate are malattached but the mucous membrane is intact. The soft palate often is short and movement is limited in submucous or occult clefts. Clefts are also classified as being unilateral or bilateral, that is, there is involvement of only one side of the lip or palate or involvement of some part of both sides of the lip or palate, respectively. Descriptions such as symmetric and asymmetric, complete and incomplete, and right and left are used in discussing clefts.

Another important feature of cleft lip and palate is the displacement of structures that are adjacent to the cleft. Dental malocclusions and nasal deviations frequently accompany the deformity, as well as conductive hearing losses. Clefts in the alveolar area disturb dental and facial growth patterns. Early feeding difficulty may cause abnormal development of lingual and labial skills. Exact causes of cleft palate are not known, but it seems to result, directly or indirectly, from multiple genetic and environmental factors that affect the embryo between the sixth and tenth week in utero.

Koepp-Baker (1971) explains the ways in which persons with cleft lip and palate are managed. Various types of treatment are used, often with a multidisciplinary approach. Surgical repair of the lip is usually done before 3 months of age and often during the first month of life. In the case of cleft lip only, lip mobility may be inhibited, but articulation is seldom affected. Palatal surgery, usually done by 18 months of age, tends to reduce the dimension of the oral cavity because the palatal vault is usually lowered and tongue movement for speech purposes seems to be limited. In such cases articulation-resonation may be affected. Secondary surgical procedures and oral orthopedic treatment may continue through the middle school years.

Surgical and orthopedic management may result in normal speech production, but if this is not the case, deviant speech patterns result (Bzoch, 1979; Dickson, 1974; Koepp-Baker, 1971; Perkins, 1977). If there is air leakage into the nasal cavity, intraoral air pressure is inadequate for normal articulation of pressure consonants and resonance is distorted. Compensatory actions are often used: (1) contraction of nasal muscles or flaring of the nares, (2) use of increased amounts of exhaled air, (3) use of the tongue to occlude the velopharyngeal port, and (4) misarticulation of phonemes, especially relative to manner and place features. Plosives are often omitted or substituted for with a glottal stop, or the air escapes through the nose causing an approximation of a nasal consonant. Fricatives and affricates may be omitted or distorted in the form of pharyngeal fricatives or nasal snorts.

Generally among the consonant sounds, fricatives, affricates, and plosives are affected the most, especially those that are nonvoiced, because these consonants require more intraoral air pressure for production. Nasals, glides, and semivowels are not as affected, although a pharyngeal tongue placement for /l/ is not uncommon. In addition to articulation deviancies, the voice often is perceived as hypernasal, primarily during production of the vowels. Articulation errors seem to influence the perception of nasality; the poorer the articulation, the more hypernasal the speech may be perceived (Dickson, 1974). In fact the presence of a repaired cleft lip tends to influence adversely the perception of nasality.

Table 10. Comparison of verbal dyspraxia with dysarthria

Verbal dyspraxia	Dysarthria
Absence of significant weakness, paralysis, or incoordination of the speech muscles; therefore, client has no difficulty with involuntary oral motor acts such as chewing, swallowing, sucking, and licking	Speech behavior and vegetative functions reflect type and severity of neurologic disease or damage present
Inconsistency in articulation performance and difficulty in predicting errors; most difficulty is with consonant clusters containing /s/ and /l/, which vary from one production to another	Speech errors are consistent and predictable
Most common types of articulation errors are substitutions and repetitions	Articulation errors are primarily distortions
Increased speaking rate results in improved articulation	Increased speaking rate results in deterioration of intelligibility
Speech production is more accurate in spontaneous speech, poorer in reading, and worst in imitative activities	Consonant clusters containing /s/ and /l/ are the most difficult to articulate, but they do not vary from one production to another
There is a discrepancy between voluntary-purposeful and spontaneous reflexive performance; the former is much more difficult	Accuracy of articulation does not vary appreciably with the situation—spontaneous speech, reading, and imitation
Rate, rhythm, and stress (prosody) of speech are adversely affected by repetitions, hesitations, and "groping" for correct articulation positions	Slow, labored speaking rate is present with evidence of strain and tension, especially for difficult consonant clusters
Articulation performance is poorer as words increase in length	Articulation performance is poorer as words increase in length

Dyspraxia can be acquired in adulthood as a result of brain damage. It also may occur in children prior to the development of speech skills. This condition is often referred to as developmental dyspraxia of speech. In both children and adults, dyspraxia may occur in isolation or in combination with dysphasia or dysarthria. In adults dyspraxia is sometimes accompanied with right hemiparesis or paralysis, whereas dyspraxic children often appear to be "essentially normal" on a neurologic examination (Rosenbek and Wertz, 1972). Rosenbek and Wertz further indicate neurologic data that suggest praxis centers in children that may involve large cortical areas of both hemispheres rather than a discrete area of the brain, as seems to be the case in adults.

Dyspraxia is a disorder that is often confused with dysphasia, but they are two different conditions in that the former is a disorder of articulation and the latter is a disorder of language. Additionally dyspraxia is sometimes confused with dysarthria. All three conditions may be present in the same person. Johns and Darley (1970) have differentiated between dysarthria and dyspraxia as shown in Table 10. The characteristics of developmental dyspraxia of speech have been described by Rosenbek and Wertz (1972) as follows:

1. Dyspraxia may occur in isolation or in combination with aphasia or dysarthria or both.
2. Speech development is delayed and deviant.
3. Receptive abilities are inordinately superior to expressive abilities.
4. Oral nonverbal apraxia often, but not always, accompanies apraxia of speech.
5. Prominent phonemic errors include omissions (errors are more often omission of sounds and syllables than substitution of sounds and syllables), substitutions, distortions, additions, repetitions, and prolongations.
6. Metathetic (transposition of two sounds in a word) errors occur frequently.
7. Errors increase as words get longer.
8. Repetition of sounds in isolation is often adequate; connected speech is more unintelligible than would be expected on the basis of single-word articulation test results.
9. Errors vary with the complexity of articulatory adjustment; most frequent errors are on fricatives, affricatives, and consonant clusters.
10. Misarticulations include vowels as well as consonants.
11. Errors are highly inconsistent.
12. Prosodic disturbances include slowed rate, even stress, and even spacing, perhaps in compensation for the problem.
13. Groping trial-and-error behavior is manifested as sound prolongations, repetitions, or silent posturing that may precede or interrupt imitative utterances.

Injury or disease can cause articulation disorders. In our modern, mechanized society there are increasing numbers of severely impaired children and adults who receive damage of such a nature as to result in speech problems. This is especially true with victims of head injuries sustained from motorcycle, automobile, bicycle, athletic, or other accidents. Damage to the brain and nerve pathways often results in speech problems caused by lack of neuromuscular control. Receptive and expressive language disorders also are common in such cases. Injuries also may damage and alter structure and function of the speech organs, and occasionally hearing is impaired. Diseases such as mumps, German measles, and infections causing extreme temperatures may cause hearing loss or brain damage that can affect speech. In the geriatric population, dysphasia, dysarthria, and dyslalia may be present as a result of degeneration of nerve centers and pathways controlling speech or as a result of major or minor cerebral insult.

SUMMARY

It is obvious from the preceding discussion that many etiologic factors may affect articulation. However, there is no general, systematic deficiency in any factor that is of sufficient size to have predictive value. No factor is consistently absent. All are found in some cases; all are absent in some cases (Powers, 1971). Again, one should look for a causal pattern, since several factors may be operating to cause an articulation disorder in a particular child or adult. Some factors that are no longer present may be related to the articulation disorder. Additionally some factors precipitate the deviancy, whereas others maintain it. The precipitating factors may no longer be operative or may not be treatable. Understanding both the precipitating and maintaining causes is important in planning a management program.

STUDY SUGGESTIONS

1. Delineate the factors that would have to be present in the articulation of a 5-year-old child to justify a diagnosis of disordered articulation in need of remediation.
2. Compare dyslalia, dysarthria, and dyspraxia from the standpoint of phonetic and acoustic properties and etiologic factors.
3. Relate the three types of articulation errors—omission, substitution, and distortion—to possible causes of each and to age levels and severity.
4. What distinctive features are likely to be defective in each type of error—omission, substitution, and distortion—in a given group of sounds?
5. How do neurophysiologic capacity, mental capacity, and environment relate in causation of articulation disorders?
6. What types of articulation errors relate most closely to orofacial anomalies? To impaired hearing? To mental retardation?

REFERENCES

Bankson, N., and Byrne, M.: The relationship between missing teeth and selected consonant sounds, J. Speech Hear. Disord. 27:341-348, 1962.

Barrett, R., and Hanson, M.: Oral myofunctional disorders, ed. 2, St. Louis, 1978, The C. V. Mosby Co.

Bernstein, M.: The relation of speech defects and malocclusion, Alpha Omega 150:90-97, 1956.

Blakeley, R.: The practice of speech pathology, Springfield, Ill., 1972, Charles C Thomas, Publisher.

Bloodstein, O.: Speech pathology: an introduction, Boston, 1979, Houghton Mifflin Co.

Bloomer, H.: Speech defects associated with dental malocclusions and related abnormalities. In Travis, L.: Handbook of speech pathology and audiology, New York, 1971, Appleton-Century-Crofts.

Bralley, R., and Stoudt, R.: A five-year longitudinal study of development of articulation proficiency in elementary school children, Lang. Speech Hear. Serv. Schools 8:176-180, 1977.

Byrne, M., and Shervanian, C.: Introduction to communicative disorders, New York, 1977, Harper & Row, Publishers.

Bzoch, K., editor: Communicative disorders related to cleft lip and palate, Boston, 1979, Little, Brown and Co.

Canter, G.: Neuromotor pathologies of speech, Am. J. Phys. Med. 46:659-666, 1967.

Carrell, J.: Disorders of articulation, Englewood Cliffs, N.J., 1968, Prentice-Hall, Inc.

Chomsky, N., and Halle, M.: The sound pattern of English, New York, 1968, Harper & Row, Publishers.

Darley, F., Aronson, A., and Brown, J.: Motor speech disorders, Philadelphia, 1975, W. B. Saunders Co.

Dickson, S., editor: Communication disorders: remedial principles and practices, Glenview, Ill., 1974, Scott, Foresman and Co.

Dworkin, J.: Protrusive lingual force and lingual diadochokinetic rates: a comparative analysis between normal and lisping speakers, Lang. Speech Hear. Serv. Schools 9:8-16, 1978.

Everhart, R.: The relationships between articulation and other developmental factors in children, J. Speech Hear. Disord. 18:332-338, 1953.

Fairbanks, G., and Bebout, B.: J. Speech Hear. Disord. 15:348-352, 1950.

Fletcher, S., and Meldrum, J.: Lingual function and relative length of the lingual frenulum, J. Speech Hear. Disord. 11:382-390, 1968.

Fletcher, S., Casteel, R., and Bradley, D.: Tongue-thrust swallow, speech articulation, and age, J. Speech Hear. Disord. 26:201-208, 1961.

Ham, R.: Relationship between misspelling and misarticulation, J. Speech Hear. Disord. 23:294-297, 1958.

Jervis, G.: Medical aspects of mental retardation, J. Rehabil. 28:34-36, 1962.

Johns, D., and Darley, F.: Phonemic variability in apraxia of speech, J. Speech Hear. Disord. 13:556-583, 1970.

Johnson, W., and associates: Speech handicapped school children, ed. 3, New York, 1967, Harper & Row, Publishers.

Kernahan, D., and Stark, R.: A new classification for cleft lip and cleft palate, Plast. Reconstr. Surg. 22:435, 1958.

Koch, H.: Sibling influence on children's speech, J. Speech Hear. Disord. 21:322-328, 1956.

Koepp-Baker, H.: Orofacial clefts: their forms and effects. In Travis, L.: Handbook of speech pathology and audiology, New York, 1971, Appleton-Century-Crofts.

Kronvall, E., and Diehl, C.: The relationship of auditory discrimination to articulatory defects of children with no known organic impairment, J. Speech Hear. Disord. **19:**335-338, 1954.

LaPointe, L., and Wertz, R.: Oral-movement abilities and articulatory characteristics of brain-injured adults, Percept. Mot. Skills **39:**39-46, 1974.

Leonard, L.: The nature of deviant articulation, J. Speech Hear. Disord. **38:**156-161, 1973.

Lillywhite, H., and Bradley, D.: Communication problems in mental retardation, New York, 1969, Harper & Row, Publishers.

Ling, D.: It is through meaningful communication that speech and language skills are acquired and perfected, Volta Rev. **75:**354-356, 1973.

Luchsinger, R., and Arnold, G.: Voice, speech, language, Belmont, Calif., 1965, Wadsworth Publishing Co., Inc.

Mason, R., and Proffit, W.: The tongue thrust controversy: background and recommendations, J. Speech Hear. Disord. **39:**115-132, 1974.

McCall, G.: The assessment of lingual tactile sensation and perception, J. Speech Hear. Disord. **34:**151-156, 1969.

McDonald, E., and Chance, B.: Cerebral palsy, Englewood Cliffs, N.J., 1964, Prentice-Hall, Inc.

McEnery, E., and Gaines, F.: Tongue-tie in infants and children, J. Pediatr. **18:**252-255, 1941.

Morley, M.: Cleft palate and speech, London, 1970, E. and S. Livingstone, Ltd.

Mysak, E.: Cerebral palsy speech syndromes. In Travis, L., editor: Handbook of speech pathology and audiology, New York, 1971, Appleton-Century-Crofts.

Perkins, W.: Speech pathology: an applied behavioral science, ed. 2, St. Louis, 1977, The C. V. Mosby Co.

Phair, G.: The Wisconsin cleft palate program, J. Speech Hear. Disord. **12:**410-414, 1947.

Powers, M.: Functional disorders of articulation: symptomatology and etiology. In Travis, L., editor: Handbook of speech pathology and audiology, New York, 1971, Appleton-Century-Crofts.

Prins, D.: Analysis of correlations among various articulatory deviations, J. Speech Hear. Res. **5:**152-160, 1962.

Prins, D.: Relations among specific articulatory deviations and responses to a clinical measure of sound discrimination ability, J. Speech Hear. Disord. **28:**382-388, 1963.

Prosek, R., and House, A.: Intraoral air pressure as a feedback cue in consonant production, J. Speech Hear. Disord. **18:**133-147, 1975.

Ringel, R.: Oral sensation and perception. In Wolfe, W., and Goulding, D.: Articulation and learning, Springfield, Ill., 1973, Charles C Thomas, Publisher.

Roe, V., and Milisen, R.: The effect of maturation upon defective articulation in elementary grades, J. Speech Hear. Disord. **7:**37-50, 1942.

Rosenbek, R., and Wertz, R.: A review of 50 cases of developmental apraxia of speech, Lang. Speech Hear. Serv. Schools **III:**23-33, 1972.

Rosenbek, R., and associates: Treatment of developmental apraxia of speech: a case study, Lang. Speech Hear. Serv. Schools **V:**13-22, 1974.

Scott, C., and Ringel, R.: The effects of motor and sensory disruptions on speech: a description of articulation, J. Speech Hear. Disord. **14:**819-828, 1971.

Skinner, P., and Shelton, R.: Speech, language, and hearing: normal processes and disorders, Reading, Mass., 1978, Addison-Wesley Publishing Co., Inc.

Snow, K.: Articulation proficiency in relation to certain dental abnormalities, J. Speech Hear. Disord. **26:**209-212, 1961.

Sommers, R., and Kane, A.: Nature and remediation of functional articulation disorders. In Dickson, S., editor: Communication disorders: remedial principles and practices, Glenview, Ill., 1974, Scott, Foresman and Co.

Spriestersbach, D.: Research in articulation disorders and personality, J. Speech Hear. Disord. **21:**329-335, 1956.

Spriestersbach, D., and Sherman, D.: Cleft palate and communication, New York, 1968, Academic Press, Inc.

Subtelny, J., Mestre, C., and Subtelny, J.: Comparative study of normal and defective articulation of /s/ as related to malocclusion and deglutition, J. Speech Hear. Disord. **29:**269-285, 1964.

Templin, M.: Certain language skills in children, Minneapolis, 1957, University of Minnesota Press.

Templin, M.: Development of speech, J. Pediatr. **62:**11-14, 1963.

Van Riper, C., and Irwin, J.: Voice and articulation, Englewood Cliffs, N.J., 1958, Prentice-Hall, Inc.

Weiss, C.: Cluttering, Englewood Cliffs, N.J., 1964, Prentice-Hall Inc.

Weiss, C.: The relationships between maximum articulatory rate and articulatory disorders among children, Central States Speech J. **XIX:**185-187, 1968.

Weiss, C.: Orofacial musculature imbalance among mentally retarded children, Br. J. Disord. Commun. **5:**141-147, 1970.

Weiss, C.: Orofacial muscle imbalance, Portland, Oreg., 1973, Anderson Printing.

Weiss, C., and Skalbeck, G.: Passive and active lingual discrimination among deaf children, Folia Phoniatr. **27:**393-398, 1975.

Winitz, H.: Articulatory acquisition and behavior, New York, 1969, Appleton-Century-Crofts.

Winitz, H.: From syllable to conversation, Baltimore, 1975, University Park Press.

Wood, K.: Terminology and nomenclature. In Travis, L., editor: Handbook of speech pathology and audiology, New York, 1971, Appleton-Century-Crofts.

GLOSSARY

addition The adding of an unnecessary sound such as /a/ between the consonant blend in the word "green" (ga̱reen).

ankyloglossia Tongue-tie, too short a lingual frenulum, or one that is attached too far forward beneath the tongue.

apraxia Inability to control movements of the articulators, mainly the tongue, voluntarily for speech purposes because of a specific motor speech involvement.

ataxia A type of cerebral palsy characterized by inability to synchronize fine movements and sometimes lack of balance.

atonia Lack of muscle tone resulting in poor voluntary muscle control.

athetosis A form of cerebral palsy characterized by uncontrolled writhing movements of the limbs.

auditory perceptual skill Skill in perceiving and understanding auditory symbols; differs from auditory acuity.

blend Two or more consonant phones positioned next to and influencing each other.

Broca area An area in the left frontal lobe thought to be responsible for motor speech, or expressive language.

cerebral insult Damage to one or more areas of the brain usually resulting in paralysis or other central nervous system related disability.

cerebral palsy A neuromuscular disability characterized by muscular weakness, paralysis, rigidity, lack of muscular control, or any combination of the preceding. It is caused by damage to the brain.

cleft palate Failure of the two sides of the palate to unite or fuse at the midline resulting in an opening in the roof of the mouth.

demyelinating disease A disease that attacks the myelin sheath, a fatty substance, which surrounds and protects nerve fibers.

dental lisp The tongue is positioned against the upper or lower central incisors during production of /s/, /z/, /ʃ/, and /ʒ/.

diadochokinetic Pertaining to the rate and accuracy with which an individual can repeat sounds in sequence, called diadochokinesis.

distoclusion A malocclusion in which the mandibular dental arch is distal to (behind) the maxillary dental arch.

dyslalia An articulation disorder that is not caused by neuromuscular damage.

dyspraxia An incomplete form of apraxia; a degree of motor speech involvement that is less than complete.

embryologic Refers to the human embryo, or first 3 months of life.

environmental factors Pertains to factors in one's environment, such as the family, home, and community.

frontal lisp A sibilant distortion or substitution caused by placing the tongue too far forward in the mouth. This term is sometimes used interchangeably with the term interdental lisp, although the latter term implies that the tongue is between the teeth.

functional disorder A nonorganic disorder.

glottal stop Approximation of plosive sounds made by stopping and releasing the breath stream at the level of the glottis. It may be a compensatory behavior in the presence of inadequate velopharyngeal closure.

in utero In the uterus; before birth.

infantile perseveration Perseveration in the use of infantile sounds beyond the developmental level at which they should have been discontinued.

intelligibility Understandability; often expressed as a percentage of contextual speech understood by the listener.

interdental lisp The tongue is positioned between the upper and lower incisors during the production of /s/, /z/, /ʃ/, and /ʒ/.

intervention Refers to intervening with a client through counseling, articulation treatment, or other measures to change speech behavior.

lalling Refers to misarticulations of /l/ and /r/.

lateral lisp The breath stream goes off one or both sides of the tongue during production of /s/, /z/, /ʃ/, and /ʒ/.

lesion Pathologic or traumatic injury to tissue, such as a lesion in the brain causing speech or language problems.

lingual lisp A term that is synonymous with frontal or interdental lisp.

lisping Distortion or substitution of sibilant sounds.

mesioclusion A malocclusion in which the mandibular dental arch is too far anterior to the maxillary arch; also called overjet.

monoplegia Paralysis of one limb only.

myopathy Disease of muscles.

nasal lisp Fricative or sibilant sounds produced (approximated) in the nasal cavity rather than in the oral cavity.

nasal snort A nasal sound that is emitted probably because the velopharyngeal mechanism is inadequate or because of habit.

neutroclusion A malocclusion in which the mandibular and maxillary dental arches are in correct anterior-posterior relationship, but individual teeth may be crowded, missing, or in an open bite relationship.

nonorganic See Functional disorder.

occluded lisp The tongue is positioned too far forward in the mouth, occluding the breath stream.

open bite A malocclusion in which the central and lateral maxillary incisors are too far forward.

oral apraxia Refers to the inability to move the articulators voluntarily for nonspeech purposes; also called nonverbal apraxia.

orthopedic Pertains to chronic diseases of the joints and spine.

otosclerosis Formation of spongy bone about the stapes and oval window.

overjet See Mesioclusion.

paraplegia Paralysis of lower limbs and lower part of the body.

Parkinson disease A disease, the principal symptoms of which are muscular rigidity, immobility of facial muscles, tremor, and deficiency in associated and automatic movements.

pharyngeal fricative Fricatives that are erroneously produced near the pharynx rather than near the front of the mouth.

phonologic system A system for studying and using English sounds. It may also refer to the anatomic and physiologic aspects of sound production.

praxis The doing or performing of action. Refers here to action of the speech structures.

quadriplegia Paralysis of all four limbs and other parts of the body.

regression Refers to the child's regressing to forms of speech of an earlier age.

rhotacism Articulation errors of the /r/ family of sounds.

semivowel A phone that has a vowel-like quality, such as /l/ and /r/.

sensorineural Refers here to hearing loss caused by nerve damage; could involve any of the other senses also.

sigmatism A term used to designate lisping.

stimulability The ability of a client to imitate a model or to be "stimulated" to reproduce accurately sounds the client misarticulates.

strident lisp A misarticulation in which /s/ or /z/ assumes a whistling quality.

structural Refers here to anatomic structures of the speech mechanism.

submucous Beneath the mucous; refers here to submucous cleft in which the bones of the hard palate fail to fuse, but the mucous membrane does, covering the underlying bony cleft.

tactile Pertaining to the sense of touch, taction.

tremor Involuntary trembling or quivering, such as in cerebral palsy.

triplegia Paralysis of three limbs, usually two legs and one arm.

CHAPTER FIVE

Case history information

"Give us the grace to listen well."
KEBLE

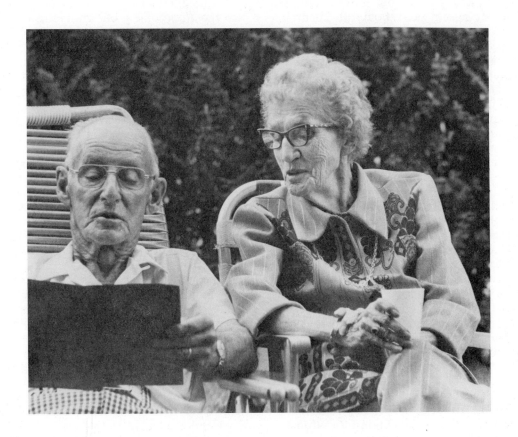

The first step in carrying out a differential diagnosis is to obtain a pertinent case history of the client and the problem—a case history that differentiates probable etiology and enables the diagnostician to formulate theories regarding the individualistic development of the problem, the client, and the related environment. The differential history should not only provide information as to why the client has the presenting problem but information also as to what areas of communication, other behavior, and mental and physical aspects should be explored in the examination and what tests and other diagnostic tools should be used.

Historical data should provide past and present information about the client, including social, emotional, psychologic, educational, intellectual, medical, dental, familial, and personality characteristics (see sequence of diagnostic procedures in Appendix). In essence a differential history should help determine why the client has the problem, what kind of person the client is, and how the client may be helped (Darley and Spriestersbach, 1978; Emerick and Hatten, 1979). These determinations, of course, preclude inaccurate collection and interpretation of the historical data. Errors in interpretation or inaccurate data reported by the informant naturally affect the significance of background information, so the diagnostician must be aware of these possibilities.

An accurate case history helps the diagnostician assess relevant variables, such as what has made the problem what it is and how it can best be modified or eliminated (Darley, 1964). The history should provide information about predisposing, precipitating, and perpetuating factors. It should provide a body of objective information that can be analyzed and synthesized to determine more exactly the actual problem, clarify how its present condition varies from the original problem, and reveal which events may have influenced the onset and development of the problem. Finally the differential history and diagnosis should employ the scientific method, which consists of (1)

collection of data, (2) objectification of data, (3) consolidation of all available data, (4) comparative analysis of data, (5) categorization of data, and (6) determination of significance of the data. Beck (1959) defines science as "a body of tested objective knowledge, obtained and unified in principle by inductive methods." Such a scientific attitude is necessary in order to obtain and process factual historical information. The scientific method usually has been thought to be the province of the "exact" and "natural" sciences, but it can be applied very successfully to the solution of behavioral and psychologic problems as well, although this is more difficult. The clinical diagnostician should become proficient in the use of such an approach if best results are to be obtained.

The term "differential history taking" is used here for several important reasons. To obtain history differentially involves more than just asking questions and recording responses. It is a dynamic process of purposeful interaction between an interviewer and an informant. It requires expert skill, training, clinical knowledge, and insight (Myklebust, 1954). It is a continuous process of evaluating historical data and clinical impressions and of formulating hypotheses and diagnoses of all the information obtained. In these ways differential history taking differs from merely taking history.

For greater efficiency in differential history taking, at least four requisites must be fulfilled: (1) the necessary information about the past status of the client must be obtained; (2) the present status of the client must be determined; (3) some idea must be formed about the future status of the client, including prognosis; and (4) the etiology of the problem must be ascertained (Doll, 1940). Myklebust (1954) adds a fifth requirement: determination of the age of onset of the disorder. In addition to these requisites, it is recommended that the client, especially if a child, be observed briefly before beginning the interview. Impressions gleaned during this initial observation can be helpful in guiding the interview.

Although simplified in this discussion, gathering historical data is not a simple matter. As mentioned previously, it presupposes considerable clinical and normative knowledge, an individualistic approach, ability to ask and answer pertinent questions, careful listening, sensitivity, objectivity, confidence, curiosity, insightfulness, trustworthiness, and ability to establish rapport, interpret significant information as it surfaces during the interview, and use it for further questioning. Gathering background information is a science and an art. It is an ongoing process, not a one-time entity, that includes a purposeful exchange of information (Nation and Aram, 1977). Additionally the diagnostician should always be cognizant of why specific questions are being asked and what they may contribute toward understanding the client. Questioning should be designed to encourage comments, conversation, and questions from the client, parents, or others involved. Much information can be gained from this kind of client participation. Awareness of the rationale helps avoid unnecessary questions. Other ways of obtaining historical data include questionnaire, autobiography, observation, and various medical, educational, and other clinical records. Ideally this type of information will be obtained and studied before the interview. This can make the interview much more productive and efficient.

In addition to interviewing the client, another effective way of obtaining historical information is to interview the person or persons most familiar and knowledgeable about the client. An interview allows the diagnostician to (1) evaluate and follow up comments immediately for important clues about the client, (2) help ease the pain of unpleasant personal matters, (3) clarify answers that are vague, incomplete, or of doubtful accuracy, (4) relieve the parents or guardians of some anxiety or guilt feelings about past experiences, (5) establish a friendly, professional relationship, and (6) pursue the pertinent behavior of the client observed previously (Milisen, 1971).

Interviewing persons other than the client is a helpful way of obtaining the necessary information about the client, but since information from such sources is based on past observation, usually by untrained observers, caution must be exercised in unequivocally accepting all the information as "fact." Moreover objectivity may not always be possible from an informant because of a relationship with the client that may have caused a bias of some kind. Also the extent and accuracy of the information obtained may have been influenced by interviewee-interviewer factors, such as rapport, cooperation, confidence, trust, memory and recall of the informant, and attitude of openness by the informant. In the final analysis the diagnostician must determine if sufficient, relevant, representative, accurate, and reliable information was obtained and if the informant's responses may have been inadvertently influenced by the diagnostician. Making these determinations probably is one of the most difficult and important tasks of the diagnostician. Given these requirements and cautions, the interview can still be one of the best ways of obtaining a complete impression of the client and of possibly explaining the reasons for the articulation problem.

GUIDELINES FOR EFFECTIVE INTERVIEWING
Beginning the interview

The interview with the client or with others should begin with general rather than specific questions. Specificity at the outset can be unnerving to the informant and can cause apprehension and defensiveness (Garrett, 1972). An appropriate way in which to begin the interview is to ask why the client came or was brought for an evaluation and what questions need to be answered. These questions should guide the diagnostician during the interview and during testing.

Establish mutual respect

An effective way of establishing an appropriate atmosphere for interviewing is to achieve a feeling of mutual respect. An attitude of mutual concern, genuine sincerity, honesty, acceptance, empathy, and humility can greatly assist the feeling of mutual respect. An open, relaxed setting should be the goal. Attitudes of superiority, rigidity, aloofness, condemnation, and superficiality definitely should be avoided. The interviewer must delve beneath superficiality and routineness in asking questions. As Kinsey, Pomeroy, and Martin (1948) have stated, the interviewer who merely asks routine questions exclusive of determining the informant's hurts, frustrations, pain, unsatisfied longings, disappointments, and tragic situations has not conducted a successful interview. The interviewer may share something of the satisfaction, pain, and bewilderment of the informant, who in return experiences the feeling or impression that things will somehow work out all right.

Excessive probing in interviewing should be avoided. An in-depth psychoanalytic approach by an unqualified interviewer can cause resentment, defensiveness, and lack of cooperation. Just exactly how far to probe in order to obtain the necessary information seems to be related to clinical knowledge, sensitivity, and experience. No specific rules or guidelines seem applicable. A sense of when to stop and when to proceed further in questioning appears to evolve with experience and a knowledge of one's own professional and personal limitations. If mutual respect and understanding are not gained at the outset, the interview is in danger of failing.

Explain the purpose of the interview

The informant should be told that a number of specific questions will be asked in order to achieve a better understanding of the client's problems and possible solutions. It is also helpful to explain the purpose or reason for seeking certain kinds of information or for asking questions in such detail. The informant should be encouraged to talk freely and openly, and an opportunity should be provided for the informant to ask questions of the interviewer and to interrupt for purposes of clarification. If the infor-

mant is convinced that the interview is one of the most important and necessary aspects of the diagnostic work up, then relevant information will be forthcoming.

Be a good listener

The importance of good listening is so obvious that mention of it hardly seems necessary. Yet virtually all of us could benefit from improving our listening skills (Nichols, 1955). One of the major roadblocks to good listening skills is that some people talk too much (Weiss and Lillywhite, 1976). People oververbalize for many reasons. They are talk oriented. They grow up with almost a fear of being silent in the presence of others. This attitude carries over into the interview, where the interviewer sometimes becomes "intoxicated with the exuberance of his or her own verbosity." The admonition that we have two ears and only one mouth means that we should listen twice as much as we talk should be remembered and followed during an interview. A good interviewer listens not only to what the informant says but also to what the informant does not say. "Listening between the lines" is an art that comes with much experience. It requires sensitivity, lack of egocentricity, patience, and perceptive listening skills.

Ask questions appropriately

A cardinal rule in an interview is to word the questions carefully. If a binary question is asked, the client will give a binary response. A vague question will probably be answered with a vague response. Likewise asking leading questions may elicit biased information. As Darley and Spriestersbach (1978) caution, the interviewer should understand why a particular question is being asked. It may also be well to provide a range of possible answers such as numbers and percentages or degrees ranging from never to always or from mild to very severe. We are reminded of the time a student diagnostician asked an adult stutterer to tell about his birth and when he said his first word. Although the intent may have been good, the questions were inappropriate for the informant-client. Effective questioning implies well-stated specific sentences, understandable vocabulary, and possible examples of answers being searched for. Carefully worded questions can be effectively used to encourage the listener to elaborate on the answer, to invite participation, and to develop an attitude of being fully involved in a search for a solution to the problem. This may be done by prefacing the questions with such phrases as, "Do you think it might be . . . ?," "Is it possible that . . . ?," and "I wonder if it could have been . . . ?" Although blunt, direct questions may sometimes be necessary in the interview, the interviewer should be aware that such an approach can limit information and sometimes "turn off" the informant.

Minimize anxiety

Even though anxiety in interviews cannot always be avoided, it can be minimized. The interviewer should assume that the informant has some concerns and that these concerns frequently are accompanied by anxiety. Rapport, relaxed environment, understanding, and arranging the interview sequence so that it progresses from low to high emotional content can limit the informant's level of anxiety. An empathic attitude by the interviewer can also help to minimize the anxiety of the informant.

Conduct an efficient interview

Efficiency in interviewing can be achieved in several ways: by phrasing questions economically, avoiding unnecessary verbal digression and "editorializing," asking relevant questions, preparing and individualizing many of the interview questions in advance, and guiding the informant back to the original question if digression or catharsis has occurred. The rate of asking questions is also important. The interviewer should not tarry, spend unnecessary time rephrasing and clarifying questions, pause excessively, or slow the speaking to an exaggerated rate in order to improve the eloquence and preciseness of articulation. For best results, the rate of questions and com-

ments should be geared to what is perceived to be the informant's ability to receive and process verbal messages.

Maintain eye contact

The interviewer should not only look at the informant but should also be interested, sincere, and understanding. Eye contact is especially important during moments when tension, emotion, and guilt are related by the informant. To look away or to look at the informant too intently at these times could be misinterpreted as negative judgments of the informant's behavior, embarrassment, uneasiness, or lack of interest. Maintaining intermittent, natural eye contact fosters effective communication and interaction and should always be practiced in an interview.

Take notes during interview

Because of the vast amount of information that can be conveyed during an interview, it is wise to take some notes. Develop some system of shorthand; otherwise it will be impossible to write down the important points shared by the informant. If too much time is spent in writing, however, eye contact and possible rapport may suffer. If necessary, the informant should be asked to repeat an answer, but the number of times repetition is requested should be limited. Another approach may be to tape-record the interview, provided the informant does not object. The presence of a tape recorder can thwart open communication and curtail sharing valuable, personal information by some informants, although most persons readily adjust to the presence of a tape recorder. Discretion should be used regarding the extent of note taking and whether or not to tape-record, but some notes should always be taken.

Ask personal questions straightforwardly

If the informant has been told of the reasons for asking a variety of casual and personal questions, there should be no problem. Personal questions should be asked matter-of-factly and quite directly. If the interviewer seems awkward, evasive, and uneasy in asking the questions, the interviewee may likewise feel uncomfortable. The interviewer must be certain that the questions need to be asked and must be able to explain or justify why it is important to obtain this requested information. Sometimes questions are asked without sufficient reason or a clear understanding as to why they are being asked (Emerick, 1969). If the information asked for does not relate to the overall management of the client, it may not have been necessary to obtain it.

Use tact in emotional situations

Not uncommonly during an interview some questions may relate to very emotional, personal experiences or may trigger a sorrowful or overwhelming experience. Such questions can elicit unexpected emotional behavior. Apology in such situations is not necessary, but patience and understanding are. Usually after a moment or two the informant will regain composure and the interview can proceed, perhaps in a somewhat different direction. If emotionality persists, the interviewer may express understanding (empathy), may excuse himself or herself from the room for a little while, or can ask another, hopefully less emotional, question. The interviewer should be careful not to show disapproval, embarrassment, or other emotional reactions.

Probe superficial responses

Occasionally an informant will provide a cursory or superficial answer to an important question. For example, the interviewer may ask what activities have been employed in the home to help the child learn to talk. Supposing the response to this question is "nothing," the response should be pursued by providing ideas of what some "teaching activities" could be before probing the original, superficial answer. It may be necessary to rephrase the question. Curt responses by the informant may be an indication of misunderstanding a question, lack of awareness, or considering the question unimportant. Answers to important questions should be pursued to the interviewer's satisfaction, but a point or topic should not be belabored.

Clarify discrepancies

It is entirely possible that discrepancies or what appear to be discrepancies will be noted. These should be clarified before the interview is concluded. The apparent discrepancy may have been a misunderstanding by the informant or by the interviewer. Discrepancies may indicate uncertainty, ambivalence, confusion, or untruthfulness. In any event clarification should be sought, if not to get a better understanding of the client's history, then to get a better understanding of the informant if it is someone other than the client. Whatever the reason, it is important not to reach conclusions prematurely or to pass judgments hastily.

Ask for interpretation of information

In addition to clarifying answers, it may also be necessary to seek interpretations. How does the informant perceive the different events? By asking "What do you mean?," "How do you feel about that?," and "How do you see the problem?," the diagnostician can obtain significant interpretations. All of the information should not be accepted at face value; some interpretations are sometimes more revealing and more valuable than the actual statement that preceded them.

Keep the purpose in mind

At all times it should be kept in mind that the purpose of the interview is to obtain the information necessary for better understanding the client, the etiology, and the possible treatment and management procedures that will be most effective. An interview is not primarily for venting feelings; neither is it intended to be therapeutic, although both of these functions may occur. The goal of obtaining answers to the questions initially determined should be accomplished by keeping the interview "on course." Additional needs of the informant can be dealt with at another time and place.

It sometimes may be necessary, however, to let the informant express strong feelings before getting back to the purpose of the interview.

Answer questions

The informant should be encouraged to ask questions during the interview. The interviewer should be prepared for questions and should answer them to the best of his or her ability. If the interviewer does not know the answer, the informant should be told that the answer will be found and provided at a later time. Situations should be handled honestly. If the answer to a question might jeopardize the interviewer-interviewee relationship, the answer should be deferred to another person or until another time. Most questions can usually be answered at the time they are asked, provided the diagnostician is knowledgeable. Also, when a response is an opinion, a personal bias, or something other than fact, this should be indicated. It is generally a good idea to terminate the interview by asking the informant if there are any unanswered questions.

Be aware of possible language or class barriers

It is important to remember that language, social level, education, or other similar barriers may exist between the interviewer and the interviewee. Most obvious of these may be present when the informant comes from a "different" ethnic, social, or age-group. The good interviewer recognizes possibilities of misunderstandings in these situations and adjusts quickly to them by using language and other behavior to fit the situation. Less obvious barriers to communication may also occur when there are not wide ethnic, age, or obvious social differences. In these situations both parties are likely to assume that they "speak the same language"—that their concepts of the problem and of each other are accurate. Rarely is this the case; as a consequence the interview may proceed with many false assumptions and inaccurate interpretations

being made. In any case, whether the differences are obvious or not, it is the responsibility of the interviewer to determine concepts and understandings as accurately as possible and to use language that is subject to minimal misunderstanding; in other words, to see that the "map-territory" relationships of the situation are as accurate as they can be (Weiss and Lillywhite, 1976). The interviewer should ensure that the relationships between the word map (verbal representation of a message) that an individual tries to draw and the territory (information, thoughts, ideas, opinions, and feelings) that the map is supposed to represent are compatible.

Indicate observations of the informant

An important aspect of the collected historical data is the diagnostician's observations and impressions of the informant. These should be noted as the interview progresses and after it is over. Darley and Spriestersbach (1978) suggest including observations on the following aspects of the informant: rapport, language behavior, knowledge, intelligence, accuracy, memory, bodily movements and facial expressions, emotional reactions, insight, rationalizing, unconscious projection, and ambivalence. If some of these aspects are questionable, the obtained information may be questionable. Personal observations about the informant can be invaluable in better understanding the historical data.

Terminate the interview effectively

This step of the interview is not always easy to achieve. The interview should be concluded by expressing appreciation and thanks to the informant for cooperating in providing helpful information. If additional information comes to mind or if other questions arise later, subsequent communication should be encouraged. It should be explained that the overall findings and impressions about the client will be discussed with the informant following diagnostic testing and interpretation. The timetable of events should be indicated at the close of the interview. If important information was not available at the time of the interview, the informant should be asked to provide it, by telephone or other means, as soon as it can be located (Emerick and Hatten, 1979). Sometimes it is beneficial to ask a parent to bring the baby book or some other source of documented information to the interview. It is a good idea to have the informant sign a release of information form that fulfills requirements of the institutional situation at the close of the interview (Nation and Aram, 1977).

Practicing these guidelines will help to ensure an effective interview. In addition the diagnostician must be careful not to provide information too soon in the interview. It is also important to remember that methods other than the oral interview are available to the diagnostician. Some of these are discussed in the following paragraphs.

Questionnaire

Another method of obtaining background information is with a questionnaire. This approach can be effective in gathering considerable information in a relatively short amount of time because it is highly structured. A questionnaire can be used to obtain data from several persons at the same time and provide a record of the information for future reference. It is also a flexible method. Its thoroughness can be modified, depending on individual needs. Specific areas can be stressed and others deleted. The questionnaire can be used as a guide for the oral interview, or it can be used as a supplement to the oral interview. It can also be completed in advance of diagnostic testing, giving the informant time to think about or research the answers before coming in for the interview and evaluation. Contents generally include any or all of the following: identifying information, statement of the problem, general development, and medical, dental, educational, communication, environmental, social, and daily history (see sample questionnaires in Appendixes C and D).

As with all methods, the questionnaire

has disadvantages. Among these are possible misinterpretations of the questions, reporting incompletely or what "sounds" best, answering the questions superficially, not answering all of the questions, and assigning equal weight to each question because it appeared on the questionnaire. Nevertheless, as a supplement to observing, interviewing, and testing, the questionnaire can provide helpful information. Also, the questionnaire should be accompanied with a release of information form to be signed and returned to the diagnostician. This will help to ensure that human rights are protected.

Autobiography

Perhaps less commonly used is the autobiography. It can be very helpful, however, with more severe problems. It can be a narrative or an oral account, depending on the age and abilities of the client. The advantages of a written account are to provide a sample of the client's language skills and allow as much time as necessary for the client to think about the contents. It also provides some insights as to how the client thinks and feels about himself in particular and about life in general. These revelations of self-perception and perceptions of others and of the world can be helpful in forming accurate concepts of the client. The autobiography can have remedial as well as diagnostic value. Because of the time involved, the autobiography is not routinely used, depending, of course, on the individual problem. Many clients also do not have the skill or the will to write anything that may be significant.

Observation

A number of different kinds of observations may be used to collect significant information about the client, family, and home environment. They can include spectator observation, participant observation, and other informant observation.

Spectator observation usually includes the diagnostician or other invited person observing the client through a one-way window. This method occurs without the client's awareness of being observed and is used in situations in which the client interacts with other children or adults, the family, or others. A good observer can note details, discrepancies between reports and observed behavior, range of behaviors, and various interactions. These observations can be made without influencing or affecting the client's behavior because of the absence of the diagnostician. However, a setting using a one-way observation window is usually somewhat artificial and thus may have inherent limitations and obvious effects on the client's normal behavior.

Participant observation on the other hand may preclude typical behavior by the client because of the presence of the diagnostician. This situation can be more structured in order to obtain more pertinent samples of behavior. The behavior of the client will naturally be affected by the type of rapport previously established and reactions to the presence of the diagnostician. Whether or not a separate situation needs to be established solely for the purpose of having some other informant observe is debatable. After all, the diagnostician is observing and interacting with the client during formal and informal testing procedures. Part of the testing situation is observation of the client's interaction, especially during the less formal activities. Observational data of other observers should be compared, consolidated, and interpreted with other existing information. Observations, including home visitations, are among the most important methods of obtaining needed information about a child with a communicative disorder.

Other clinical records

Medical, dental, communicative, educational, psychosocial, nutritional, and other data can provide much needed additional information about the client. Information about illnesses, diseases, tests, hospitalizations, surgeries, and medical treatment can reveal valuable information about why the client has a communicative disorder, age of onset, communicative intervention procedures, and prognosis. Similarly, dental,

educational, nutritional, and other records about the client's historical development should be explored and considered in diagnosis and treatment. Each piece of information helps to complete the historical puzzle of the client. Time spent in obtaining historical and other diagnostic data will greatly facilitate diagnostic and remedial procedures.

With this basic foundation of how background information may be gathered, let us proceed to look at what information should be collected. Again, the type and extent of information necessary will vary with the age of the client, type of disorder, severity of disorder, age of onset, and other factors. An individualistic approach certainly must be practiced during this phase of clinical management.

Communicative information

The most important clinical records to a speech-language pathologist are those pertaining to communication. Some basic questions that should be asked include the following:

1. Excluding crying, was the client a quiet, average, or very vocal infant?
2. Were there normal baby sounds in the first year, such as cooing, gurgling, babbling, pitch inflection, and attempts to imitate sounds of parents?
3. When were the first words, other than "mommy" and "daddy," spoken? What were they?
4. Were words added regularly thereafter?
5. When did naming people and objects begin?
6. When did two-word combinations begin to appear?
7. Were the words easy or difficult to understand?
8. Did struggle behavior accompany the speech efforts?
9. Was speech treatment ever provided? If so, when, how long, for what, and with what degree of success? Who was the clinician?
10. Has any progress occurred in speech during the last 6 months?
11. Is the client aware of a speech difference? If so, how is it shown?
12. What has been done to help the client talk better?
13. Has the client's speech ever been better than

it is now? If so, in what way and when did it change?

14. At what age was the client thought to have an articulation disorder? By whom?
15. Does the speech cause the client to show concern about it?
16. What is the parents' estimate of severity of the speech problem?
17. Are there other family members with speech problems? Who? What kind?
18. Has adverse attention been called to the speech problem by family or by others? If so, in what way?
19. Has the client's speech ever been evaluated? If so, when and by whom?
20. Does the client prefer to use speech or gestures?
21. What percentage of the time is the client understood by other members of the family? By persons who are not around the client much?

These are some questions that should be pursued. The list certainly is not exhaustive, but it should provide a core of basic information about communicative development. Most of this information must come from parents, but a school speech-language clinician or teacher can also provide some of it.

Hearing information

Also important to articulation is information pertaining to hearing. Some questions that might be asked include:

1. During the first year of life, did the client startle, blink, turn to search for sound source, or change immediate activity in response to sudden, loud, or different sounds?
2. Did the client, at a young age, imitate gurgling and cooing sounds or show response to noise-making toys?
3. Did the client respond to his or her own name prior to 1 year of age?
4. Do people have to raise their voices to get the client's attention?
5. Does the client frequently say "huh" or "what" when someone is speaking?
6. Does the client respond inconsistently to sound?
7. Does the client have a history of ear infections?
8. Did the mother of the client have any prob-

lems during pregnancy, such as rubella or Rh blood incompatibility?

9. Is there a familial history of hearing problems? If so, who, what kind, and what degree of severity?
10. Is the client overly careful to watch the speaker's face?
11. Does the client turn the head so that one ear is toward the sound source?
12. Does the client ever complain of the ears hurting? How often?
13. Does the client consistently talk in an overly soft or loud voice?
14. Has the client been exposed to considerable loud noise over extended periods?
15. Does the client ever complain of ringing in the ear, dizziness, or nausea? How often?
16. Have there been considerable upper respiratory and middle ear infections?
17. Has there been treatment for otitis media (middle ear infection)? If so, how often and what kind?
18. Does hearing acuity seem to fluctuate from time to time? If so, how often and to what extent?

These and other questions should be asked in order to determine if the client has or has had significant hearing problems. Parents usually can provide most of this information, but the client's teacher, speech clinician, clinic, and family physician may be very helpful.

Developmental information

Some of the more typical questions that relate to developmental landmarks are:

1. When did the client:
   a. First hold up his head?
   b. First roll over?
   c. First crawl?
   d. First sit without support?
   e. First pull self to a standing position?
   f. Get his first tooth?
   g. First walk unaided?
   h. Gain bowel control?
   i. Gain bladder control?
   j. Dress self?
   k. Feed self?
2. What was the client's:
   a. Birth weight?
   b. Weight at age 6 months?
   c. Weight at age 1 year?

d. Present weight?

e. Present height?

3. At what age did the client establish handedness? What is the handedness?
4. Does the client fall or lose balance easily? If so, in what way and how often?
5. Does the client seem awkward or uncoordinated?
6. Does the client have difficulty in chewing or swallowing? If so, how often and how severe?
7. Has the client ever drooled, other than when teething?
8. Does the client have difficulty in moving the tongue or lips for speech purposes?
9. Did the client ever walk on his toes?

Answers to these questions should assist in determining if the client had any developmental delay that might explain, in part, the reason for the articulation disorder. The family physician and medical records can help provide this information, but most of it usually will have to come from the parents.

Medical information

Medical information includes prenatal, natal, and postnatal history including illnesses, diseases, hospitalizations, surgeries, and medications. Some questions to be asked include:

1. Did the mother have any illnesses, accidents or complications or take medications during pregnancy with the client? If so, what kind and extent?
2. What was the length of the pregnancy with the client, and what was the birth weight?
3. What was the duration of the delivery?
4. Were there any complications at birth? Any unusual conditions?
5. Were there any unusual conditions shortly after birth?
6. What diseases or serious injuries did the client have and were there any complications?
7. Was the client ever hospitalized? If so, why?
8. What is the present condition of the client's health?
9. Does the client have any physical problems? If so, what are they?
10. What is the name of the family physician?
11. Is the client receiving any medication or under medical treatment now? If so, what kind and for what reason?

12. Did the client ever suffer a severe head injury or high fever? If so, when, what kind, severity, or extent of fever?

This kind of medical information can be helpful in specifying etiology and diagnostic and remedial procedures. It can be obtained in several ways: questionnaire, medical records, school records, interviews with family physician or by telephone, and interviews with parents and client.

Educational information

Also important in understanding the total problem of the client is the educational information. Some questions that should be included are:

1. Did the client ever attend a day-care center or nursery school? Were there any problems?
2. Did the client attend kindergarten? Were there any problems?
3. At what age did the client begin school?
4. What kind of grades did the client achieve?
5. Was the client ever retained a grade in school? If so, which grade? Why?
6. Did the client ever skip a grade? If so, which one?
7. Was the client frequently absent from school? If so, why?
8. What are or were the client's poorest subjects? Best subjects?
9. How does or did the client feel about school and the teachers?
10. How far did the client go in school?
11. Has the client ever attended any special classes or received special instruction? If so, why, when, for how long, where, results?
12. What were the educational levels and performances of the parents and the other siblings?

Educational background information can provide helpful data for better understanding the client and for planning communicative treatment for the client. It can be obtained by questionnaire from school personnel and parents or by interview with each.

Psychosocial information

This category includes a wide range of areas including various interpersonal and personal behaviors, home and family relationships, history and environmental conditions, and other social characteristics. Among the questions that can be asked are:

1. How does the client relate to others?
2. Are there any disciplinary problems?
3. Are there or have there been problems in eating or sleeping?
4. Is the client nervous, fearful, happy, or unhappy? If so, in what ways?
5. Is the client overactive? Lethargic?
6. How does the client get along with others at home?
7. What is the neighborhood like?
8. What are the names and ages of the other children in the family?
9. Does the client have any personality problems? What kind and how extensive?
10. What interests, hobbies, or other activities does the client have?
11. What are the occupations of the parents?
12. What are the educational levels of the parents?
13. What are the ages of the parents?
14. What are the ages of the siblings?
15. What is the health of the parents and siblings?
16. What are leisure time activities of the family?
17. What ethnic, social, or other related aspects of the family need to be considered?
18. What other psychosocial information might be helpful in better understanding the client?

Many more questions could be asked regarding the psychosocial aspects of the client. The number and range of questions should be determined individually. Most of this information can be obtained from the parents by interview or questionnaire or both, but school records and interviews with teachers are often helpful.

Dental information

Occasionally dental information, past and present, is related to the client's communicative problem. However, relating dental history and status to disordered articulation should be done with caution. It might be well to pursue the following questions:

1. Has there been any unusual dental treatment or oral surgery?

2. Have any dental prostheses ever been worn? If so, did they affect the client's articulation? How?
3. Has the client ever undergone orthodontic treatment? If so, for what kind of malocclusion?
4. Has the term "tongue thrust" ever been used in regard to the client? If so, by whom?
5. Are there any dental problems present now?
6. Are there any other oral structure deviations present?

Dental information usually can be obtained from the parents. Additional information may be obtained from the client's dentist. A rating scale may be useful in determining if the particular dental information, or any other specific historical information for that matter, is significantly related to the present speech disorder. The higher the numeric rating, the more likely the dental or other data are related to disordered articulation. The following rating scale could be used:

0   Insignificant; the information probably is unrelated to the problem
1   Possibly significant; the information may be but probably is not related to the problem
2   Mildly significant; the information appears to be related somewhat to the problem and should be considered in managing the client
3   Significant; the information definitely appears to be related to the problem and must be considered in managing the client

Nutritional information

The awareness of the role of nutrition in normal development has increased considerably during the past few years. Its importance should not be overlooked when gathering historical data. Some of the questions that might be included are:

1. What are the nutritional habits in the home? Regularity of meals? Type of diet?
2. What are the parental attitudes toward nutrition?
3. Does it appear that the nutritional needs of the client are being met? If not, what is lacking?

4. Have the parents ever received nutritional counseling?
5. Does it seem as if nutrition could be related to the client's communicative problem? If so, in what way?

The diagnostician should be aware of the potential problems resulting from inappropriate diet and carefully explore the nutritional habits of the client. Parents must be relied on for most of this kind of information, but it must be realized that they often are not reliable informants in this area, because of either lack of knowledge or unwillingness to give accurate information. The nutritionist, school nurse, teacher, and family physician or clinic may be of help.

Identifying information

This information should be collected for future reference and correspondence and for obtaining a more complete idea about the client. It includes:

1. Date
2. Name
3. Age
4. Birth date
5. Sex
6. Address
7. Parent's name, address, and age
8. Telephone number
9. Statement of problem
10. Marital status
11. Occupation
12. Referral source
13. Name of physician
14. Name of school

ANALYSIS AND INTERPRETATION

After the pertinent information is collected, it must be analyzed and interpreted. This is a further step in the scientific method, and an important one. What does the information mean? How is it relevant? How is it applicable? Is it accurate? Does it contain identifiable trends and patterns that can be readily assimilated and categorized? How can it be used as a guide to the examination and testing that follow? Only after all of the available information is collected, analyzed for significance, and interpreted is the diagnostic process of gathering historical information complete (Nation and Aram, 1977). However, the overall diagnostic workup is not complete until the examination and testing are done, the test scores calculated, and the entire examination interpreted.

Several points should be remembered during *analysis* and *interpretation* of the information. First, effectively comprehending the significance of the available information requires not only clinical knowledge and understanding but also clinical experience and thoroughness. The beginning clinician may initially experience some difficulty in sorting out all of the relevant data and then synthesizing the salient information. Significant information is not always readily apparent, so that considerable time may have to be spent in extrapolating the data. Even with extensive experience, the diagnostician will have histories to analyze and interpret that do not appear to present recognizable patterns or that may actually seem contradictory. It is important to look beneath the superficiality or contradictory nature of some statements made by the informant, since these statements may only be the "tip of the iceberg" of significance. Thoroughness cannot be sacrificed if the analysis and interpretation are to be correct.

Second, analysis and interpretation are ongoing. They should occur continually from the onset of collecting historical data to the conclusion of testing and examination. If interpretations are reserved until after the data are collected and analyzed, significant information may be overlooked or excluded. Interpreting in situ helps to guide the direction of the case history and other diagnostic processes. Hasty, superficial interpretation, however, can lead to faulty conclusions and interfere with further diagnostic procedures.

Third, the interviewer should be particularly aware of personal biases—those of the informant as well as those of the diagnostician. It is all too easy to distort the facts with prejudice. It is important to differentiate between what the informant said and what the informant was thought to have said or was expected to say. Prejudice can invalidate the interpretation of the historical data. An attitude of objectivity helps to overcome biases while ensuring some measure of accountability. The interviewer should not let biases cause him or her to reach conclusions prematurely or erroneously; the data should be analyzed carefully and objectively. The interviewer should also be aware that the informant may be biased or prejudiced and thus distort the information given.

Fourth, the fact that collection, analysis, and interpretation of historical information are interrelated should be recognized. In fact the processes may sometimes occur simultaneously. These processes, along with examination and test results, are utilized to solve problems—to answer questions that the informant and the client have and to try to determine cause and effect. It should be kept in mind that the "sum of the parts may be greater or different than the whole" insofar as analyzing and interpreting the findings. Conclusions reached when combining collection, analysis, and interpretation may be different from conclusions reached when considering each process separately. Considering the processes collectively may result in a more accurate diagnosis.

Interpretation is the final and probably the most crucial task in the diagnostic workup. Errors in interpretation can have far-reaching effects; therefore, much care and effort must be given in categorizing common symptomatology, in weighing salient information, and in relating the most essential information to possible etiology and treatment. Test data must also be considered before the final diagnosis is made. If there is ever any doubt concerning the accuracy or appropriateness of symptomatology, etiology, and some notions about treatment, then definite conclusions should not be made at that time. It is better to reach tentative conclusions than to formulate a definite diagnosis when a degree of uncertainty exists. It may be that more informa-

tion is needed. This may be obtained by repeating or extending some of the previous steps or perhaps by referral to another specialist for examination and testing, such as a psychologist, physician, audiologist, or special educator. A philosophy of tentative diagnosis and trial diagnostic treatment may be conservative, but it may also be more appropriate since it can add further information. The fact that interpretation is the final aspect of gathering historical and other diagnostic data does not mean that it must be permanent.

SUMMARY

Five methods of obtaining historical information, (1) interview, (2) questionnaire, (3) observation, (4) autobiography, and (5) other clinical records, have been discussed. A combination of some of these methods, if conducted effectively and interpreted appropriately, can provide the background information necessary for guiding examination and testing, helping to determine the diagnosis, and assisting in planning the communicative treatment. However, clinical examination and testing, counseling the client and family, determining the base performance of the client, writing a comprehensive clinical report, ascertaining effective approaches to treatment, and making a statement about prognosis are also integral parts of the entire diagnostic workup. The historical data can also be helpful in determining if and to whom additional referral should be made. With experience the diagnostician will find shortcuts and time-saving methods of history taking. There may be a tendency, especially among beginning clinicians, not to be aware of the necessity of a thorough, complete, *differential* case history. Without it the remaining tasks in management of the articulation disorder are much more difficult.

STUDY SUGGESTIONS

1. What are the different methods of obtaining case history information? Select the method you think is most effective and defend it.
2. What are some questions that the diagnosti-

cian might typically ask the informant about communicative development?

3. What are ten guidelines for conducting an effective interview?
4. Besides obtaining case history information, what must the diagnostician do with the information?

REFERENCES

Beck, S.: The simplicity of science, Garden City, N.Y., 1959, Doubleday & Co., Inc.

Darley, F.: Diagnosis and appraisal of communication disorders, Englewood Cliffs, N.J., 1964, Prentice-Hall, Inc.

Darley, F., and Spriestersbach, D.: Diagnostic methods in speech pathology, ed. 2, New York, 1978, Harper & Row, Publishers.

Doll, E.: Some things we know in clinical psychology, J. Appl. Psychol. **24:**20, 1940.

Emerick, C., and Hatten, J.: Diagnosis and evaluation in speech pathology, ed. 2, Englewood Cliffs, N.J., 1979, Prentice-Hall, Inc.

Emerick, L.: The parent interview: guidelines for student and practicing speech clinicians, Danville, Ill., 1969, The Interstate Printers & Publishers, Inc.

Garrett, A.: Interviewing: its principles and methods, ed. 2, New York, 1972, Family Service Association of America.

Kinsey, A., Pomeroy, W., and Martin, C.: Sexual behavior in the human male, Philadelphia, 1948, W. B. Saunders Co.

Lillywhite, H., and Bradley, D.: Communication problems in mental retardation: diagnosis and management, New York, 1969, Harper & Row, Publishers.

McDonald, E.: Articulation testing and treatment: a sensory-motor approach, Pittsburgh, 1964, Stanwix House, Inc.

McReynolds, L., Kuhn, J., and Williams, G.: Articulatory-defective children's discrimination of their production errors, J. Speech Hear. Disord. **40:**327-338, 1975.

Milisen, R.: Methods of evaluation and diagnosis of speech disorders. In Travis, L., editor: Handbook of speech pathology and audiology, New York, 1971, Appleton-Century-Crofts.

Myklebust, H.: Auditory disorders in children, New York, 1954, Grune & Stratton, Inc.

Nation, J., and Aram, D.: Diagnosis of speech and language disorders, St. Louis, 1977, The C. V. Mosby Co.

Nichols, R.: Ten components of effective listening, Education **75:**292-302, 1955.

Rosenbek, R., and Wertz, R.: A review of 50 cases of developmental apraxia of speech, Lang. Speech Hear. Serv. Schools **III:**23-33, 1972.

Weiss, C.: Weiss Comprehensive Articulation Test, Hingham, Mass., 1978, Teaching Resources.

Weiss, C. E., and Lillywhite, H. S.: Communicative disorders: a handbook for prevention and early intervention, St. Louis, 1976, The C. V. Mosby Co.

Winitz, H.: From syllable to conversation, Baltimore, 1975, University Park Press.

Winitz, H.: Articulation disorders: from prescription to description, J. Speech Hear. Disord. **42:**143-147, 1977.

Young, E., and Hawk, S.: Moto-kinesthetic speech training, Stanford, Calif., 1955, Stanford University Press.

GLOSSARY

autobiography A brief written account by a client of significant aspects of the client's own life.

case history A written account of as much significant information about the client and the disorder as is available. It is used as a basis for management of the problem.

client The individual with a communication problem needing diagnosis and management; also referred to as "case" or "patient."

diagnostician Used here to refer to the speech pathologist or audiologist charged with the task of making a diagnosis.

differential case history A compilation of information about the client that will help the diagnostician to differentiate this particular problem from others, which leads to a differential diagnosis.

differential diagnosis A sorting out or differentiating of factors peculiar to the particular problem being considered as different from other types of problems.

editorializing As used here, refers to an interviewer inserting personal opinions and comments when they are unnecessary or irrelevant.

etiology The cause or causes of a disorder.

examination As used here, refers to assessment of anatomic, physiologic, and functional performance of the speech mechanism and the administration of speech and other tests necessary to arrive at a diagnosis.

extrapolating data To infer or project certain factors about the problems on the basis of data already known.

eye contact Genuine, interested, sincere contact with another person by looking directly and naturally at him without looking too constantly or too infrequently and not looking away during stress or embarrassment.

malocclusion Irregularity or abnormality in the closure or relationship of the lower and upper teeth and jaws.

map-territory relationship A term from general semantics used to denote a concept that a person tries to represent meaning, another person, situation, or condition (territory) by means of a verbal "map" of that territory.

observation As used here, the diagnostician, clinician, or student observes the client in various situations and in different ways to obtain significant information about the client.

otitis media Infection in the middle ear.

perpetuating factors Conditions or events that tend to maintain (continue rather than diminish) a disorder.

precipitating factors Conditions or events that appear to bring about or cause a disorder to surface; not a basic cause of the disorder.

predisposing factors Conditions or events that seem to make an individual vulnerable or predisposed to the communication disorder.

presenting problem The communication problem of the person that appears to come forth or present itself.

prosthesis An appliance used to assist or partially restore some damaged part or function of the body, such as an artificial limb, hearing aid, or speech appliance.

questionnaire An organized set of written questions designed to elicit specific types of information about the client or problem.

symptomatology Refers to the symptoms of diseases; in speech pathology the symptoms of communication disorders.

testing As used in this book, it refers to the various tests, mostly formal, used to determine various communication weaknesses and levels.

unconscious projection As used here, an interviewer's observations of what and how an informant unconsciously reveals or projects information and behavior. It may also include the unconscious projection of thoughts, feelings, and opinions about the client by the interviewer.

CHAPTER SIX

Assessment and diagnosis of articulation

"A man is hid under his tongue."
ALI IBN-ABI-TALIB

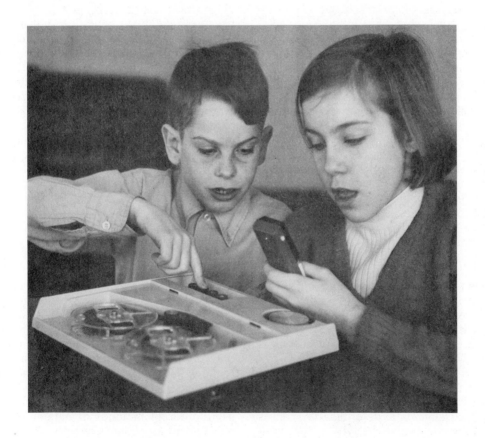

The second major stage of articulation management is assessment and diagnosis. Following the collection of a thorough differential case history, a careful assessment should be completed as a basis for diagnosis and for planning appropriate and effective treatment. It should also provide a basis for making a statement about prognosis and for providing a framework for counseling the client and family.

PRINCIPLES OF ASSESSMENT

In assessment of articulation leading to the diagnosis of an articulation disorder, if one is present, the physiologic (kinetic and cosmetic), acoustic, phonologic, and perceptual aspects of speech should be considered, that is, what articulation looks like, sounds like, and seems like to the diagnostician. The assessment process includes some assumptions that may or may not be entirely valid: (1) the client's production of a specific phoneme at that particular time is a true reflection of inclusive articulation ability for that sound; (2) the performance is reflective of all other speech situations; (3) the responses on single-word picture tests can be generalized to contextual speech; (4) there is a phonetic rationale for testing phonemes in the initial, medial, and final positions; (5) the diagnostician is proficient in translating the perceived articulation patterns into some kind of code such as the International Phonetic Alphabet; and (6) speech is considered a sequence of discrete elements, like beads on a string.

The assessment stage of management also presupposes that identification of the problem has previously occurred (see Appendix B). Assuming that the problem has already been detected, the remaining major tasks confronting the diagnostician are to describe the patterns of misarticulation, analyze and interpret the collected data, establish baseline data, determine the causes if possible, determine the type of treatment required, make a statement about prognosis, outline recommendations, counsel the appropriate persons, and write a diagnostic report.

In order to accomplish these major tasks, the diagnostician must first plan the assessment procedures. This planning should include a review of the historical information, selection of testing instruments and procedures, and determination of a procedural sequence. It is usually helpful to outline on paper the activities or areas to be included in the assessment and the order in which to proceed. For example, it would be unwise to begin assessment of a young child with an oral examination. Such a beginning might cause the child to become fearful or even cry, thus affecting the subsequent activities. Careful planning is imperative.

Another important consideration for the diagnostician is establishment of rapport, because a child can be enticed but not coerced to perform a task (Goodenough, 1949). To entice the child the diagnostician must know what kind of person the child is and adjust approaches and procedures to "fit" that particular child. Each person is different from all others and will respond in different ways. Although some of the same general assessment procedures and materials are used with most clients, the specific approach and application should be adjusted to suit different needs. In fact the diagnostician should routinely consider an individualistic diagnostic approach.

Besides knowing how to assess and interpret articulation behaviors, the diagnostician must also know how to assess and interpret the areas that may be related to articulation development, such as the neuromuscular system, language, auditory acuity, memory, discrimination, and conceptualization; oral sensation-perception; oral diadochokinesis; and tongue thrust. Interpreting the significance of these areas may require the assistance of persons in other disciplines.

The diagnostician should be skilled in using different methods of obtaining samples of articulation behavior. Since the method and setting in which speech samples are obtained, not to mention the diagnostician, can significantly affect the sample, several different settings and methods may need to be considered. Some of the available methods include pictures, objects, observations, conversation, oral reading, imitating, storytelling, games, and asking questions. Some of the possible settings are the clinic room, waiting room, classroom, playground, home, and mother's lap. The setting may involve a one-to-one relationship; the client playing alone or with someone else; the client talking to the parents, another child, or other adults; or the client interacting with other members of the family in the clinic or home. Besides the variety of available methods and settings, the diagnostician must also realize that assessment, regardless of the method and setting, is complicated by the fact that there is no satisfactory method for assessing articulation without using human listeners (Moll, 1968).

To help conduct an objective assessment and obtain valid results, Darley and Spriestersbach (1978) offer several procedures and reminders:

1. Keep the purpose clearly in mind
2. Carefully record the client's responses (on paper and on tape)
3. Analyze the misarticulations in regard to error, consistency of error, response to stimulation, and common factors
4. Conduct the test and other procedures without observers in the room, if possible
5. Do not work too fast
6. Keep the client motivated
7. Remember that the diagnostician is in charge
8. Use a straightforward approach
9. Answer questions
10. Ask for repetition, if necessary
11. Remember that the test is merely a tool
12. The client, not the test must be central

The range and extent of what assessment involves varies among clinicians, but the end result may be the same—to arrive at an accurate diagnosis of the articulation disorder.

Another principle that is important in diagnosis pertains to *philosophy*. Every diagnostician should develop a philosophy of assessment; one that inculcates the scientific method in a flexible and perhaps tentative manner. The philosophy may be relatively simple or it may be rather complex, but each diagnostician should have one. It should be continuously reexamined, modified, and improved as one's clinical knowledge, experience, listening skills, and expertise develop. Such a philosophy helps to ensure that every client with a disorder is looked upon as a challenge, a problem to be solved by the application of scientific problem-solving techniques.

A philosophy should be based on proved methods and techniques and on an experientially based frame of reference. It should incorporate a rationale that can support the selection of methods, techniques, and diagnostic tools and an attitude that is individualistic in nature, since persons with articulation disorders are not a homogeneous population that can be dealt with in the same way (Powers, 1971). This type of clinical attitude can help assure a logical, systematic approach to obtaining representative speech samples and interpreting them correctly. A point of view that considers the importance of clinical knowledge will also ensure the use of appropriate tools for assessing articulation and areas that may be related to articulation. If the diagnostician possesses these philosophic principles, diagnostic workups will more likely be valid.

GENERAL CHARACTERISTICS OF PERSONS WITH ARTICULATION DISORDERS

Requisites for conducting a good assessment are knowledge and awareness of the general characteristics of persons with articulation problems. Although there are a great many behavioral differences, a number of likenesses are present among persons with disordered articulation. Furthermore, not all of the characteristics have been clearly related to articulation disorders. Nevertheless an awareness of these characteristics should assist in the challenging process of obtaining, analyzing, synthesizing, and interpreting pertinent behavior of this heterogeneous population.

As a group, persons with defective articulation appear to have poorer *speech discrimination abilities* (Winitz, 1969; Powers, 1971); however, this contention is not undisputed (Kronvall and Diehl, 1954; Prins, 1963). Speech discrimination may be very individualistic; it may be good in some persons and poor in others. More research needs to be done in this area, especially in looking at discrimination abilities in regard to sounds misarticulated. As Spriestersbach and Curtis (1951) indicated, children with defective articulation may have poor auditory discrimination abilities for only the phonemes they misarticulate and have no difficulty in discriminating sounds that they produce correctly. Future studies should also attempt to assess the client's self-discrimination abilities rather than ability to discriminate other speakers. Even though some persons with articulation problems do not have poor speech discrimination abilities, ear training seems to be beneficial in facilitating carry-over and maintenance. We suggest routine assessment of all of the parameters of audition—acuity, memory, discrimination, and conceptualization.

A characteristic common to articulation testing is *inconsistency of test results*. Winitz (1969) stated that variability in test results can be attributed to the client, the diagnostician, the diagnostic test, and the interaction between the client and the diagnostician. A phoneme misarticulated at one time, in one context, or in one emotional state may be correctly articulated at another time or in another phonetic context (Oller, 1973). Because of this variability it is important to assess a client's articulation performance in a variety of contexts, including contextual speech (Milisen, 1971; McDonald, 1964). Determining the contexts in which a typically defective sound is produced correctly enables the clinician to identify a starting point for intervention (Van Riper, 1963; Weston and Irwin, 1971).

As mentioned earlier, disordered articulation commonly relates to a *hierarchy of sound development* that is reasonably orderly and predictable. That is, later-developing sounds generally are misarticulated more frequently than earlier-developing sounds (Templin, 1957; Ingram, 1976). Roe and Milisen (1942) found the following sounds most often misarticulated in order of frequency /θ,s,t,ð,dʒ,tʃ,r,v,k,d,ʃ,g,f,p,l,b,ŋ,w/. Many speech-language clinicians report that /s,z,r,l/ and the consonant clusters are among the most frequently misarticulated sounds.

Misarticulation according to type includes the following sequence in order of frequency: consonant clusters, single consonants, diphthongs, and vowels. Wellman and associates (1936) said that nasal consonants are easier to produce then plosives, plosives are easier than fricatives, and fricatives are easier than consonant clusters. Pendergast and associates (1969) found nonvoiced consonants to be defective more frequently than voiced consonants. More errors were associated with place of articulation in the oral cavity than with either manner or voice-nonvoice (Bricker, 1967). These findings suggest general agreement regarding misarticulations according to type. One additional point should be remembered; consonants occur in speech nearly twice as often as vowels or diphthongs.

As mentioned previously, misarticulations regarding the *sound position in words* are least common in the initial position, followed by those in the medial position, and finally in the final position. The influence of one sound on another in context is an important factor that should always be assessed. In fact the effects of context on articulation may be more important than the position of the misarticulated sound. Concerning the type of misarticulation, omissions are thought to be the most difficult to correct (also the most devastating to intelligibility), followed by substitutions and then distortions.

Familiarity with *articulation norms* is essential, as mentioned in Chapter 3. Knowledge of phonemic development provides some guidance not only in deciding which sounds to begin treatment with but also in determining whether an articulation problem exists or not. Moreover the diagnostician should also be familiar with the standards that were used in specifying norms for each sound. If the norms were based on 90% correct production of the children tested compared with 75% or 51% correct production, these normative guidelines can be confusing. Either could be used as long as interpretation of results is based on awareness of the criteria used.

Mean length of utterance tends to be shorter among persons with articulation disorders (Templin, 1957); however, this behavior is highly individualistic and should be assessed for adequacy with each client. Mean length of utterance may be a reflection of the client's personality or language capabilities rather than of an articulation disorder. An inferior mean length of utterance should be noted and incorporated into the plan of treatment.

Intelligibility is poorer among this population. This statement appears so obvious that mention of it almost seems superfluous. Nevertheless impaired intelligibility can seriously interfere with articulation testing and analysis and should, therefore, be considered when deciding on the assessment protocol. Sometimes poor intelligibility can completely preclude a valid assessment. Although closely associated with articulation, intelligibility is not synonymous with it. In some persons several phonemes can be misarticulated yet intelligibility will be quite good. In others only one or two sounds may be in error and intelligibility will be seriously affected, suggesting that much more is involved in intelligibility than number of misarticulations. Compensation, rate and loudness of speech, frequency of occurrence of the faulty sounds, and such factors strongly influence intelligibility (see Appendix F). Also isolated sounds or words may be quite intelligible and connected speech just the opposite, as in persons with certain types of motor speech disorders.

Oral diadochokinesis, oral sensation-perception, and other motor and sensory factors may be impaired in persons with articulation disorders. Although the research findings are inconclusive, problems in these areas may exist in some cases (McCall, 1969; Weiss, 1968; Artley, 1948). Therefore, they should be assessed before a differential diagnosis is made. Likewise reading, writing, and listening skills should also be considered in the diagnostic workup.

The role of *maturation* is a concept important to articulation development (Sayler, 1949; Roe and Milisen, 1942; Everhart, 1960). Females develop articulation skills slightly earlier than males because they mature earlier. They also have fewer articulation disorders (Templin, 1957). We know that maturation assists articulation development up to a point, but sometimes it is difficult to differentiate between the role of maturation and the role of environment in acquisition of articulation. Environmental factors can enhance or interfere with a child's articulation development, as can immaturity. Yet one should not necessarily expect to find a child with an articulation disorder to be less mature than some other child.

An aspect that varies considerably among persons with articulation problems is *level of awareness*. Some persons appear to be keenly aware and sensitive to their deviant articulation, whereas others seem to be unaware of or at least unconcerned with their speech differences. A number of factors could influence the level of awareness, some of which are mentioned in Chapter 1.

Defective articulation usually has *multiple etiology* (Powers, 1971). This characteristic should remind the diagnostician to conduct a thorough assessment in order to determine the different causes and, if possible, to alleviate them if they are still present. Dichotomizing etiology into organic or nonorganic categories should be avoided because it tends to narrow the approach to assessment. The diagnostician may become preoccupied in trying to decide into which category to place the disorder and overlook the possibility of its having both organic and nonorganic etiologies. It is also important to remember that articulation is not always normal when all conditions for its development are favorable, and vice versa, thus complicating the process of making a differential diagnosis.

Individuals with disordered articulation tend to have a higher percentage of *tongue thrust* than normal speakers (Fletcher, Casteel, and Bradley, 1961). However, the relationship is still unclear. In addition the area of tongue thrust continues to be controversial and in need of more scientific research. Nevertheless tongue thrust seems to be more prevalent among persons who misarticulate sibilants and should be assessed if there is any evidence indicating its possible presence in the client. If present the diagnostician must determine whether it is benign or detrimental.

Stimulability among persons with defective articulation may vary considerably. Some persons are more stimulable than others, especially persons with nonorganic etiologies. Since stimulability may relate to articulation change, it is one characteristic that is important not only in diagnosis but also in case selection (Sommers, Cox, and West, 1972). Because it relates to predictive testing, stimulability may provide valuable information in deciding which children might outgrow their misarticulations without intervention (Carter and Buck, 1958; Steer and Drexler, 1960).

Misarticulations are describable and can usually be imitated. An effective way to describe them is by looking at their distinctive features and noting which features are readily distinguishable and describable, including the presence or absence of phonologic rules. If the misarticulations can be described, they should be. It is also helpful to imitate the specific misarticulations in order to "feel" how the client is misarticulating them and to show the client what the misarticulation looks and sounds like. This activity increases the awareness of both the diagnostician and the client.

One final characteristic worthy of mention is the *tendency of people to resist change*. Although this characteristic may be more important in treatment than in diagnosis, it nevertheless has implications for the diagnostician. Concomitant with the tendency of the client to resist change may be the difficulty in becoming motivated, in being cooperative, and in providing representative samples of communication. This tendency should be taken into consideration especially when assessing younger clients.

These and other characteristics present a serious challenge for the diagnostician. Awareness of their possible existence should facilitate a thorough, appropriate diagnostic workup and subsequent differential diagnosis.

ASSESSMENT OF ARTICULATION

Several different methods of obtaining speech samples have been mentioned. One or a combination of these can be used to obtain a representative sample of the client's articulation behavior. The essential point to remember is that the method used must provide a representative sample. If only a limited number of different speech contexts are sampled, the diagnostician will probably be unable to describe adequately the client's articulation, specify the correct level of functioning, and determine the most effective treatment approach.

Assessment of error patterns should be done in order to analyze the organization of the phonologic system. This is best accomplished through the use of distinctive features to describe the errors (McReynolds and Engmann, 1975). In addition the diagnostician should look for phonologic processes and rules that describe the client's speech, such as patterns of simplification, omission of medial and final stops, backing errors, and other morphophonemic errors (Ingram, 1976; Weiner, 1979). Phonologic assessment relates articulation more closely to language in that it attempts to assess communicative competence and cognition. In fact its original intent was to analyze linguistic behavior.

Categorization of phonologic processes can also be done according to syllable structure, feature contrast, and harmony. Syllable structure analysis includes deletions and reductions of sound clusters; feature contrast involves the processes of fronting, gliding, vocalization, denasalization, and affrication; and harmony includes analysis of velar, alveolar, and labial assimilation and devoicing of final consonants. Although helpful in analyzing articulation, this system, like most, is incomplete by itself.

The type of test selected should depend on the purpose or reason for testing a specific client. If the primary purpose is *detection* of children (or adults) who have misarticulations, then fairly informal methods can be used. Detection testing is done to find out which persons are behind developmental norms or have articulation deviations of omission, substitution, distortion, or addition. It involves a yes or no decision; either articulation development is on target or it is not. Ways of detecting the presence of misarticulations are to engage the client in conversation, question and answer, naming objects in the room or in a book, imitating the diagnostician saying words containing key sounds, repeating words in sequence such as days of the week and numbers, and observing the client's verbal interactions with someone else. Detecting persons with inappropriate articulation is usually a quick procedure for the trained and experienced diagnostician, taking no more than a couple of minutes with each person. After all, the purpose is detection, not diagnosis. At the same time speech samples of the subject should be obtained until a definite "yes" or "no" can be determined. The probing should be continued until the conclusion is certain.

Unlike most of the procedures and methods used in detection, *assessment* of someone's articulation is considerably more time-consuming and complex. The diagnostician must make every attempt to determine misarticulations, missing rules and features, phonologic processes, levels, trends or patterns, inconsistencies, and cosmetic peculiarities in the client. Etiologies should also be ascertained, if at all possible. However, not until after all of the information has been collected and analyzed should a diagnosis be made.

The assessment process typically proceeds with the administration of an articulation test battery. The test battery selected should provide a range of articulation behaviors obtained in a variety of contexts, using procedures such as the following: The diagnostician begins by bringing the client into a relatively small, comfortable room with appropriately sized furniture, usually a table and two or three chairs, good lighting, adequate acoustics, limited "clutter" and other distractions, a one-way observation window, and an intercom system with good fidelity. Although many situations are not ideal, an attempt should be made to approximate this setting as nearly as possible. Next rapport is established through casual conversation or questioning. After rapport is established, the diagnostician explains (to the younger client) that "we are going to play a game" or "look at some pictures." The instructions, as indicated in the test manual, are carefully given to the client and further explained, if necessary. The diagnostician is seated either across from or next to the client while the pictures from the test are presented in a fairly expeditious manner. The diagnostician should be seated next to the client during the oral examination. All phonetic and cosmetic deviations are written on the appropriate response form for later scoring, analysis, and interpretation. Whenever a key word is not elicited, it should be provided for the client within 10 seconds from the time the stimulus was first presented.

The final stage of articulation testing is to engage the client in conversation if old enough. A topic of interest should be probed and pursued so that the client will talk openly and freely. During this time any misarticulations or morphophonemic errors that were not present previously should be noted. Any other differences, such as changes in articulation pattern, cosmetic features, or intelligibility, should be recorded. If possible this sampling of conversational speech should be tape-recorded and used later for analysis of intelligibility as well as for analysis of the client's most representative articulation.

If the client is uncooperative or very taciturn, the parent, sibling, or another child should be brought into the room to interact with the client. At this point the diagnostician should go into the adjacent observation room and continue articulation assessment.

In older clients the sentence form of an articulation test may be used. Again the instructions are carefully given to the client, and, as in testing of younger clients, the diagnostician obtains a tape-recorded representative sample of conversational speech for eventual analysis and interpretation. Five minutes of conversational speech is usually sufficient.

Articulation testing should progress as rapidly as the client will proceed with occasional positive reinforcement but with little digression. Asking for repetitions may sometimes be necessary but hopefully can be kept to a minimum. Familiarity with the test and with testing procedures will facilitate efficiency and effectiveness.

Another possible assessment procedure involves *prediction*. The clinician usually is unable to schedule all of the referred children with communicative disorders; therefore, information relative to which persons may outgrow their disorders and which will not is valuable. Unfortunately we have no way of knowing definitely which children will and which will not outgrow their misarticulations spontaneously. Van Riper and Erickson (1968) have developed a test that tends to predict which first-grade children might outgrow their misarticulations. Administration of such a test may help in selecting the caseload.

As with other assessment tools, a predictive test should be carefully administered according to standardized procedures. Accurate judgments of right or wrong productions are critical in predicting which children will outgrow their errors. The diagnostician does not need to specify the type or degree of misarticulation, only whether or not the speech production (specific phoneme or phonologic process) was correct or incorrect. Predictive testing usually includes minimum scores or percentages that need to be obtained in order for the child to be excluded from treatment because of the possibility of outgrowing the articulation errors.

Some articulation tests appear to be especially appropriate for *analysis* and *interpretation*. However, most of them can be readily used for these purposes. In the "Diagnostic Battery for Articulation" we have included the Arizona, Templin-Darley, and Weiss tests as useful tools in analyzing and interpreting articulation data. Although McDonald's test would serve well in these areas, we elected to list it for purposes of research. Even though all of these tests can be useful in analysis and interpretation, they, by themselves, are not enough. Articulation usually must be assessed in additional contexts. Analysis of the articulation information can be done in several ways. We have already alluded to place of articulation, manner of articulation, and voicing as one system of analysis. Another way to analyze articulation is in terms of initial, medial, and final position errors. The diagnostician can also look for the absence of phonologic processes and rules. Ingram (1976) and Weiner (1979) provide a fairly extensive system for analyzing phonologic processes.

Another system utilizes articulation age norms to compute an articulation age and frequency of occurrence of misarticulated phonemes for calculating an articulation score. Simply counting the number of misarticulated phonemes is another method. A system for looking at the effects of abutting consonants, overlapping movements, and assimilation helps analysis of phonemes in regard to their position within syllables, as prevocalic, intervocalic, or postvocalic. Discrepancies between articulation of isolated words and conversational speech can also be analyzed; this is also referred to as analysis of inconsistencies in speech production. Conspicuousness of the misarticulations should be considered. Sounds can be conspicuous because of their acoustic component or because of their cosmetic features.

Performing these different analyses will take time; however, it will be time well spent, because it is important to ascertain the total articulation problem. Furthermore, not all methods need to be employed. Ways of utilizing some of these methods will be discussed later in this chapter.

The final assessment procedure relates to *research*. Articulation testing may be part of a research design pertaining to the effectiveness of assessment procedures or the effectiveness of a certain therapeutic process. The Deep Test of Articulation (p. 121) is sufficiently thorough to sample virtually all phonemic contexts. Therefore, it lends itself well to research in phonology. Because the test assesses abutting and overlapping sounds, it is sometimes more difficult to administer to the client. For example, if the two pictures are "sun" and "tub," the client must say them quite rapidly in succession in order to achieve the intended purpose of producing abutting and overlapping consonants. If there is even a slight pause between "sun" and "tub," the desired response of "suntub" will not have been obtained. If this requisite is overcome, the test can be a useful tool in research activities.

The following summary of a battery for detecting, assessing, predicting, analyzing, interpreting, and researching articulation can be used as a guideline in test selection.

Diagnostic battery for articulation

Detection: Informal testing procedures—quick, easy, and effective in detecting misarticulations

Assessment: Weiss Comprehensive Articulation Test (p. 122) and Goldman-Fristoe Test of Articulation (p. 121)—sufficiently thorough to permit an adequate sample of articulation

Prediction: Predictive Screening Test of Articulation (p. 126)—tends to predict which children might not outgrow their misarticulations

Analysis and interpretation: Templin-Darley Tests of Articulation (p. 122), Fisher-Logemann Test of Articulation Competence (p. 120), phonological process analysis (p. 122), and Weiss Comprehensive Articulation Test— each of these tests provides a different but appropriate method for analyzing and interpreting the obtained articulation information

Research: Deep Test of Articulation (p. 121)— provides the most in-depth information regarding phonemic context from which base rate can be determined and progress measured, such as in clinical research

Since this battery provides a range of tests that can be used to meet the needs of five different categories, not all categories would necessarily be assessed. Test selection would depend on the specific purpose at that time. Also there are articulation tests available other than the ones mentioned that could be used in meeting the purpose of each category, or one test that might serve several purposes. For example, if the purpose is assessment, then detection testing would be excluded because the individual has already been identified. Analysis, interpretation, and research might also be accomplished by the same tests used for assessment, again reducing the need for using several different tests. The important point for the diagnostician to remember is why the test is being given at all, which implies using the best possible test or test battery for that particular client and diagnostician.

Moreover test selection is contingent on specific case history data, presenting behaviors of the client, results of testing of areas related to articulation and of the speech mechanism, concerns of the family, and any other pertinent information. Test selection is an individual matter and will naturally vary with the diagnostician's training, experience, and preference. It is not necessary to use several different tests to assess articulation as long as the assessment is appropriate and complete, that is, it adequately samples the client's speech. The diagnostician must remember to listen for one phoneme at a time, determine what the client can and cannot do, look for missing phonetic rules or distinctive features, and remember that the important variable in testing articulation is not the test, but rather the client and the tester.

How to administer the articulation test should be described in the manual of the test selected. Some tests also provide guidelines regarding degree of severity. Other ideas on diagnostics can be found in Darley and Spriestersbach (1978) and in Emerick and Hatten (1979). Not only should the directions be followed explicitly, but familiarity with the test is essential before using it. The diagnostician should be able to use the test selected with ease and efficiency and to record the responses appropriately and accurately. Again well-developed visual observation and listening skills and familiarity with the test are indispensable for noting valid articulation behavior.

ASSESSMENT OF STIMULABILITY

Closely related to administering the articulation test for analysis of specific phonemes and phonologic processes is the assessment of stimulability. Testing of stimulability requires the client to imitate or model the clinician producing the phonemes that were misarticulated during articulation testing. Imitations may be of the phoneme in isolation, in syllables, in words, or in sentences. We suggest having the client imitate the misarticulated sounds in isolation and in words. Three repetitions should be elicited in isolation and three in words containing each error. Then the percentage correct should be calculated for each sound and a total or composite percentage calculated for all of the error sounds. In this way a stimulability score is recorded for each sound as well as an overall stimulability score for all defective sounds. Even though each repetition is scored either right or wrong, the diagnostician can also determine if the client showed any improvement during subsequent repetitions or imitations. Improvement, even though still unacceptable, might be suggestive of more positive stimulability in one client than in another

who showed no improvement on succeeding productions.

Ability of young children to imitate phonemes correctly has been used to suggest favorable probability for spontaneously outgrowing the misarticulations (Carter and Buck, 1958). Additionally stimulability scores have been used in selection of target sounds for treatment and in determination of therapeutic progress. Low stimulability scores indicate unfavorable prognosis, but high stimulability scores do not necessarily indicate favorable prognosis (Pollack and Rees, 1972). A client may achieve a high stimulability score, yet progress in treatment may not be rapid. This may be related to the concept that high stimulability scores reflect good phonetic skills (motoric skills) but not necessarily phonologic competence (cognitive skills) (Turton and Clark, 1971). Ease of production may also be an important variable here. The client who easily produces misarticulated sounds may show faster progress in treatment than the one who displays effort or difficulty in imitating sounds. Generally the higher the stimulability score, the more favorable the prognosis for improvement or for a more rapid rate of improvement.

ASSESSMENT OF INTELLIGIBILITY

The understandability of oral speech is one of the most important factors in articulation. It should be routinely assessed during contextual speech, assuming of course that the client is talking in sentences rather than in isolated words. If contextual speech is not present in the client, intelligibility can be determined for isolated words. Degree of unintelligibility is perhaps the most important indicator of articulation severity.

Although determined quite subjectively, intelligibility scores can be equated with levels of articulation development and degree of speech handicap. Many factors influence intelligibility. Because of the multiplicity of factors involved, Casteel (1970) devised a "Grid for Diagnosing Intelligibility" (Appendix F), which considers such factors as (1) articulation, (2) redundancy,

(3) syntax, (4) mean length of utterance, (5) juncture, (6) rate, (7) prosody, (8) pronunciation, (9) intensity, (10) rhythm, and (11) quality. We might add to this list signal-to-noise ratio (amount of background noise in comparison to the loudness level of the speaker's voice), morphology, and inflectional and stress patterns of the speaker. By rating the degree of adequacy or inadequacy of each factor, the diagnostician can determine which factors are contributing most to unintelligible speech.

Particular aspects of articulation per se may influence intelligibility. For example, perceptual judgments are increasingly impaired as the number of phonemic errors increases (Jordon, 1969). The understandability of articulation is further influenced as the misarticulations become more consistent, depart more from the target sounds, and include increasing numbers of more frequently occurring sounds. In some instances intelligibility may be so poor as to interfere with the diagnostician's obtaining valid articulation results because the client's responses could not be understood.

Notwithstanding these multiple influences and relative subjectivity of intelligibility, assessment of it is an important aspect of the diagnostic workup. As mentioned in the Weiss Comprehensive Articulation Test (W-CAT) (Weiss, 1978), intelligibility can be calculated by randomly selecting 100 consecutive words from the client's tape-recorded contextual speech sample. This recorded sample should be played back as the diagnostician, or preferably a panel of three persons (who do not necessarily need to be speech-language pathologists) listens to the sample and counts the number of unintelligible words. This number is then subtracted from 100 (the number of words spoken), yielding the intelligibility score for that client. If the client's speech is so unintelligible that words cannot be differentiated from syllables (that is, whether "uh uh" is one two-syllable word or two one-syllable words), the number of syllables should be counted and the percentage of intelligibility calculated based on this system.

If the tape-recorded sample is assessed by someone other than the diagnostician who obtained the speech sample, the score may tend to be slightly lower than the client's actual level of understandability because of the absence of visual clues. Also intelligibility should not be initially and subsequently determined by the clinician providing treatment because of the accommodation effect. Although a somewhat variable phenomenon among listeners, perception of intelligibility is a factor that must receive ample attention in diagnosis and treatment.

FORMAL ARTICULATION TESTS

Although there are important commonalities among persons with articulation disorders and among the disorders themselves, there are also important differences that must be considered by the diagnostician when appropriate tests are being selected. These include age, sex, degree of severity of the disorder, purpose of the referral, needs of the client, causal pattern of the disorder, concerns of the family, personality and attitude of the client, level of intellectual functioning, motor coordination, and educational, emotional, and environmental factors. The rationale underlying test selection and other procedures must always be kept in mind. Assessment should specify not only the nature of the disorder but also the conditions that brought it about. The task is complicated because articulation is a learned process, even though there may be some innate capacity for speech, as some psycholinguistic literature suggests, that is superimposed on fundamental physiologic and perceptual processes. Nevertheless articulation can be considered a "whole" process and a basic aspect of oral communication, but it must be separated into "parts" for analysis and categorization.

Previously we have mentioned certain tests that we believe are useful for various aspects of assessment, but the diagnostician still must make selections for each testing situation. These selections will be based partly on client characteristics but also on test characteristics. Information about the tests that should help in making a decision includes: (1) length, (2) standardization, (3) thoroughness, (4) ease of administration, (5) appropriateness, (6) client appeal, and (7) cost. Some of these factors will be discussed in the following review of formal articulation tests.

Arizona Articulation Proficiency Scale

The Arizona Articulation Proficiency Scale (AAPS) was standardized for reliability on 105 children and for validity on forty-five children (Fudala, 1961). The major difference between this and some of the other diagnostic tests is in quantification. The AAPS provides an articulation score based on a weighted phonemic value according to frequency of occurrence of both consonants and vowels. Schissel and James (1979) question the assumptions underlying the scoring, but the test still has been found useful.

The picture stimuli used to elicit responses are individually presented on five-by-eight black and white cards. The test samples most sounds in the initial and final positions only and eight consonant blends. Scoring is rather traditional; only the errors are recorded as follows: − for omissions, X for distortions, and the substituted sound for substitutions. It appears to be sufficiently thorough and easy enough to administer to satisfy the needs of most examiners. Time of administration is no more than 30 minutes. The cost is comparable to that of other articulation tests.

Administration includes presenting the picture stimuli cards preceded by the instruction, "I am going to show you some pictures, and I would like you to tell me what they are." If the child does not name the picture, it is generally most expedient for the examiner to name it and ask the child to repeat it. Subjective judgments of the child's speech are made, based on the perception of the listener. The AAPS has a 24−sentence form from which the older client is asked to read sentences aloud. The sentences contain phonemes in key words. The AAPS also has a survey form for screening the most commonly misarticulated sounds. Finally the test provides guidelines for assessing stimulability, severity of articulation deviations, and interpretation of AAPS total score.

Developmental Articulation Test

The Developmental Articulation Test (DAT) was constructed by Hejna in 1963. It is designed to assess consonant sound production on a developmental scale. Twenty-six cards provide black and white pictorial stimuli for sampling all of the single consonants in all positions and a number of double-consonant blends in the initial position in words. The developmental norms are based on the age at which 90% of the children in the standardization sample had mastered a particular sound. Information on standardization procedures is not available. As with other articulation tests, this one can be administered to children as young as 2½ years of age. Administration includes presenting each card containing a picture and asking the child to identify it. If the child is unable to identify a picture, the diagnostician says the word for the child to repeat. Scoring the responses is the same as for the AAPS. The obtained score provides a developmental composite of the child's articulation.

Since the DAT does not include standardization data or vowels, it might serve best as a screening test rather than as a diagnostic test. Its cost is somewhat less than that of the other articulation tests. Ease of administration and comparative brevity, 15 minutes, combine to make this a popular screening test of articulation.

Fisher-Logemann Test of Articulation Competence

The purpose of this test is to provide a distinctive feature analysis of the client's phonologic system (Fisher and Logemann, 1971). The distinctive features of consonants analyzed are voicing, place of articulation, and manner of articulation. Analysis of vowels includes the distinctive features of tongue height, place of articulation, degree of tension, and lip-rounding.

Test material consists of 109 colored picture stimuli displayed on thirty-five cards that test twenty-five consonants, twenty-three consonant blends, twelve vowels, and four diphthongs presented in a vertical (upright rather than flat on the table) manner. Analysis is by phoneme according to syllabic function: prevocalic, intervocalic, and postvocalic. This test also includes a short form for screening and a sentence form for older clients. Instructions are simple; the client is asked to look at pictures and tell what is seen. Prompting phrases are included for those pictures that may not be readily identified. Interpretation requires considerable familiarity with the test as well as knowledge of distinctive feature analysis. The following protocol is used for recording responses: correct response, no entry; omission, enter a dash; substitution, enter symbol for substituted sound; distortion, use allophonic transcription. Validity and reliability measures are not reported in the manual. The age range is from 3 years to adult, and the cost is comparable to that of other articulation tests. This test takes up to 20 minutes to administer, as do most articulation tests.

Goldman-Fristoe Test of Articulation

This test provides a systematic means of assessing an individual's articulation of consonant sounds in words and, to some extent, in context (Goldman and Fristoe, 1969). It is the feature of having the client paraphrase two picture stories that distinguishes it from some of the other articulation tests. It also includes a stimulability assessment of each misarticulated phoneme in syllables, words, and sentences all on a color-coded response form according to initial, medial, and final position. Forty-four single-item, large colored pictures on an easel presentation provide the stimuli. Instructions are, "You are going to see some pictures here. I want you to tell me what you see as I turn the cards."

Norms are based on samples obtained from 38,884 schoolchildren. Test-retest and intrarater agreement ranges from 70% to 100%. Recording of responses is the same as that for the DAT, and, like the DAT, this test does not sample vowels and diphthongs. The cost is comparable to that of other articulation tests. Administration time is approximately 20 minutes.

Deep Test of Articulation

This test, developed by McDonald (1964), attempts to sample articulation in many different phonetic contexts, hence it does "deep" testing. It assesses abutting and overlapping consonants and their effects on each other. In fact it tests each phoneme in approximately thirty different contexts. In this manner it helps to identify contexts in which a misarticulated phoneme may be correctly articulated. It is perhaps the most thorough test of articulation presently on the market. It also has a sentence form and a screening form.

Administration instructions of the picture form are as follows, "We are going to play a word game with pictures." (Show picture of cup and cake.) "When we say the names of these pictures together we say cupcake—you try it." The objective is for the client to say a "funny big word" without pausing between the two words. The test includes combinations of twenty-five consonants and ten vowels on small, colored pictures. Two pictures are presented simultaneously until a specific phoneme is sampled in thirty different contexts and the percentage of correct responses is calculated for each one. Standardization procedures were followed in this test, which helps to make it a good, in-depth testing instrument for use also in conducting clinical research. Length of administration must be taken into consideration, especially if a client has a number of misarticulations or other communication problem. The cost is comparable to that of other articulation tests. Administration time varies with the number of misarticulations each client has.

Photo Articulation Test

The Photo Articulation Test (PAT) was developed by Pendergast and associates (1969). It consists of seventy-two small, colored photographs, nine pictures on each of eight sheets, which tests all consonants, vowels, and diphthongs. The last three pictures test connected speech. The authors also suggest using these pictures in speech treatment. Test instruction is, "I am going to show you some pictures, and I want you to tell me what they are as I point to them." Recording responses is similar to that of other articulation tests, except that distortions are rated as to severity. Standardization procedures were followed, and the validity and reliability scores were high. Norms are based on 684 white children. The cost is comparable to that of other articulation tests. Age range is from 3 to 8 years, and testing time is approximately 20 minutes.

Phonological process analysis

The phonological process analysis was published by Weiner (1979). This type of analysis differs from more traditional articulation testing in that it is not sound specific and it is not a test. It is a system designed to provide a better understanding of speech patterns of children with communication problems by sampling both single words and contextual speech. The stimulus items are arranged according to phonologic process rather than sound. The responses are then recorded and analyzed in regard to the phonologic process and the underlying rules. It is a structured, step-by-step approach that is intended to facilitate analysis of unintelligible speech. Action pictures are used to elicit the speech samples. Test time is approximately 45 minutes.

This system of analysis is based on the assumption that the child has an adult speech system but expresses it by using a set of adjustment rules called phonologic processes. The three major processes that are analyzed include (1) syllable structure, (2) harmony, and (3) feature contrast. For a thorough discussion of these processes, the reader is referred to Weiner (1979). No information is provided about standardization procedures, validity, and reliability. The cost is minimal.

Templin-Darley Tests of Articulation

The Templin-Darley Tests of Articulation include the Diagnostic Test (Picture and Sentence Forms), Screening Test, and Iowa Pressure Articulation Test (Templin and Darley, 1969). The last test assesses the adequacy of the velopharyngeal mechanism by sampling the pressure consonants. The Diagnostic Test is designed to obtain a detailed sample of the client's articulation. It is thorough, consisting of fifty-seven semicolored cards containing several pictures on each card. The pictures elicit 141 speech sounds. The Screening Test includes fifty items.

Carrier phrases are included in the Diagnostic Test to facilitate eliciting correct responses. Testing procedures and recording of responses are essentially the same as for the other tests mentioned, except that a check is used for noting correct productions. Scoring and interpretation are accomplished by counting the number of sounds correctly produced and then comparing them with the norms. This test also encourages determination of intelligibility in contextual speech.

Norms were determined by testing 480 children aged 3 through 8 years. Reliability and validity were also established. Because it is a thorough test, administration may take up to 45 minutes, not counting completion of the Analysis Sheet. Its cost is comparable to that of other articulation tests.

Weiss Comprehensive Articulation Test

The last articulation test to be mentioned, although there are others, is the Weiss Comprehensive Articulation Test (W-CAT) (Weiss, 1978). This test incorporates several methods for quantifying articulation abilities, such as articulation score, articulation age, intelligibility score, auditory-visual stimulability score, and number of misarticulations. Different methods of quantification are recommended for clients of different ages. Interpretations are provided for each category. The test also includes guidelines for testing areas related to articulation in an attempt to help determine etiology, need for treatment, prognosis, and baseline from which to measure and report progress.

The W-CAT has eighty-five single-item, colored drawings that are presented in an upright manner accompanied with a different carrier phrase for each picture. The pictures sample twenty-four consonants, fourteen vowels, ten diphthongs, and twenty-two consonant blends. The last ten pictures assess not only consonant blends but also contextual speech. The diagnostician is encouraged to administer the test in its entirety or any parts thereof, as in screening. The single-page response form has ample space for recording the misarticulations in either the traditional initial-medial-final method or by using a distinctive feature system of analysis. Space is also provided for recording performances in related areas and for comments regarding nonsegmental and cosmetic aspects of misarticulation. In addition to the picture test, the W-CAT has a thirty-eight–seminonsensical sentence test for clients who can read. Standardization procedures were followed, and the test-retest reliability score was high. Normative data were collected on 4000 children between the ages of 3 and 8 years. Cost and administration procedures are similar to those of other articulation tests. Administration time is approximately 20 minutes.

SPECIAL TESTS AND OBSERVATIONS

Special tests and observations may be conducted when the diagnostician believes that special or additional information is needed. These procedures may include (1) clinician-made tests, (2) informal assessment, (3) screening tests, (4) conversation, (5) question and answer, (6) observation, (7) naming, (8) imitating, (9) serial verbalizations, (10) reporting by adults, (11) recording informal test results, and (12) predictive tests. These tests and observations can be instrumental in formulating a differential diagnosis as well as providing an overall judgment of "articulation defectiveness."

Clinician-made tests

Clinicians not uncommonly construct their own articulation tests. These tests typically sample each consonant phoneme in three different positions and usually in three different words. The tests usually are arranged according to the developmental order of sounds. They generally provide a good sample of the client's articulation performance, with the exception of contextual speech. Construction of an articulation test sometimes is a requirement for a college or university course in speech-language pathology. Because developing a clinician-made test and finding pictures of similar size and quality for each target sound are quite time-consuming, clinicians usually prefer to purchase a commercially available test.

Informal assessment

As a precursor to diagnostic testing, the diagnostician also has recourse to less formal testing procedures. These procedures may be used for the purpose of identifying persons with articulation disorders when more formal approaches are not indicated. Informal testing may be the method of choice because a young or otherwise uncooperative client cannot be tested formally. In the final analysis effective testing of articulation is really determined by the diagnostician. If the diagnostician's observational and recording skills are well-developed, test selection is less important. However, personality of the diagnostician can influence articulation performance (Shriberg, 1971). In fact formal testing is often unnecessary for the diagnostician skilled in informal testing. Informal assessment refers to the use of nonstandardized measures and other informal procedures.

Screening tests

A number of different approaches can be used in screening or detecting persons with articulation disorders. The purpose of screening is to identify persons who may have an articulation disorder, but not to describe it or make a diagnosis. The procedures are generally informal, although formal screening tests are available and include such activities as saying one's name and address, counting, naming colors, describing pictures, and repeating a sentence such as, "I should just choose that treasure," or "Mother, see Robert sitting over there by the little girl," and others. The purpose of screening is to detect those persons having defective articulation as quickly as possible, such as entire classrooms or school populations. The amount of time spent with each individual is just long enough to determine whether or not speech is deviant, usually no more than 2 or 3 minutes per person. Once this has been determined, the diagnostician can contact school officials and the family and proceed with more extensive testing. Screening of school populations typically includes the other areas of communication: language, voice, fluency, and hearing.

Conversation

Engaging the client in conversation can provide the most representative sample of articulation as long as the client is cooperative and responsive. Among the topics that may be useful for discussion are hobbies, television programs, movies, pets, toys, games, friends, sports, brothers, and sisters. The diagnostician may choose to structure some play activities while engaging the child in conversation. Older clients generally present no problems in using this conversational approach. If the younger client continues to be unresponsive, the parent, sibling, or another child should be invited to join in the conversation and play while the diagnostician leaves the room to observe through a one-way window. This provides another means of assessing the child's articulation during contextual speech. The conversational approach can be time-consuming, especially if all of the phonemes are to be sampled, and it requires refined listening and recording skills, but it can be very effective.

Question and answer

This technique is commonly used both as a supplement to formal testing and as a means of obtaining background data. If the questions are open-ended and the client cooperative, questions and answers can provide many samples of articulation. Questions that can be answered briefly or with a binary response should be avoided but may be needed with the young child. Furthermore a child may become disinterested if the interrogation is excessive. Questions such as, "What did you see on the way here this morning?" "Can you tell me something about some of the kids you like to play with?" "What are the names of your brothers and sisters?" and "Who are your classmates?" often can be developed into further comments and conversation. Questioning is usually most effective as an adjunct to other forms of assessment but not as the sole method of obtaining samples of articulation.

Observation

As mentioned previously, several different methods of observation can be employed to gain valuable information about a client's articulation abilities. These methods usually include either *spectator or participant* observations. No matter which method is used, the diagnostician must be perceptive and have astute observational skills, auditory as well as visual. It cannot be overemphasized that one of the most important skills a diagnostician must possess is discerning listening skills, since listening and seeing are what the competent diagnostician is constantly doing. Of course observation implies knowing what and what not to look for, sufficient training, experience, and knowledge to sort out the important from the insignificant. The ego must not be involved. Concentration should be on the client, not on the self. Whether the diagnostician is a spectator or participant observer, the setting must be conducive to communication. The client must have some incentive to talk and react and someone with whom to do so. As with other types of informal appraisal, the observations should be recorded on paper and on tape for later analysis and interpretation.

Some activities in which younger clients can be engaged for observation include structured play activities, building things, response to a story just read, blackboard activities, talking about pictures, and looking at books. As mentioned earlier, spectator observation may be the only feasible method of obtaining information about some clients' articulation.

Naming

Naming is an efficient way of obtaining samples of articulation. It does not provide a representative sample of contextual speech, but it does provide a good sample of sounds in isolated words. It utilizes a key word approach in assessing articulation. Materials can include objects in the room, colors, and pictures. The concept of naming, as used here, differs from naming as it is used in diagnostic testing. Here naming is more random; it utilizes objects within the client's present environment, particularly the names of objects, furniture, and persons that might contain the more commonly misarticulated sounds when named. Also, naming is an activity that occurs quite early in a child's development so that it can be used with minimal confusion with young children. If a client's misarticulations are quite consistent, naming can be effective in identifying specific misarticulations even though it may sample only a minimum number of phonetic contexts.

Imitating

Undoubtedly the most direct approach for eliciting samples of articulation is imitation. The diagnostician says words containing phonemes to be analyzed and asks the client to repeat them. Again this technique requires the cooperation of the client. Roe and Milisen (1942) reported fewer misarticulations when clients imitated words than when they said the words spontaneously. Their data suggest that imitation may not provide a typical sample of articulation. However, it may give a more positive indication of errors. If a child cannot produce a phoneme when seeing and trying to imitate a model, it is quite certain that the phoneme is a definite misarticulation and cannot be produced when there is no model. Perhaps

the effects of imitation can be minimized by deemphasizing the word to be imitated, especially the key phoneme, or by covering the mouth when presenting the stimulus word. If the client is unaware of the reason for repeating words, a more representative sample may be obtainable. This technique is used mostly for informal appraisal, although it is used in formal testing when a client cannot correctly identify a stimulus picture.

Serial verbalizations

Serial verbalizing such as counting, saying the days of the week, months of the year, seasons, and letters of the alphabet, and naming colors can provide spontaneous samples of rote speech. Since these serial verbalizations contain many of the sounds in our language, saying them should indicate which ones are articulated correctly and which ones are misarticulated. Furthermore this type of subpropositional communication is generally fun for the younger client because it is relatively easy. It is also easily supplemented with repetitions of jingles and nursery rhymes if additional speech samples are necessary.

Reporting by adults

This method can be used in both formal and informal testing. As used here, reporting by adults (parents, teachers, and other persons) results in impressions about the client and the client's articulation, that is, impressions rather than scientific evidence. Adults may express concern about the client's intelligibility, stimulability, number of errors or misarticulations, reactions to being teased, difficulty in talking, conspicuousness of accompanying cosmetic habits, consistency of articulation, or what help the client had previously received and the consequent results. These "impressions" can be very helpful to the diagnostician in formulating an appropriate, formal diagnosis and sometimes in knowing something about the articulation disorder, such as type, severity, and possible etiology.

Informal appraisal should be an integral part of the assessment and should be utilized. As much information as possible should be obtained about a client. The time spent in collecting this information is time well spent. The more pertinent data available about a client, the greater the possibility of reducing the length of time required for effective treatment. Most experienced diagnosticians become adept at informal testing and rely heavily on such procedures in assessment. There is a danger in relying too much on formal standardized tests and trying to use one or more with every client. These tests often are too confining and remove spontaneity. They also are not infallible and are not for all clients. Informal testing often is the only means of assessment possible.

Recording informal test results

The diagnostician must not only have quick, discerning listening and seeing abilities but also an efficient method of recording what is heard and seen. Formal tests always provide recording forms, but methods of recording what is heard and seen in various informal test situations usually must be devised by each diagnostician. Often this will be an individual's system of noting errors by phonetic transcription as they occur plus taking notes concerning those things that cannot be recorded phonetically. Forms can be devised to make it easier to note errors, but these may be slower and may interfere with client-diagnostician interaction. We advise experimenting with several methods and then developing skill with the one that serves best. There is a danger in relying on memory too much and recording too little. Too much data can be omitted in this way.

Predictive tests

For years speech-language pathologists have wrestled with the problems involved in case selection. Knowing which persons would and which would not spontaneously outgrow their disordered articulation would greatly facilitate their dilemma. In an effort to predict spontaneous improvement, several investigations have been conducted

(Carter and Buck, 1958; Steer and Drexler, 1960; Van Riper and Erickson, 1968). Results of these efforts have been encouraging. The end result of one such study was the Predictive Screening Test of Articulation (PSTA) by Van Riper and Erickson (1968).

Theoretically the PSTA identifies those children at the first-grade level who will correct their misarticulations by third grade. If the individual achieves a score of 34 or more out of the total of forty-seven responses, treatment might be deferred because the child might spontaneously outgrow the articulation deviation. The authors report a reliability score of 0.89, which suggests some degree of test consistency. Administration of this test is easy. The test items are presented and the responses circled and tallied. Test time is approximately 7 minutes, and the cost is minimal.

Most experienced clinicians also make predictive judgments based on factors usually not directly related to testing, such as the pattern of the child's misarticulations. Do they follow the developmental hierarchy, but at a delayed age level? If so, is the delay a major one or is maturation likely to take care of it? Is the pattern of errors typical of siblings or parents who "grew out of it" without help? Children in many families typically develop adequate speech at a delayed rate compared with accepted norms. Is there an ethnic, cultural, or community explanation for the deviant articulation that might indicate leaving it alone? The answers to any of these questions may give the clinician a basis for a good subjective judgment concerning whether or not to intervene.

OTHER TYPES OF ANALYSES

Categorizing is a process of looking for similarities and differences in order to separate or combine. It may include sorting out all misarticulations according to sound class, position of error, common feature patterns of all misarticulations and phonologic processes, and classifying sound errors according to severity, frequency of occurrence, consistency, ease of production, or conspicuousness.

Knowing the *consistency of articulation* can be of value in making a statement about etiology, prognosis, and where and how to begin treatment. An analysis of consistency usually includes a comparison between articulation of isolated words and contextual speech. However, sampling many different phonemic contexts is helpful in determining consistency more realistically, but it can be time-consuming. Increased variability during contextual speech could be suggestive of verbal dyspraxia, whereas increased numbers of oral inaccuracies during contextual speech might mean that a dysarthric problem exists.

Cosmetic distractions are occasionally part of the articulation disorder. An eye blink, a nasal squint, an unusual lip posture, or some other facial tic should be noted and analyzed in terms of consistency, phonemic context, and degree of conspicuousness. A cosmetic distraction may be the result of a habit, neuromuscular incoordination, psychologic factors, or speech struggle behavior or a possible indication of inadequate velopharyngeal closure. It may not be directly related to speech, but because it distracts speech, a cosmetic distraction might become part of the communication problem. It is assessed by observation.

As mentioned previously, additional analyses the diagnostician can make are simply to count and total the *number of articulation errors,* calculate *articulation age* based on articulation norms, and determine the *articulation score* based on frequency of occurrence of phonemes. These scores, either individually or in total, can provide a level of articulation functioning for a specific client. Examples of how these scores are derived are included in the Weiss Comprehensive Articulation Test (W-CAT). Advantages of utilizing such a quantifiable system are that it provides numeric data, an objective way of determining baseline data and measuring progress, and a score that is easily interpreted by professionals other than speech-language pathologists. All of

these scores can be derived from data obtained by administering the W-CAT.

ASSESSMENT OF SPEECH STRUCTURES

Inextricably related to assessment of articulation is assessment of the peripheral oral structures. No diagnostic workup is complete without having done one. Assessment of the speech structures must consider both structure and function. Structural assessment should include the face, mouth, pharynx, nasopharynx, nasal passages, and larynx. Assessment of structural function should include all of the movable structures comprising the speech mechanism: lips, tongue, mandible, soft palate, pharyngeal muscles, and vocal folds. These structures should be assessed during speech and nonspeech functions, which is accomplished by asking the client to perform some activity while the diagnostician observes and takes notes.

Assessment of structures

The face and head should be examined for any unusual features of the hair, skin, eyes, nose, and chin. These features may include deviations in coloration, texture, size, symmetry, scarring, tissue excess, or tissue deficiency. Deviations in these structures may only be indirectly related to articulation, if at all, but they may be very helpful in the total assessment or in detecting other possible problems or syndromes that the client may have. Early detection and referral to appropriate disciplines are good preventive procedures. If one is going to err in an assessment, the error should be in the direction of being overly thorough.

Observation inside the mouth should include all of the structures, although the movable structures will be assessed later when adequacy or inadequacy of function is considered. The diagnostician should note any deviations of the teeth, alveolar ridge, tongue, height and width of the hard palate, dental arch alignment, depth and width of the pharynx, and any deviations of the laryngeal structures. If significant deviations are noted, examination by a physician or dentist may be indicated. Obviously not all of the structures are of equal importance insofar as articulation is concerned, but they should all be observed, using a flashlight and tongue depressor, in order to make a differential diagnosis.

The speech structures should be assessed by carefully observing the client at rest and during speech and vegetative functions. The diagnostician must possess an adequate frame of reference regarding normality of these structures and functions, so that in comparison deviations can be readily detected and analyzed. The diagnostician must be able to establish rapport with the client, convey an attitude of competence and confidence, and evoke cooperation from the client. As mentioned earlier, the assessment should not begin with an oral examination. Clinical knowledge, sincerity, genuine interest, and an understanding of behavioral principles will enable the diagnostician to complete this task.

Nasal cavity clearance is primarily important to nasal resonance (usually hyponasality) and in production of the three nasal consonants. Inadequate clearance may be related to a deviated nasal septum, hypertrophied turbinates, growths, adenoids, or upper respiratory problems causing mucosal swelling or excessive mucus. Nasal cavity clearance can be assessed by having the client breathe and blow through the nose while alternately occluding one naris and then the other. Any obstruction in airflow can readily be detected. If the child cried prior to this examination, the perceived airflow may have been invalidated because of mucosal swelling and proliferation of mucus caused by crying. Having the client blow the nose prior to this procedure is recommended.

Irregularities pertaining to the *teeth and dental arches* are observed by looking inside the mouth. Intraoral inspection with the assistance of a flashlight and tongue depressor can provide information about the occlusal relationship and dental caries. Determining the significance of dental irregularities is difficult to do. Using a rating scale, such as the one proposed by Darley and Spriestersbach (1978) and indicated on p. 104, may assist in determining their significance. Nevertheless each client must be considered individually. Besides dental arch alignment and dental caries, the diagnostician should note other aspects of the teeth such as oral hygiene, size of teeth, discoloration, and any other unusual dental characteristics.

The *sinuses* can affect resonance. A change in resonance usually occurs with a head cold or other upper respiratory infection. Any change in these cavities can affect the quality of resonance; however, the change is usually transitory and treatable by a physician. Assessment of altered resonance because of changes in the sinuses is quite subjective. It is assessed by listening to the client talk and checking case history data such as the presence of a cold, upper respiratory problems, or sinus cavity deviations. A resonance change caused by sinusitis is untreatable by the speech-language pathologist; however, if it is perceived the patient should be referred to a physician.

The *alveolar ridge and hard palate* are involved in virtually every sound in the English language. Fortunately, except for a gross deviation of these structures, they usually do not interfere with articulation. An unusually rough or prominent alveolar ridge may distort the quality of sibilant sounds or be related to a tongue thrust. A markedly narrow (sometimes related to finger- or thumb-sucking, past or present) or low palatal vault can crowd the tongue and cause distortions of front consonants, but these structures usually are inconsequential as etiologic factors in articulation disorders unless there has been traumatic damage resulting in cleft of the palate or alveolar ridge. These structures are assessed through intraoral inspection.

Two other structures that could affect speech, mainly in regard to resonance but also concerning production of the nasal and pressure consonants, are the *tonsils* and *ade-*

noids. Occasionally their removal results in irreversible hypernasality and weak production of pressure consonants. As previously stated, the tonsils are located between the anterior and posterior pillars or fauces on either side of the back of the oral cavity. If they are enlarged they can obstruct oral airflow and restrict velar movement. The diagnostician must look inside the mouth and observe the tonsils while the client is at rest and while phonating /a/. It might also be helpful to observe them during gag. If the tonsils are of such size that they nearly contact each other at the midline of the oral cavity during rest, then they probably are too large (hypertrophied) and are interfering with speech. Coloration is important from a medical standpoint. A bright red color indicating inflammation or a grayish color suggesting abscess should be cause for referral to a physician.

Adenoids, which are located in the nasopharynx, are not as easily visualized. An intraoral dental mirror or a fiberoptic instrument can be used for viewing the adenoids. If they are hypertrophied, a marked degree of hyponasality may be present. Enlarged adenoids have been associated with middle ear infections. Their indiscriminate removal can cause the opposite resonance disorder—hypernasality (Gibb, 1958). A cautious preventive approach would be to assess the velopharyngeal mechanism thoroughly for possible signs of subtle inadequacy prior to considering an adenoidectomy in order to prevent irreversible hypernasality. A selective adenoidectomy might be a satisfactory compromise between no surgery and complete surgery. Normal atrophy of both the tonsils and adenoids generally occurs with maturation, so that by around 16 years of age they have essentially disappeared in most persons.

Unfortunately structural assessments are rather subjective. We cannot definitively state what constitutes adequate nasal cavity clearance, acceptable dental occlusion for speech, relatively smooth alveolar ridge, or nonrestricting hard palate. Nevertheless judgments have to be made and they usually are based on the clinician's past experiences. Sometimes it is helpful to place judgments of each structure on a continuum of severity from one (insignificant) to four (definitely significant). It is very helpful for students in training or beginning clinicians to examine as many persons as possible who have no known structural abnormality in order to recognize "normal" structures compared with "abnormal" structures. How else can the clinician formulate a personal reference system regarding the presence of a large or small tongue, long or short palate, normal or abnormal occlusion, and deep or shallow pharynx?

Assessment of functions

Functional assessments are likewise subjective. Moreover they include looking for subtleties, because a millimeter can make a difference. Factors such as rate, range, precision, and timing of the movable speech structures should be assessed through visual inspection, again with the assistance of a flashlight and tongue depressor. A nasal listening tube and intraoral dental mirror are also useful. These functions should similarly be assigned a numeric value regarding the relative importance of the deviation (scale of one to four). The movable structures are the cheeks, fauces, hyoid, larynx, lips, lower jaw, pharynx, soft palate, uvula, and tongue. The importance of these different "articulators" varies, depending on the client and the type of articulation disorder.

Cheeks tend to serve only an indirect function. Their primary function is to provide lateral walls for reinforcing the lateral dental arches of the oral cavity for sustaining intraoral breath pressure and resonance. Only rarely are they directly involved in articulation. An example would be buccal speech of the laryngectomee. Looking for deviations in muscle tonus, asymmetry, scarring, discoloration, and unusual contraction should be part of the diagnostic workup, even though deviations may be more medically significant than communicatively significant.

The *fauces* or *pillars* may provide insight

into velopharyngeal physiology. They form the archway between the oral and pharyngeal cavities, moving toward the midline of the back part of the mouth and backward during phonation and swallowing. The rate, range, precision, and timing of pillar movement can only be subjectively assessed in a clinical setting.

Hyoid physiology again assumes a rather passive role in articulation as the hyoid bone moves upward and forward or upward and backward as a result of contraction of the muscles attached to it. This V-shaped bone at the root of the tongue furnishes leverage and anchorage for the muscles of the jaw, tongue, pharynx, and larynx. It may be considered a "facilitator" of articulation. If excessive muscle tension is noted about the area of the hyoid, this could affect laryngeal physiology and articulation, especially if there is muscle asynergy or imbalance between the agonistic and antagonistic muscles attached to it. Assessment of the hyoid function is difficult, even in a clinic.

Although movable, the *larynx* is not directly observable except by an instrument such as the laryngoscope. Again the diagnostician must rely on subjective means for assessing adequacy such as listening to vocal quality, looking at the client's neck for excessive tension, and noting abnormal head and neck postures. Vocal qualities such as roughness and breathiness indicate to the diagnostician something about the structure and function of the vocal folds. The larynx relates to articulation insofar as it affects the passage of air over the vocal cords determining subvocalic air pressure and the voicing of the voiced consonants, vowels, and diphthongs. Excessive tension, lack of tension, inappropriate pitch level, and vocal abuses and misuses can usually be judged somewhat more objectively than other aspects of laryngeal physiology, particularly pitch level and number and kinds of vocal abuses (Wilson, 1979; Boone, 1978; Moncur and Brackett, 1974). Exploring laryngeal physiology by altering pitch, loudness, posture, effort, or tension may provide some valuable diagnostic information.

Examination by an otolaryngologist should always precede intervention.

The *lower jaw or mandible* is important to articulation in terms of providing adequate intraoral clearance and modification for both articulation and resonance. If the lower jaw does not or cannot open widely enough, speech can be impaired. Adequacy of mandibular movement should be assessed during speech and nonspeech activities. Asymmetry, restriction, and slow movement should be noted. Excessive overjet (prognathism) or receding jaw (micrognathism) can directly affect articulation. Sometimes the tongue and lips can compensate for mandibular problems; however, compensatory abilities are individualistic traits. Function can be assessed by having the client open and close the jaw in rapid succession, lateralize the jaw, and produce labiodental sounds, such as /f/ and /v/. Temporomandibular joint problems are occasionally present to restrict mandibular movement. These joint problems should be referred to a dentist (oral surgeon). As with many aspects of the speech mechanism, there is a paucity of normative data with which to make comparisons (Bell, 1968).

Muscles of the *pharynx,* particularly of the lateral and back walls, can do much to modify the size and configuration of the pharynx. Since this structure is primarily concerned with velopharyngeal closure, it is most directly related to resonance and production of pressure consonants. In viewing the pharynx the diagnostician should note height, width, depth, amount of lateral and back wall movement, and of course timing of this movement in relation to velar movement and onset of speech production. For example, if the lateral walls begin to move later than the soft palate or after the onset of speech, speech could be affected.

Intraoral inspection of the pharynx is not enough. Other ways of assessing function of the pharynx should also be used such as a nasal listening tube, modified stethoscope, and alar flutter (Weiss, 1974); roentgenography (Subtelny, Koepp-Baker, and Subtelny, 1961; Skolnick and associates, 1975);

electromyography (Basmajian, 1961); electrical capacitance (Cole, 1971); ultrasound (Ewanowski, Watkin, and Zogyebski, 1974); airflow (Hardy, 1965); and fiberoptics (Croft and associates, 1978). More recently computerized tomography has been used to assess the velopharyngeal mechanism (Weiss and associates, 1980). Oral manometry might also provide some helpful information. Some of these methods and techniques require rather expensive and sophisticated equipment that is not always readily available to the diagnostician; however, not all of these procedures need to be used.

Two techniques that can be effectively used in a clinical setting are the alar flutter test and the nasal listening tube (Fig. 6-1). The alar flutter consists of compressing and releasing the alar cartilages of the client while producing high vowels in isolation, words, and sentences. It is important that none of these phonemic contexts contain the nasal sounds. If there is a positive flutter (perceptible change in resonance between compressed and released nares), then the mechanism may be functioning inadequately. By placing one end of the listening tube to the client's nose and the other end to the diagnostician's ear, perceptible changes in resonance and nasal airflow can be noted, again during production of pressure consonants in various phonemic contexts, but excluding the nasal sounds. By using these two simple techniques, the diagnostician can obtain inferential information about velopharyngeal physiology.

Like the pharynx, the *soft palate or velum* is mainly concerned with closure of the velopharyngeal mechanism. As such, it is related to the production and resonation of essentially all phonemes. The diagnostician will want to note the extent, rate, and timing of velar movement during phonation. Look for any deviation to one side or the other of the soft palate. Note if there is localized contraction during phonation such as a noticeable depression in the center of the soft palate. Also look for scarring, discoloration, and clefts or fistulas. Does the soft palate become tense for production of /k/ and /g/? Is its range of motion more or less than that of the average soft palate, compared with observations of others? Does it seem to be long enough? These and other questions should be asked in determining the adequacy or inadequacy of the soft palate. The information is obtained through intraoral inspection (make certain that the jaws are parted no more than 1 inch, the tongue is not protruded, and the head is not tilted backward to avoid restriction of velar movement); historical informa-

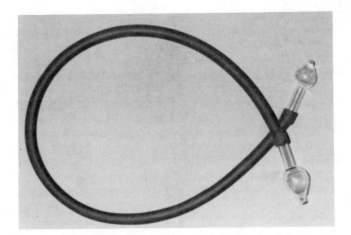

Fig. 6-1. Nasal listening tube for assessing velopharyngeal closure.

tion such as presence of chronic nasal regurgitation, postoperative cleft palate, and paresis; and scientific instrumentation, which can aid the assessment of the soft palate if necessary.

Importance of the pharynx and velum functioning in concert should be emphasized. Together these two structures provide the circle of muscles necessary to effect the sphincteric closure of the velopharyngeal port. Although determination of adequacy or inadequacy of this mechanism is readily possible, the diagnostician cannot always be certain why. For example, if the client has hypernasality or weak production of pressure consonants, which structure is defective, or are both structures functioning inadequately? Conversely, if one part of the velopharyngeal mechanism is not functioning adequately, how can a particular client still have normal resonance and articulation? Even though difficult, an attempt should be made to determine cause and effect so that the most appropriate treatment procedures can be instigated, and although the degree of resonance and articulation distortion may not be indicative of the degree of inadequacy of this mechanism, quantification of the perceived nasality and articulation distortion should be routinely practiced (zero—normal nasality of speech distortion—to +3—severe hypernasality or speech distortion).

The *uvula* really is insignificant to articulation per se. However, it can provide helpful information about other aspects of the velopharyngeal mechanism. For instance, deviation of the uvula might be indicative of neuromuscular or structural involvement. A bifid uvula could suggest the possibility of a submucosal cleft, and the absence of an uvula might be a microform that is of importance to genetics. It does not contribute to velopharyngeal closure, but it might enhance snoring, for those who are particularly concerned about noise pollution.

The most important structure of the speech mechanism is the *tongue*. This mobile, multifunctioning articulator usually has great compensatory ability. It is involved in articulation and resonance for most phonemes. Rate, range, precision, and timing of its movements should always be assessed.

Rate of tongue movement is assessed by administering a test of oral diadochokinesis or maximum articulation rate. The client is asked to repeat syllables such as /pʌ/, /tʌkʌ/, and /pʌtʌkʌ/ in rapid succession. Each activity should be practiced once and then produced while the diagnostician tape-records, counts, and times the repetitions. The amount of time consumed to produce the required number of repetitions is then compared with available norms. The client must be instructed to repeat the nonsense syllables as rapidly as possible until told to stop. If the repetitions are so fast that each one cannot be counted accurately, then they should be tape-recorded and played back at a slower speed in order to facilitate counting. However, if the repetitions are that fast, it is doubtful that rate is impaired in that client.

Range of tongue movement is assessed more subjectively by having the client engage in various oral gymnastics: protruding and retracting the tongue, elevating and lowering it, grooving it, and lateralizing it by pushing out the cheeks. Each activity should be attempted at least twice. These gross lingual movements provide some information about tongue dexterity, but they do not necessarily correlate with fine lingual adjustments necessary for consonant production. Oral gymnastic activities could reveal the existence of an ankylosed tongue and neuromuscular involvement. The important decision to be made here is whether or not the range of lingual movements is adequate for speech or adequately stimulable for eventually acquiring normal speech.

Timing of tongue movement is closely related to precision. If the tongue shows faulty timing, then it will not arrive within that acceptable positional range in time, causing distorted articulation. Faulty timing could also relate to leaving a target position too late, which would consequently affect contiguous sounds. The tongue, as well as the other articulators, must function in a synchronous manner for normal articulation to occur. Asynergistic movement (faulty timing and coordination) of the tongue in relation to the other articulators must be scrutinized by the diagnostician through inspection and other approaches such as radiography when possible. Because of its subtleness, a timing problem may not always be detected.

Precision of tongue movements is important to articulation. The diagnostician should note "overshooting" or "undershooting" of the tongue or a "searching" pattern in trying to locate the correct placement for a sound. Replication of tongue position for speech and nonspeech movements can provide information about the efficiency of kinesthetic feedback. Judging precision of articulation physiology is not only very subjective but very difficult. Looking for imprecise tongue movements during contextual speech and listening for slurring and other types of oral inaccuracies are the two most effective techniques available to the diagnostician. Lack of lingual precision may be associated with central or peripheral nervous system involvement, moderate mental retardation, or heightened emotional states.

Additional aspects of the tongue that should be noted include tongue size and other structural deviations such as deviated lingual raphe (midline depression), fissured tongue, geographic tongue, asymmetric tongue posture or size, abnormal tongue position or carriage at rest or during speech, unusual coloration, scarring, tremors, or fibrillations (especially when the tongue is protruded and the eyes are closed), and poor tongue sensitivity. A diagnostic summary of the different aspects of the tongue and other structures of the speech mechanism follows.

Summary of battery for assessment of speech structures

  I. Head and face
    A. Size and symmetry
    B. Texture of hair
    C. Scars
    D. Grimaces
    E. Control of facial expression
    F. Coloration
    G. Distance between eyes
    H. Drooping of eyelids
    I. Intranasal clearance—passageway and nares
    J. Deviated septum
    K. Size of mouth
    L. Nasal "squinting" during production of pressure consonants
  II. Lips
    A. Size and shape
    B. Symmetry—during rest, smile, and movement
    C. Mobility—occlude, pucker, retract, lateralize
    D. Strength (see Testing for Orofacial Muscle Balance)
    E. Rapid repetition of lip movements
  III. Teeth
    A. Size
    B. Coloration
    C. Number—excessive or deficient
    D. Hygiene
    E. Caries
    F. Spacing
    G. Prostheses
  IV. Tongue
    A. Size
    B. Shape
    C. Symmetry
    D. Mobility and strength
      1. Rate—repeating /pʌ/, /tʌkʌ/, /pʌtʌkʌ/, etc. in rapid succession
      2. Range—grooving, pointing, protruding, lateralizing and pushing against the cheeks, and elevating the tongue
      3. Timing—assuming correctly timed target positions during contextual speech
      4. Precision—repeating tongue tip and /r/ sound positions accurately
    E. Coloration
    F. Tremors or fasciculations
    G. Sensation-perception—tactile threshold sensitivity, tactile localization, two-point discrimination, oral stereognosis, and kinesthesis
    H. Attachment of frenulum
    I. Tongue thrust
  V. Lower jaw
    A. Size in relation to upper jaw and tongue
    B. Symmetry of shape and movement
    C. Mobility—rate and range of opening and closing in rapid succession

D. Position in relation to upper jaw—
   overjet or receding
VI. Upper jaw and hard palate
   A. Size—length and width
   B. Height
   C. Scars
   D. Occlusion (if malocclusion is present,
      list the type)
   E. Coloration
   F. Cleft
   G. Fistula
   H. Configuration of alveolar bone
   I. Configuration of palate
VII. Velopharyngeal mechanism
   A. Size of soft palate
   B. Mobility of soft palate and degree of
      movement
   C. Mobility of lateral pharyngeal walls
      and degree of movement
   D. Mobility of posterior pharyngeal wall
      and degree of movement
   E. Symmetry of movement
   F. Synchrony of timing of movement
   G. Coloration
   H. Scars
   I. Cleft
   J. Fistula
   K. Adequacy of closure
   L. Movement of posterior pillars in
      direction of pharynx
   M. Size and condition of tonsils and
      adenoids, if present
   N. Uvula—bifid
   O. Deviation in movement of uvula
   P. Type of gag reflex
VIII. Breathing
   A. Rate
   B. Rhythm
   C. Pattern—clavicular or diaphragmatic
   D. Phonation sustained steadily for 10
      seconds

ASSESSMENT OF OTHER FUNCTIONS RELATED TO ARTICULATION

Auditory abilities are important to articulation and should routinely be assessed. They include auditory acuity, discrimination, memory, and conceptualization. Without auditory acuity, or the ability to hear, normal articulation is practically impossible. Some ideas on how to assess these auditory functions follow.

Auditory acuity, or the reception-perception of environmental sounds and noises, is extremely important to articulation acquisition. The range of normal hearing encompasses a frequency range from approximately 20 to 20,000 Hz and an intensity range from 0 to 140 dB. If auditory acuity is significantly impaired, articulation is affected. However, "significantly impaired" in one individual may not always be the same for another (Rose, 1971).

A typical battery for assessing auditory acuity might include pure tone testing with an audiometer to determine thresholds, impedance testing of the eardrum and middle ear structures to measure impedance and transmittance of sound vibrations, and speech reception threshold to determine the intensity level required to perceive speech. Excellent procedural descriptions are provided in Newby (1972) and Martin (1975).

Auditory discrimination, or the ability to discriminate from among different auditory stimuli and in different environments, may be assessed in several different ways using several different instruments and tests. Stimuli may include digits, phonemes, words, sentences, nonsense syllables, environmental noises, and rhythmic patterns. Some tests of auditory discrimination include the Auditory Discrimination Test by Wepman (1958), the Goldman-Fristoe-Woodcock Test of Auditory Discrimination by Goldman, Fristoe, and Woodcock (1970), and the Short Test of Sound Discrimination by Templin (1943). Auditory discrimination may be assessed by having the client say "same" or "different," "yes" or "no," or "right" or "wrong" when given a sound, syllable, or word stimulus or by identifying a picture of the correct stimulus. However, auditory discrimination abilities might best be determined in regard to self-discrimination, rather than discrimination of someone else, as we have previously suggested. The discrimination tasks should include the phonemes that are misarticulated by the client and an analysis thereof. For example, if a child substitutes /θ/ for /s/, phonemes may be presented in pairs, such as /say/ and /they/ or /bathe/ and /base/ and then the differences between them analyzed. It would be better if the client could produce the phonemes correctly and incorrectly in these tasks and decide instantaneously if the production is correct or incorrect. Discrimination of nonmisarticulated sounds may be irrelevant and unnecessary, except perhaps for gross discrimination training of right and wrong productions. Problems in auditory discrimination should be noted for future consideration in specifying the etiologies and treatment approach.

Auditory memory, or the ability to remember auditory stimuli, may be related to misarticulations in some persons. If a sound or sound sequence cannot be remembered, it is not likely that it can be correctly learned. Memory tests include sentences, words, digits, nonsense syllables, and rhythmic patterns. Some tests include memory for rhythmic patterns such as the Basic Concept Inventory by Englemann (1967), the Short Term Auditory Retrieval and Storage Test by Flowers (1972), repeating digits forward and backward and memory for sentences from the Stanford-Binet Intelligence Scale by Terman and Merrill (1973), and repeating sentences from the Wechsler Preschool and Primary Scale of Intelligence by Wechsler (1967). Administration generally includes having the client repeat the presented stimuli. Any performance below average, based on test norms, should be noted for future consideration.

Auditory conceptualization is a term that denotes perception, central auditory processing, assimilation of auditory input, and the ability to recognize and interpret auditory stimuli. It involves the linguistic or cognitive functions of the auditory system. If a client cannot assign meaning to incoming messages, it is doubtful that articulation can develop normally. Auditory conceptualization is assessed by administering tests such as the Lindamood Auditory Conceptualization Test (Lindamood and Lindamood, 1971) or the Flowers-Costello Test of Central Auditory Abilities (Flowers and Costello, 1970).

Whereas the previous four areas pertained to assessment of the auditory system, the following areas pertain to a variety of functions. *Verbal sequencing,* or the ability to say polysyllabic words in proper sequence, may relate to articulation. Children between 4 and 7 years of age can usually repeat words such as "linoleum," "aluminum," "persistence," and "reliability" correctly one out of three times. It is understandable that as the words increase in length, children will have progressively greater difficulty saying them, but most children should be able to repeat at least one trial correctly. Persons above age 7 years should be able to repeat these words correctly two out of three times. Inability to do so could be indicative of verbal dyspraxia. Polysyllabic words are assessed by asking the client to look and listen carefully while the diagnostician says the stimulus word each time before the patient repeats. Three trials are given in a normal manner. Scoring is either all correct or all wrong.

Oral sensation-perception of the tongue, lips, and even soft palate can influence the functioning of these structures. Five dimensions of sensation-perception commonly assessed are: (1) tactile sensitivity, (2) tactile localization, (3) oral stereognosis, (4) kinesthesis, and (5) two-point discrimination (see pp. 144 and 145). *Tactile sensitivity* is assessed by gently stroking the tongue at different locations with a wisp of cotton, asking the client if the tongue was touched. *Tactile localization* is assessed similarly, except that the client is asked to point to the exact location of each stimulus. For both of these activities several stimuli should be presented. *Oral stereognosis* is assessed by placing geometric shapes inside the mouth and then asking the client to identify the stimulus shape from multiple choices. *Kinesthesis* is grossly appraised by having the client replicate elevated tongue tip and tongue protruded positions. Kinesthetic feedback is assumed to be adequate if the replications do not vary more than 2 or 3 mm. *Two-point discrimination* is assessed by placing a two-point object (spaced 2 mm apart), such as a dial caliper, on various locations of the tongue. Then by alternating between a two-point object and a one-point object and asking the client if one or two points were felt, the diagnostician can make a determination about the adequacy or inadequacy of two-point discrimination. For additional descriptions of how to assess these areas, the reader is referred to the test manual of the Weiss Comprehensive Articulation Test.

Orofacial muscle imbalance (OMI) or tongue thrust may occasionally be present to interfere with the production of the sibilants and other linguadental and lingua-alveolar sounds. Orofacial muscle imbalance can be assessed by having the client swallow solids and by noting, by parting the lips while swallowing, if the tongue is thrusting against or between the front or side teeth. It should also be noted if the masseter muscles contract during swallowing of solids by placing the index fingers near the angle of the mandible; if there is any associated malocclusion when the teeth are in approximation; if there is excessive use of the lips in chewing and swallowing; and what the lip strength is, by placing a button tied to a string behind the lips, attaching it to a small scale, and noting the registered amount of pressure when it "popped" out of the client's mouth. This should be done three times and the derived scores averaged. If these characteristics, plus defective articulation, are unfavorable, the client may have a detrimental tongue thrust.

Vocal phonics, or word-attack skills in reading, is sometimes defective among persons with articulation problems. Since this skill seems to be related to articulation, it should be assessed routinely. Van Riper (1963) developed a method for assessing a client's ability to analyze a word into its component graphemes and then synthesize it again. Inability to do this could interfere with normal articulation development. Again, significant findings in this or any other area do not suggest cause and effect, merely a possible relationship.

Language abilities should routinely be screened in persons with articulation problems. Although variably defined, language includes such parameters as vocabulary, syntax, morphology, semantics, phonology, and most recently pragmatics, which is tangentially related to articulation. Bates (1976) defines *pragmatics* as the rules governing the use of communication in context. Pragmatics may also be regarded as the effectiveness in communication, or communication competence. It is this relationship between words, expressions, or symbols and their users and patterns of usage that is the core of communication.

Pragmatics must be considered in the development, diagnosis, and treatment of communication disorders. This important aspect of a child's communication development considers such factors as: (1) how much of the information provided by the child is appropriate, (2) how appropriate is the communication in regard to time and place, mean length of utterance, frequency, intensity, and rate of speaking, (3) how appropriate is the communication in relation to what was said previously and to the present situation, and (4) how appropriate is the communication act in terms of who can say what, in what way, where and when, by what means, and to whom. Determining what the child is doing to communicate and which rules of social interaction are being used or misused within a particular situation or community can provide helpful information about the child's communication competence. If the child's communication is inappropriate in social situations, then improving articulation or language skills alone will not result in normal communication.

The diagnosis of pragmatics necessitates an examination of the usage of the child's communication in various situations, since different rules are followed in different situations. For example, a child speaks differently to the same people under different circumstances. The diagnostician must determine what the linguistic demands of a particular situation are. This can be accomplished by setting up different communication situations, by asking questions, and by noting the responses. There are five aspects of situational context that influence how a person communicates: (1) the people that are present, (2) what was said just before, (3) the topic of conversation, (4) the task that is to be accomplished through communication, and (5) the times and places in which communication occurs (Prutting, 1979). If communication is not appropriate in regard to these five aspects, pragmatics is impaired. However, attributing levels of delay or degrees of impairment to faulty pragmatics is not an easy task because normative data and objective procedures are not clearly defined at this time. Rules and concepts of pragmatics are learned skills (Prutting, 1979). For example, the young child's first attempt at answering the telephone might well be to say, "Who is this?" after picking up the receiver rather than saying "Hello." Or the child might respond to the question, "Is your mommy there?" with "Yes," rather than by calling his mother to the telephone. Obviously the child has not yet learned certain rules or subtle pragmatic concepts. Also a child can make grammatical sentences that make no sense. For example, if you ask why a child kicked a cat and the child's answer is, "Because I like apple pie," the answer is grammatical but inappropriate. A more appropriate response from the standpoint of pragmatics might have been "angry," even though it is grammatically incomplete.

Ways in which communication competence can be measured and fostered include structuring different situations, changing situational demands, asking different questions, and altering linguistic demands. Although our understanding of it is still incomplete, pragmatics should be considered when diagnosing a child's overall communication abilities. The fact that pragmatics is learned, continues to develop throughout life, and has not been readily amenable to standardized procedures of assessment presents even greater challenges for the diagnostician.

The past two decades have witnessed a proliferation of tests in language. Some tests assess specific dimensions of language such as syntax or morphology (Lee, 1966; Berry, 1966), whereas others are more general in nature (Crabtree, 1958; Mecham, 1967). Screening tests are becoming more prevalent. Because of time constraints, the diagnostician concerned with articulation should do no more than screen the language of the client seen for an articulation assessment. Screening need not provide more than just a "yes" or "no" response regarding the presence of a language delay or disorder.

The final areas to be assessed, usually informally, are *client cooperation* and *motivation,* family cooperation and motivation, and client and family attitudes. These psychosocial variables can be determined through interviewing, observing, and case history information. Sometimes other persons, such as grandparents, neighbors, friends, and relatives, can provide additional information about the client's desire for assistance. All of the negative characteristics should be identified for future modification. A negative attitude in the client at the outset of assessment or treatment does not necessarily suggest diagnostic or therapeutic failure but should be noted. Poor attitude, cooperation, and motivation can be positively altered in some persons and eventually contribute to therapeutic success through the application of carefully selected behavioral procedures. If the diagnostician wants to use a more formal approach in this area, attitude and other psychosocial scales are available to the trained clinician. Although important considerations, these psychosocial malbehaviors should not discourage the clinician from attempting assessment, just as poor motivation should not dissuade the clinician from attempting treatment.

ASSESSMENT OF SPECIAL PROBLEMS

Before concluding this chapter, some mention should be made of special problems. Although the general concepts discussed in this chapter may be applicable when assessing special articulation problems, specific modifications usually are necessary.

Articulation problems associated with cerebral palsy

The expression "cerebral palsy speech" is probably a misnomer because cerebral palsy covers a wide range of handicapping conditions caused by central nervous system damage and motor, hearing, and mental impairment. Many kinds of cerebral palsy cause a variety of articulation problems covering the whole continuum of severity, and many persons with cerebral palsy have no speech problems at all. Nevertheless, when articulation is affected, speech is generally slurred, sluggish, and sometimes difficult to understand. Pitch, inflection, volume, and resonation may also be affected. These characteristics are readily observable when the person with cerebral palsy is talking in connected speech; however, they may not be as easily perceived, or perhaps not necessarily present, during production of isolated words. Hence, for the most valid sample of articulation, the client's speech should be assessed in context as well as by one-word articulation tests. If impairment is severe, one word at a time may be all that can be produced.

Additional aspects of assessment include testing for rate, range, and precision of articulator movement, stimulability in various contexts, compensatory capabilities of less involved speech structures, and respiratory and postural habits (Crickmay, 1966). Often faulty respiration is a major cause of poor articulation in the person with cerebral palsy. These areas must be carefully assessed in order to ascertain treatment goals, since not all persons with motor speech disorders may be able to learn normal articulation or learn articulation in a "normal" manner. The final goal may be improved intelligible articulation and respiration but not necessarily normal speech. Such factors as phrasing, number of words spoken per breath, and bodily postures may also need to be modified from what is commonly acceptable. Perhaps more so than with nonorganic disorders, persons with cerebral palsy and other organic problems must be thoroughly assessed in terms of capabilities. Such thoroughness implies extensive exploratory activities during the assessment.

Articulation problems associated with verbal dyspraxia

Verbal dyspraxia, another motor speech disorder caused by central nervous system damage, should also be assessed in a special, thorough contextual setting. Single-word testing tends to overlook the variability in articulation, difficulty in sequencing, effortful articulation, and dysprosody so frequently observed among persons with verbal dyspraxia (Darley, Aronson, and Brown, 1975; Rosenbek and Wertz, 1972). However, single words may be all that can be produced. The emphasis in diagnosis should be on the preceding characteristics as well as noting if the client has difficulty with nonspeech movements of the articulators; imitation of later-developing consonants, when asked; self-monitoring skills; and memory for articulation movements and positions. There should also be an absence of muscle weakness. The assessment emphasis and procedures must be somewhat different for this special group since the disorder is very complex and requires much skill in observing and recording articulator function.

Articulation problems associated with cleft palate

Another special articulation problem relates to cleft palate, or inadequate velopharyngeal closure. Clients with inadequate closure often demonstrate hypernasality and misarticulations that are rather unique, although in some minor clefts and repaired clefts there may be no problems. The articulation errors, when present, may consist of (1) weak production of pressure consonants, (2) pharyngeal fricatives, (3) laryngeal and pharyngeal stops, (4) pharyngeal /l/, and (5) distorted articulation related to the use of the tongue blade for tongue tip sounds and to tongue carriage that is somewhat posterior and superior in the mouth (Bzoch, 1979).

Assessment should emphasize sampling the sixteen pressure consonants and the high vowels in words and contextual speech. Tongue position and function for these sounds should be carefully observed, and inadequate velopharyngeal function resulting in nasal escape of air and hypernasality during their production should be noted. Place and manner of articulation are commonly in error and need to be analyzed. These and other faulty compensatory habits should be considered during assessment since they tend to differentiate defective articulation-resonance of persons with a cleft palate from defective articulation of persons without a cleft palate.

Articulation problems associated with mental retardation

Another special problem concerns clients who are mentally retarded. These persons typically have more difficulty with later-developing sounds and sound clusters and with contextual speech rather than with isolated words (Lillywhite and Bradley, 1972). They also tend to omit phonemes more commonly than intellectually normal clients with articulation disorders.

Assessment should consider parameters related to articulation such as language, sensation-perception, discrimination, memory, spatial relationships, closure, and motor and memory skills (Carrow, 1972). Special techniques and methods are an important consideration for this population primarily because they do not have specific distinctive patterns of articulation, making them difficult to test. However, difficulties in testing and types of speech patterns vary with the client and the client's level of intellectual and neuromuscular functioning.

The preceding are the major populations that require special consideration when assessing articulation. Other groups include persons who are autistic, dysphasic, hard of hearing, deaf, and combinations of any of the above. Assessment may range from giving formal articulation tests to giving no tests at all. These groups require special diagnostic skills, knowledge, and consideration, and results of assessment may not be reliable until one has had specialized training and experience in these areas.

ANALYSIS, INTERPRETATION, AND RECOMMENDATIONS

Having collected the articulation data from the assessment and related information, the diagnostician is ready to complete the final stages of the diagnostic workup. These stages require the diagnostician to analyze and interpret the data, arrive at a diagnosis, and recommend the course of treatment, in other words, to put together the pieces of the diagnostic puzzle.

Analysis

A rather scientific approach can be implemented to analyze the obtained data. This stage requires the nonjudgmental organization of the "facts" (Nation and Aram, 1977). It requires skill in scoring, objectifying, comparing with norms, and organizing the data in terms of possible solutions and what supports those solutions, what does not support the hypothesized problem, and what is still missing.

Knowledge and familiarity of the diagnostic tests used will facilitate scoring, which in turn will tend to objectify the articulation behavior. This behavior can be described, quantified, or qualified but should not be judged during this stage of analysis. When tests are not readily amenable to objective analysis, the diagnostician may either select a different test or devise a system for scoring and quantifying the obtained data. This is especially important when only informal testing is possible. A system of distinctive feature analyses (Appendix L) can be effective in analyzing the articulation data.

Comparing the data with norms provides another method of analysis. In this way the diagnostician can determine how a specific client is doing in comparison with the "average" person of that age. Comparison with norms eventually aids in the decision of whether or not the client under question has normal, accelerated, or delayed articulation development.

Organizing the data is the next task. The diagnostician must decide what data are available and how helpful they are in interpreting specific aspects of the client's articulation. The data may be organized in regard to type of phonemes, phonetic categories, distinctive features, and even non-segmental aspects of speech. Organization is a means of categorizing similar data for later interpretation. Whatever system is helpful should be used in organizing the data to determine its significance. There are many possible systems that can be used to ascertain relevance of the obtained data; as yet none has demonstrated a decided superiority.

Interpretation

One of the most important steps for the diagnostician is to interpret the data. This problem-solving task is critical to making appropriate recommendations and planning effective treatment. Misinterpretation can be devastating. The clinical results must be carefully interpreted to explain such aspects as formulating a diagnosis, stating a diagnosis, suggesting possible etiologies, offering a prognosis, and formulating a treatment plan or possibly a need for more data. Decisions must be made not only as to whether or not an articulation disorder is present, but also regarding its severity and type. The diagnostician must know what all the obtained data mean and how to interpret them to the client and family. Emerick and Hatten (1979) stated that interpretation includes (1) identifying types of errors, (2) discovering location of error in context, (3) discerning patterns of misarticulation, if present, and (4) scrutinizing variability of performance. Such an interpretation not only considers which phonemes are defective, but also how they are misarticulated. In a sense this stage really "pulls it all together." It synthesizes and interprets all of the data and impressions obtained from each of the assessment steps. Furthermore

it places all of the pertinent information in its proper perspective in regard to all other aspects of the client, such as personality, attitude, ability, motivation, needs, and concerns. In other words all of these speech data are only one part of the whole person, a perspective that should never be forgotten.

Recommendations

The final stage of the diagnostic workup requires formulation of recommendations both in a written report and orally to the client and family. Recommendations may be for additional testing and assessment, particularly by other professional disciplines, or specific steps to be followed in treatment.

Some typical recommendations for additional assessment might include referral for a psychologic evaluation, dental consultation, audiologic or otologic examination, educational testing, physical examination, or neurologic testing. Assessment of one or more of these additional areas may provide the additional information needed to arrive finally at a diagnosis and form a treatment plan, if necessary.

Common recommendations regarding treatment may include time of commencement, location, type of treatment, type of setting (group or individual sessions), length of sessions, sex of the clinician, homework considerations, specific parameters of communication to be considered in treatment, goals, priorities, procedures, and prognosis. All of these considerations must be based on carefully and accurately made interpretations. This information should be given orally to the client or parents or guardians, depending on age and maturity of the client, and in the diagnostic report, which is the final stage of the diagnostic workup.

SUMMARY

Assessment of articulation is an often difficult and always challenging task. It requires a philosophy and understanding of basic principles of behavioral management, familiarity with articulation tests, knowledge of general characteristics and pertinent history of persons with articulation problems, understanding formal and informal testing procedures; cognizance of assessing competencies and structures related to articulation, acquaintance with articulation problems of persons with special problems, and ability to score, analyze, and interpret the collected data and organize it in a scientific, meaningful manner. Finally assessment requires that the diagnostician have established frames of reference and standards with which to compare the anatomic, physiologic, and acoustic correlates of articulation. Implicit in all these requirements are well-developed visual and auditory observation skills by the diagnostician, skills that nevertheless might need to render a diagnosis as tentative while extending the diagnostic process beyond the initial workup and into the therapeutic process, as in diagnostic therapy.

STUDY SUGGESTIONS

1. Relate the phrase "what articulation looks like, sounds like, and seems like" to specific aspects of assessment and to each other.
2. Define and show the relationships among identification, assessment, evaluation, and diagnosis of articulation disorders.
3. Relate "sound position in words," "articulation norms," and "a hierarchy of sound development" to disordered articulation and assessment.
4. Describe the "general characteristics" of persons with articulation disorders and show how each may cause the disorder itself, be caused by it, or be unrelated. How do these characteristics relate to assessment?
5. Describe and compare three formal articulation tests that you think might be useful and explain why.
6. Describe ways in which "informal appraisal" procedures can be used to supplement formal testing.
7. Discuss the factors that should be considered in determining what tests and procedures you would use with a particular client.
8. Relate "pragmatics" to specific aspects of articulation, articulation deviations, and articulation disorders.

REFERENCES

Artley, A.: A study of certain factors presumed to be associated with reading and speech difficulties, J. Speech Hear. Disord. **34:**151-156, 1948.

Basmajian, J.: Electromyography of the pharyngeal constrictors and levator palati in man, Anat. Rec. **139:**561-563, 1961.

Bates, E.: Pragmatics and sociolinguistics in child language. In Morehead, D., and Morehead, A., editors: Normal and deficient child language, Baltimore, 1976, University Park Press.

Bell, R.: Development of the mandible with reference to micrognathism, McGill Dent. Rev. **30:**47-52, 1968.

Berry, M.: Berry-Talbott Language Tests, Rockford, Ill., 1966.

Blakeley, R.: Myth articulated, J. Calif. Speech Hear. Assoc. **14:**2-7, 1965.

Bloomer, H.: Speech defects associated with dental malocclusions and related abnormalities. In Travis, L., editor: Handbook of speech pathology and audiology, New York, 1971, Appleton-Century-Crofts.

Boone, D.: The voice and voice therapy, Englewood Cliffs, N.J., 1978, Prentice-Hall, Inc.

Bricker, W.: Errors in the echoic behavior of preschool children, J. Speech Hear. Research **10:**67-76, 1967.

Bzoch, K., editor: Communicative disorders related to cleft lip and palate, ed. 2, Boston, 1979, Little, Brown and Co.

Carrow, E.: Auditory comprehension of English by monolingual and bilingual preschool children, J. Speech Hear. Disord. **15:**407-412, 1972.

Carter, E., and Buck, M.: Prognostic testing for functional articulation disorders among children in the first grade, J. Speech Hear. Disord. **23:**124-133, 1958.

Casteel, R.: Grid for diagnosing intelligibility (unpublished), 1970.

Cole, R.: Electrical capacitance measures of oropharyngeal functions. In Bzoch, K., editor: Communicative disorders related to cleft lip and palate, Boston, 1971, Little, Brown and Co.

Crabtree, M.: The Houston Test for Language Development, Houston, 1958, Houston Test Co.

Crickmay, M.: Speech therapy and the Bobath approach to cerebral palsy, Springfield, Ill., 1966, Charles C Thomas, Publisher.

Croft, C., and associates: The occult submucous cleft palate and the musculae uvulae, Cleft Palate J. **15:**150-154, 1978.

Darley, F., editor: Evaluation of appraisal techniques in speech and language pathology, Reading, Mass., 1979, Addison-Wesley Publishing Co., Inc.

Darley, F., and Spriestersbach, D.: Diagnostic methods in speech pathology, ed. 2, New York, 1978, Harper & Row, Publishers.

Darley, F., Aronson, A., and Brown, J.: Motor speech disorders, Philadelphia, 1975, W. B. Saunders Co.

Emerick, L., and Hatten, J.: Diagnosis and evaluation

in speech pathology, ed. 2, Englewood Cliffs, N.J., 1979, Prentice-Hall, Inc.

Englemann, S.: The basic concept inventory, Chicago, 1967, Follett Corp.

Everhart, R.: Literature survey of growth and development factors in articulation maturation, J. Speech Hear. Disord. **25:**39-69, 1960.

Everhart, R.: The relationship between articulation and other developmental factors in children, J. Speech Hear. Disord. **18:**332-338, 1960.

Ewanowski, W., Watkin, K., and Zogyebski, J.: One-line monitoring of velar and lateral pharyngeal wall movements during speech production, Paper presented at ACPA meeting in Boston, 1974.

Fisher, H., and Logemann, J.: The Fisher-Logemann Test of Articulation Competence, Boston, 1971, Houghton Mifflin Co.

Fletcher, S.: Norms for diadochokinetic rate, Research project, Crippled Children's Division, University of Oregon Medical School, 1961.

Fletcher, S.: Time-by-count measurement of diadochokinetic syllable rate, J. Speech Hear. Disord. **15:**763-770, 1972.

Fletcher, S.: Casteel, R., and Bradley, D.: Tongue-thrust swallow, speech articulation, and age, J. Speech Hear. Disord. **26:**201-208, 1961.

Flowers, A.: Short Term Auditory Retrieval and Storage Test, Dearborn, Mich., 1972, Perceptual Learning Systems.

Flowers, A., and Costello, M.: Flowers-Costello Test of Central Auditory Abilities, Dearborn, Mich., 1970, Perceptual Learning Systems.

Fudala, J.: Arizona Articulation Proficiency Scale, Los Angeles, 1961, Western Psychological Services.

Gibb, A.: Hypernasality (rhinolalia aperta) following tonsil and adenoid removal, J. Laryngol. Otol. **72:**433-451, 1958.

Goldman, R., and Fristoe, M.: Goldman-Fristoe Test of Articulation, Circle Pines, Minn., 1969, American Guidance Service, Inc.

Goldman, R., Fristoe, M., and Woodcock, R.: Goldman-Fristoe-Woodcock Test of Auditory Discrimination, Circle Pines, Minn., 1970, American Guidance Service, Inc.

Goodenough, F.: Mental testing: its history, principles and applications, New York, 1949, Holt, Rinehart and Winston, Inc.

Hardy, J.: Airflow and air pressure studies. In Proceedings of the Conference: communicative problems in cleft palate, ASHA Report #1, 1965.

Hejna, R.: Developmental Articulation Test, Ann Arbor, Mich., 1963, Speech Materials.

Ingram, D.: Phonological disability in children, London, 1976, Edward Arnold.

Jordon, E.: Articulation test measures and listener ratings of articulation defectiveness, J. Speech Hear. Res. **3:**303-319, 1960.

Kronvall, E., and Diehl, C.: The relationship of auditory discrimination to articulatory defects of children with no known organic impairment, J. Speech Hear. Disord. **19:**335-338, 1954.

Lee, L.: Northwestern Syntax Screening Test, Evanston, Ill., 1966, Northwestern University Press.

Lillywhite, H., and Bradley, D.: Communication problems in mental retardation, New York, 1972, Harper & Row, Publishers.

Lindamood, C., and Lindamood, P.: Lindamood Auditory Conceptualization Test, Hingham, Mass., 1971, Teaching Resources Corp.

Martin, F.: Introduction to audiology, Englewood Cliffs, N.J., 1975, Prentice-Hall, Inc.

McCall, G.: The assessment of lingual tactile sensation and perception, J. Speech Hear. Disord. **34:**151-156, 1969.

McDonald, E.: A Deep Test of Articulation, Pittsburgh, 1964, Stanwix House, Inc.

McReynolds, L., and Engmann, D.: Distinctive feature analysis of misarticulations, Baltimore, 1975, University Park Press.

Mecham, M.: Utah Test of Language Development, Salt Lake City, 1967, Communication Research Associates.

Milisen, R.: Articulatory problems. In Rieber, R., and Brubaker, R., editors: Speech pathology, Amsterdam, 1966, North Holland Publishing Co.

Milisen, R.: Methods of evaluation and diagnosis of speech disorders. In Travis, L., editor: Handbook of speech pathology and audiology, New York, 1971, Appleton-Century-Crofts.

Milisen, R., and associates: The disorder of articulation: a systematic clinical and experimental approach, J. Speech Hear. Disord. (Suppl. 4), 1954.

Moll, K.: Speech characteristics of individuals with cleft lip and palate. In Spriestersbach, D., and Sherman, D., editors: Cleft palate and communication, New York, 1968, Academic Press, Inc.

Moncur, J., and Brackett, I.: Modifying vocal behavior, New York, 1974, Harper & Row, Publishers.

Morris, H., Spriestersbach, D., and Darley, F.: Articulation test for assessing competency of velopharyngeal closure, J. Speech Hear. Disord. **4:**48-55, 1961.

Nation, J., and Aram, D.: Diagnosis of speech and language disorders, St. Louis, 1977, The C. V. Mosby Co.

Newby, H.: Audiology, New York, 1972, Appleton-Century-Crofts.

Noll, J.: Articulatory assessment. In Speech and the dentalfacial complex, ASHA Reports **2:**283-296, 1970.

Oller, D.: Regularities in abnormal child phonology, J. Speech Hear. Disord. **38:**36-47, 1973.

Pendergast, D., and associates: Photo Articulation Test, Danville, Ill., 1969, The Interstate Printers & Publishers, Inc.

Pollack, E., and Rees, N.: Disorders of articulation: some clinical applications of distinctive feature theory, J. Speech Hear. Disord. **37:**451-461, 1972.

Powers, M.: Functional disorders of articulation: symptomatology and etiology. In Travis, L., editor: Handbook of speech pathology and audiology, New York, 1971, Appleton-Century-Crofts.

Prather, E., Hedrick, D., and Kern, C.: Articulation development in children aged two to four years, J. Speech Hear. Disord. **40:**179-191, 1975.

Prins, D.: Relations among specific articulatory deviations and responses to a clinical measure of sound discrimination ability, J. Speech Hear. Disord. **28:** 382-388, 1963.

Prutting, C.: Process /'prȧ/,ses/ n: the action of moving forward progressively from one point to another on the way to completion, J. Speech Hear. Disord. **44:**3-30, 1979.

Roe, V., and Milisen, R.: The effect of maturation upon defective articulation in elementary grades, J. Speech Hear. Disord. **7:**37-45, 1942.

Rose, D., editor: Audiological assessment, Englewood Cliffs, N.J., 1971, Prentice-Hall, Inc.

Rosenbek, J., and Wertz, R.: A review of 50 cases of developmental apraxia of speech, Lang. Speech Hear. Serv. Schools **III:**23-33, 1972.

Sayler, H.: The effect of maturation upon defective articulation in grades seven through twelve, J. Speech Hear. Disord. **14:**202-207, 1949.

Schissel, R., and James, L.: A comparison of children's performance on two tests of articulation, J. Speech Hear. Disord. **44:**363-372, 1979.

Shriberg, L.: The effect of examiner social behavior on children's articulation test performance, J. Speech Hear. Disord. **14:**659-672, 1971.

Skolnick, L., and associates: Patterns of velopharyngeal closure in subjects with repaired cleft palate and normal speech: a multi-view videofluoroscopic analysis, Cleft Palate J. **12:**369-375, 1975.

Sommers, R., Cox, S., and West, C.: Articulatory effectiveness, stimulability, and children's performance on perceptual and memory tasks, J. Speech Hear. Disord. **15:**579-589, 1972.

Spriestersbach, D., and Curtis, J.: Misarticulation and discrimination of speech sounds, Q. J. Speech **37:** 483-491, 1951.

Steer, M., and Drexler, H.: Predicting later articulation abilities from kindergarten tests, J. Speech Hear. Disord. **25:**391-397, 1960.

Subtelny, J., Koepp-Baker, H., and Subtelny, D.: Palatal function and cleft palate speech, J. Speech Hear. Disord. **26:**213-224, 1961.

Templin, M.: Study of sound discrimination ability of elementary school children, J. Speech Hear. Disord. **8:**127-132, 1943.

Templin, M.: Certain language skills in children, Minneapolis, 1957, University of Minnesota Press.

Templin, M., and Darley, F.: The Templin-Darley Tests of Articulation, Iowa City, 1969, Bureau of Educational Research and Service, The University of Iowa.

Terman, L., and Merrill, M.: Stanford-Binet Intelligence Scale, Boston, 1973, Houghton Mifflin Co.

Turton, L., and Clark, M.: Linguistic theory and the child, Acta Symbolica **2:**42-47, 1971.

Van Riper, C.: Speech correction, principles and methods, Englewood Cliffs, N.J., 1963, Prentice-Hall, Inc.

Van Riper, C., and Erickson, R.: Predictive Screening Test of Articulation, Kalamazoo, Mich., 1968, Continuing Education Office, Western Michigan University.

Wechsler, D.: Wechsler Preschool and Primary Scale of Intelligence, New York, 1967, Psychological Corp.

Weiner, F.: Phonological process analysis, Baltimore, 1979, University Park Press.

Weiss, C.: The relationships between maximum articulatory rate and articulatory disorders among children, Central States Speech J. **19:**185-187, 1968.

Weiss, C.: The speech pathologist's role in dealing with obturator-wearing school children, J. Speech Hear. Disord. **39:**153-162, 1974.

Weiss, C.: Weiss Comprehensive Articulation Test, Hingham, Mass., 1978, Teaching Resources.

Weiss, C., and associates: The feasibility of computerized tomography in assessing the velopharyngeal mechanism, 1980.

Wellman, B., and associates: Speech sounds of young children, University of Iowa Studies in Child Welfare **5**(2):1936.

Wepman, J.: Auditory Discrimination Test, Chicago, 1958, Language Research Associates.

Weston, A., and Irwin, J.: Paired-stimuli in modification of articulation, Percept. Mot. Skills **32:**390-397, 1971.

Wilson, D.: Voice problems of children, ed. 2, Baltimore, 1979, The Williams & Wilkins Co.

Winitz, H.: Articulatory acquisition and behavior, New York, 1969, Appleton-Century-Crofts.

GLOSSARY

alar flutter Fluttering movement of the nasal alae (nostrils).

alveolar ridge As used here, the maxillary ridge of mucosa circling inside the upper teeth.

ankylosed tongue Unusually short lingual frenulum that restricts movement of the tip of the tongue, commonly referred to as tongue-tie.

asynergistic movements Faulty timing and coordination of the articulators, as used here; may also refer to other organs and functions of the body such as swallowing and gagging.

auditory conceptualization Ability to perceive, assimilate, understand, and form concepts of messages received through auditory channels.

auditory discrimination The ability to discriminate, one from another, stimuli such as phones, phonemes, digits, nonsense syllables, words, and environmental noises.

auditory memory Ability to recall (remember) units of sound, phones, phonemes, numbers, etc. received through auditory channels.

aural rehabilitation Rehabilitation or retraining of deficiencies resulting from hearing loss or other auditory problems.

autism An individual's retreat from, or failure to enter into, normal personal and social relationships with other human beings.

bifid A split or failure to grow together of an organ of the body, usually referring to bifid uvula.

buccal speech A method of speaking by using buccal (cheek) muscles to simulate phonation, sometimes used by individuals who have had the larynx removed.

central auditory processing Understanding, interpreting, and organizing (processing) messages reaching appropriate brain centers through auditory channels.

clavicular breathing In which most movement related to breathing is observable above the chest area in the region of the clavicle. Usually thought to be "shallow breathing," in which the lungs are not fully utilized.

cosmetic Pertaining to improvement of a person's appearance, as in the case of "cosmetic surgery" to improve appearance after initial repair of cleft lip or palate.

deviated septum Irregularity or separation of the bony partition between the nasal cavities.

diaphragmatic breathing In which most movement related to breathing is observable in the lower chest area and the diaphragm. Usually thought to be "deep breathing" utilizing the lungs and diaphragm more fully than in clavicular breathing.

dysprosody Inability to control inflectional patterns, rate, stress, and rhythm of speech.

electric capacitance Capacity of a condenser for the storage of electric energy.

faucial arch An archway between the pharyngeal and buccal cavities formed by the faucial pillars, which are two sets of vertical muscles on either side of the oral cavity.

fiberoptics A technique used to view directly the larynx and velopharyngeal mechanism by use of high-intensity light in a tube of small diameter.

fistula An opening into or through body tissue, such as an opening remaining in the hard or soft palate after palate surgery.

grapheme A letter of an alphabet.

hyoid bone A U-shaped bone at the base of the tongue. It gives leverage and anchorage to the muscles of the jaw, tongue, pharynx, and larynx.

hypertrophy An overgrowth, such as enlarged tonsils and adenoids.

intervocalic During vocalization, as opposed to prevocalic or postvocalic.

intraoral breath pressure Breath pressure inside the oral cavity.

kinesthesis Muscle sense ability, such as where in space the tongue is at a given time.

kinetic Relating to the motion of material bodies and the forces and energy associated therewith. As used here, relating to the movement and energy of the speech organs.

labiodental Pertaining to the lips and teeth functioning together in articulating phonemes, such as /f/ and /v/.

lingual frenulum A membrane extending from the floor of the mouth to the midline of the inferior surface of the tongue blade. It may restrict movement of the tongue tip if exceedingly short or if extending too far toward the tongue tip.

masseter muscles Muscles that control the action of the mandible.

modified stethoscope A stethoscope with nasal "olives" on the ends of the tubing, used for listening to nasal air escape.

nasal listening tube Twelve- to 18-inch tubing with glass or plastic "olives" attached to each end; one olive is held in the client's nostril and the other in the clinician's ear to hear or feel nasal air escape.

nasal septum Bone and cartilage divider separating the nasal cavities.

nasal squinting Observable restriction of the nares sometimes developed by an individual to help occlude the nares when too much air is felt to be escaping through the nose.

nasopharynx The upper part of the pharynx that joins the nasal passages.

oral stereognosis The ability to perceive and recognize the form and nature of objects by the sense of touch within the oral cavity.

orofacial muscle imbalance More commonly called tongue thrust. The tongue "thrusts" between or strongly against the upper anterior incisors during swallowing and speaking.

overshooting tongue The tongue overreaches its mark, such as in attempting to reach the alveolus it protrudes all the way between the teeth. May pertain to lateral movement also. May be a symptom of orofacial muscle imbalance or of dyspraxia.

peripheral speech mechanism All speech organs that are removed from (away from) the center of control, the central nervous system, specifically the organs of voice, resonation, and articulation.

postvocalic After vocalization. Actions of the

vocal mechanism above the larynx in producing speech.

prevocalic Before vocalization. Preparation or activity preceding the vocal act of producing voiced sound in the larynx.

roentgenography An X-ray technique that reveals tissue in "layers" or "slices" for better visualization.

subvocalic air pressure Pressure of air from the lungs through the respiratory tract up to and through the vocal bands.

tactile localization Ability of the tongue to know where it was stimulated.

tactile sensitivity Sensitivity of the tongue to touch.

temporomandibular joint A joint at the base of the temple on each side providing for hinging action of the mandible.

tongue thrust *See* Orofacial muscle imbalance.

turbinate One of three thin bones (conchae) projecting downward into each nasal passage from the upper and outer wall of the passages.

two-point discrimination The ability of the tongue to discriminate and recognize the nature, or name, of an object at two points on the tongue; a function of stereognosis.

ultrasound The use of high-speed sound to determine the site and mass of lesions or the extent of excursions of muscles.

undershooting of the tongue The tongue falling short when attempting to make contact with another articulator, such as teeth, hard palate, etc. Often a characteristic of dyspraxia or paresis.

velopharyngeal mechanism Composed of the velum and pharynx acting in conjunction to control airflow and sound flow into the nasal passages.

velopharyngeal port A port or gateway formed by action of the pharynx and velum to control the flow of air and sound through the mouth and nasal passages.

vocal phonics Word attack skills. Analysis of a word by separating its component phonemes and then synthesizing it into a word; "sounding out" a word.

CHAPTER SEVEN

A philosophy of articulation treatment

"Words learned by rote, a parrot may rehearse."
COWPER

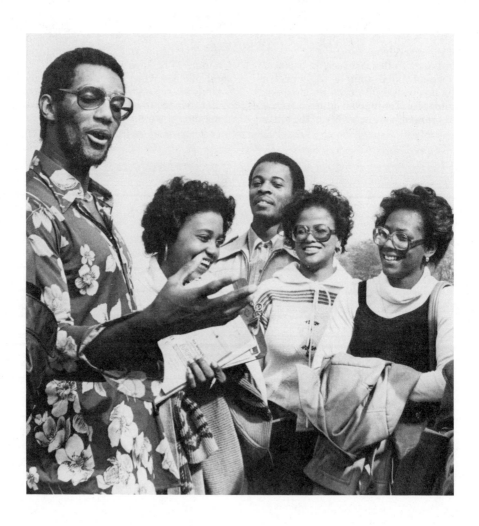

Articulation is more than a mechanical act implemented by specific muscular action (Dickson, 1974). Therefore, it is necessary to discuss the relationship between articulation treatment and language treatment, the relationship of articulation treatment to other aspects of communication, and the wide range of communication patterns within normal limits. We continue by considering the factors important in determining need for formal articulation intervention. General principles and rationale for articulation treatment, special considerations for treatment, management options, and general stages of treatment are also presented.

RELATIONSHIP BETWEEN ARTICULATION TREATMENT AND LANGUAGE TREATMENT

It is important to discuss the relationship between articulation treatment and language in general because articulation is actually a part of the total language system. You may recall that language is comprised of four integral subsystems: semantics, syntax, phonology, and morphology (Byrne and Shervanian, 1977). A fifth subsystem known as pragmatics should also be added. *Semantics* deals with the meaning of utterances. *Syntax* is concerned with the word order of utterances and thus is the study of the arrangement of words and the rules for ordering words; it is the study of the formation of words. *Phonology* involves the sound system of language and can be defined as the study of the sounds that comprise language and the rules for using sounds. *Pragmatics* considers the rules governing the use of communication in context in terms of its effectiveness. *Morphology* includes the formation of words such as plurals, past tense, or possessives. It has been called the grammar of language.

Winitz (1969) explains that the way speech sounds are used is part of the language subsystem known as phonology; therefore, when articulation errors occur, the individual is using a sound system that is at variance with the adult system. Recent linguistic literature has led to a view of articulation as an integral part of the whole language system and of looking for patterns of misarticulations rather than considering each error as being unrelated to other errors (Shewan, 1978). Articulation treatment, then, may be considered one level of language treatment, but it is confined to the phonemes of language. Thus it is often differentiated from language treatment involving the other four language subsystems, namely semantics, syntax, morphology, and pragmatics. Articulation treatment is not to be confused with treatment of morphologic errors, such as incorrect use of plurals, past tense, or possessives, nor is it involved with syntactic errors, such as incorrect noun-verb agreement. Different treatment approaches are needed for these types of errors. For example, it is not recommended that articulation treatment be implemented for correction of omission of /s/ and /z/ if these omissions occur only in plural nouns or singular verbs or possessive nouns. Articulation treatment also is not designed for teaching word meaning; a different language treatment approach is suggested.

The preceding statements do not mean that semantics, syntax, morphology, and pragmatics are not involved in articulation treatment, since the various subsystems of language cannot be completely separated. When teaching correct articulation patterns, the sounds are taught in the context of correct word forms, syntactic structures (phrases and sentences), word meaning, and appropriate relationship between words and expressions. Therefore, other areas of language may be learned incidentally although they would not be the focus of the treatment program.

RELATIONSHIP OF ARTICULATION TREATMENT TO OTHER ASPECTS OF COMMUNICATION

Just as articulation is intrinsically related to language, it is an important component of communication. Communication has been defined by Skinner and Shelton (1978) as "the transmission and exchange of information." It takes many forms, including speaking, listening, writing, and using gestures. As these authors point out, the speech and hearing communication process is the primary mode of communication among human beings. Because it involves at least two people, a speaker and a listener, it is a complex interaction. The information-giver selects and produces symbols to convey an idea, and the receiver perceives and interprets the message and responds accordingly (Byrne and Shervanian, 1977).

Communication processes include, in addition to the five subsystems of language, paralanguage or nonverbal communication, for example, gestures, facial expressions, body posture, voice pitch, inflection, voice quality, and fluency. Communication also involves speech production, hearing, and cognition (awareness, perception, conceptualization, differentiation, and thought, which enables comprehension, interpretation, and symbol usage). Interpersonal relations are another component of communication. How a speaker's message is interpreted by the listener depends on the previously named factors and probably others. The speaker's articulation skills influence the accuracy with which a message is understood. Certainly articulation contributes greatly to the intelligibility of a speaker's message, that is, how much of the message is understood. Consequently a person with an articulation disorder may have a communication handicap. According to Powers (1971), the severity of the communication handicap of a person with an articulation disorder is related to degree of intelligibility, number and type of different misarticulated sounds, particular sounds that are misarticulated, consistency of error sounds, and personal and social speech standards and attitudes. If management of an articulation disorder improves articulation skills, communication with others will be enhanced.

During articulation treatment other aspects of communication cannot be ignored since articulation of sounds does not occur in isolation but overlaps with the other parameters of speech production. For example, appropriate speaking rate, correct pronunciation of words, appropriate inflection patterns, and appropriate loudness levels should be incorporated into the practice material. Correct articulation patterns need to be incorporated into everyday communication situations under the guidance of the speech-language pathologist.

WIDE RANGE OF COMMUNICATION PATTERNS WITHIN NORMAL LIMITS

Before discussing the need for articulation treatment, it must be emphasized that there is a wide range of communication patterns, including articulation, that falls within the normal limits of acceptability. As Silverman (1976) indicates, "Most speech pathologists are in agreement that every speech difference is not a speech defect." Byrne and Shervanian (1977) state that identifiable standards of language usage exist against which oral communication of individuals can be compared. They further discuss three major dialectic regions in the United States, which include Eastern, Southern, and General American. Distinctive articulation patterns are used by members of each dialect, for example, dropping of /r/ (or the "floating /r/") by Eastern speakers and use of diphthongs instead of vowels by Southern speakers as well as other differences. There are also differences among speakers within the three regions related to ethnic, cultural, and socioeconomic groups. For example, the substitution of /θ/ for /f/ is generally acceptable in the black language – speaking community. The substitution of /r/ for /l/ by English-speaking Japanese or of /j/ for /dʒ/ by speakers of Swedish origin are not considered to be articulation disorders but normal bilingual ethnic differences.

Factors other than dialect influence judgment of normalcy of communication patterns. Sometimes differences are accepted by some occupational communities but not by others. Additionally different situations for the same speaker may influence which articulation patterns are used (Eisenson and Ogilvie, 1977). A black speaker may use standard American speech when talking with a teacher but use black English when talking with peers. A college professor will probably use quite precise enunciation in giving a formal lecture and "slur" articulation when talking at home with family members. The age of the speaker also influences whether a misarticulation is within normal limits, for example, it is acceptable for a 4-year-old child to substitute /w/ for /r/. Generally, *normal* dialectic, situational, and age differences in articulation patterns are acceptable and thus are considered normal.

NEED FOR TREATMENT

Not every person who misarticulates is in need of articulation treatment. First, need for treatment is related to social, cultural, ethnic, and occupational aspects of the individual's environment. Evaluation criteria for the adequacy of communication skills are based on social acceptability. Similarly two criteria used by Perkins (1978) for determining the extent to which misarticulations are a problem relate to cultural speech standards and vocational goals. When dealing with children, one must assume that the child needs a language system that is useful in many expanding and changing environments, a system or systems to be used at home, away from home, with the same social group, and with others. Along these same lines the probable or desired life-style or occupation of a person should be considered when determining need for treatment since articulation deficits may or may not become a barrier to social and professional opportunities (Byrne and Shervanian, 1977).

At least two studies have shown that even a person who has the so-called "minor" articulation disorder of lisping is perceived more negatively by listeners. Both studies used male speakers. In the study by Silverman (1976), a speaker was rated more negatively by college students when reading a passage with a simulated lateral lisp than when reading without a lisp. Similar results were reported by Mowrer, Wahl, and Doolan (1978), except the speakers simulated

frontal lisps. They concluded that speakers with frontal lisps are rated more negatively on speaking ability, intelligence, education, masculinity, and friendship. In the latter study attorneys and businessmen served as judges. Even though neither study used a cross section of judges and only male speakers were used, they do lend support to the consideration of social factors in determining need for correction of articulation disorders.

A second factor in determining need for articulation treatment is attitudes of peers, family, and other important people in the person's environment. One criterion that Perkins (1978) mentioned relative to the extent to which articulation errors constitute a problem is how satisfied the speaker is with his or her speech. When referring to children, Johnson and associates (1967) agreed that self-evaluation by the child is important and added that parent and teacher views must be considered as well. The speaker's attitude ranges from acknowledgement of the speech problem, rejection and insistence that the problem does not exist, to overconcern with it. Important persons in the individual's environment sometimes react to articulation errors by rewarding them and sometimes by penalizing them. Such reactions must be considered in determining need for treatment.

The preceding discussion leads to two questions that must be considered when determining need for treatment. Is an articulation deviancy a problem if the client, family, teacher, or other important persons do not perceive it as one even though the speech-language pathologist does? Speech-language pathologists must be acutely aware of imposing their values on those of their clients. The misarticulations can be described in relation to normative data and other criteria and may be considered deviant, but if the primary persons in the client's environment do not desire treatment, then treatment should be deferred. Conversely is there a problem if the client, family, teacher, or others perceive it as such but the speech-language pathologist does not consider it to be a disorder? In this case the clinician may need to provide services or refer the client elsewhere. One of the authors once enrolled a kindergarten child in a public school speech program for mis-articulation of /r/ because of student and parental concern, even though the sound would likely have developed without formal intervention. In this instance the attitudes of the parent and child were the overriding consideration. However, if the clinician believes that he or she cannot help the client, treatment should not be undertaken.

A third factor in determining need for treatment is the nature of the articulation deficiency itself, that is, the causes, severity, and effects on communication. Certainly an important criterion for determining the extent of the problem is how intelligible the speaker is. Additionally the frequency with which articulation errors occur, type of error (distortion, substitution, omission, and addition), stimulability for correct production, and consistency of errors are important considerations. The more unintelligible the person is, the more conspicuous the speech is, the more frequently errors occur, the more consistent the errors are, and the less stimulable correct sound production is, the more severe the articulation disorder is and the greater the need for formal intervention.

Age is also a critical factor in determining need for treatment, as explained in Chapters 3 and 6. Although some errors may normally persist until age 7 or 8 years, this does not mean that articulation treatment should not be instituted earlier in many cases. As Johnson and associates (1967) state, ". . . the help they need should not be postponed until everyone else of their age level has developed adequate speech by adult standards." Such a postponement may handicap a child in an educational system, family, or community that rewards good oral communication skills and may result in embarrassment, teasing, and frustration for the child. In other words developmental age levels of particular phonemes must be considered in determining need for

intervention, but other factors must also be taken into consideration.

GENERAL PRINCIPLES OF ARTICULATION TREATMENT

Some general principles to be followed in administering articulation treatment will now be discussed. These principles are not universally adhered to by all speech-language pathologists but are general guidelines that we believe provide a good rationale for treating articulation disorders.

Eliminate or minimize the effect of the maintaining causative factors

This principle is contingent on a thorough evaluation of the client as presented in the previous two chapters. In adhering to this guideline, the maintaining causes are of primary concern. Those that precipitated the disorder but are no longer operative are likely not critical. Of course there are instances when the precipitating and maintaining causes are not fully determined, and it is not always essential to do so (Dickson, 1974). Many times the articulation disorder may be the result of multiple causative factors or of unknown etiology. In the latter instance articulation treatment will truly be symptomatic treatment.

Nonetheless, before planning a remedial program, the speech-language pathologist should investigate what changes can be made to eliminate, minimize, or compensate for the maintaining causes. If there is a physical deviancy that significantly contributes to the disorder, it needs to be corrected to the extent possible, for example, cleft palate repair, clipping the lingual frenulum, and orthodontic treatment. The improvement to be expected from correcting facial and oral cavity structural deviancies is uncertain and must be considered on an individual basis. Certainly such changes will not guarantee correct articulation. In some cases it may be more feasible to teach the individual to compensate for the deviancy, except for cleft palate, which must be treated. Depending on one's professional background and philosophy and the age of the client, the speech-language pathologist may choose to correct tongue thrust swallow before initiating formal articulation treatment. Unfavorable parental, sibling, and teacher attitudes and interactions with the client may be alleviated through counseling. We have mentioned only a few examples of eliminating or minimizing causes prior to or during articulation treatment. Each case must be considered individually and handled accordingly.

Write behavioral goals and procedures

One of the most important contributions that operant philosophy has made is in writing specific behavioral goals, objectives, and procedures. These goals, objectives, and procedures enable the clinician to observe and measure progress in treatment (Mager, 1962; Mowrer, 1978). However, if they are not measurable or if they are written with vague wording, they serve no purpose. Therefore, it is important for every clinician to become proficient at writing clear, concise, quantifiable goals, objectives, and procedures that delineate exactly what the client is supposed to do, under which specific conditions it is to be done, and precisely how well the task is to be accomplished (criterion level). In fact we recommend indicating in the section on procedures the type of reinforcement to be used, that is, positive, negative, or punishment, and the reinforcement schedule, that is, continuous, fixed interval or ratio, and variable interval or ratio. The reinforcement schedules are typically indicated in percentages. Another part of the process may include the rationale underlying each procedure and baseline data. Such rigorous programming tends to instill an attitude of thoroughness, orderliness, and systematic progression. Once the clinician has mastered the art and science of writing behaviorally stated goals and objectives, he or she should be able to apply this skill in writing individual educational programs (IEP), lesson plans, and other protocol for indicating why and how treatment will be conducted for a specific client. An example of behaviorally stated goals, objectives, and procedures is included in Appendix N, along with a sample format of an individualized educational program.

Use different treatment approaches

Historically clinicians have not utilized different treatment approaches much for different clients. There is a great temptation to continue using the approach that has worked in the past, and this may be sound clinical reasoning. But now with the pressures for performing these tasks in less amount of time, pressures because of the present era of accountability, and pressures to help more severely handicapped persons and individuals with multiple handicaps, we are faced with the challenge of improving our therapeutic armamentarium. To help meet this challenge we suggest using a differentiated treatment approach and selection of the approach that seems to be most efficient and effective in remediating a specific articulation disorder. A combination of common sense, clinical experience, and research findings has led us to suggest specific treatment approaches for specific problems, as listed in Appendix P.

Teach the distinction between the error and the standard production

We have referred to speech or auditory discrimination on several occasions. Part of the problem in this area resides in the fact that its importance is not substantiated at this time. Nonetheless some clinicians have noted marked increases in carry-over and maintenance when they went back and included speech discrimination activities in treatment. Conversely some clinicians have observed limited success in achieving carry-over and maintenance when speech discrimination was not specifically taught. As Winitz (1969) and Weiner (1979) have suggested, learning a "new" sound (correctly producing a previously incorrect sound) probably is not possible until the client has distinguished between the correct production and the incorrect production. Whether or not this discrimination between correct and incorrect productions requires special sessions on speech discrimination is debatable. We prefer that some special attention be directed to speech discrimination and self-monitoring because all too often we observe clients struggling in treatment because they do not "hear" their misarticulations. Perhaps what we are actually suggesting is to teach auditory conceptualization of the target sounds, since self-monitoring abilities probably cannot be mastered at the motoric level but rather must be mastered at the cortical level. Whatever one's philosophy of speech discrimination training, the client must be made aware of the difference between correct and incorrect productions. If speech discrimination activities are included, they should be arranged in a hierarchic order of difficulty and should require the client to be an active participant, especially in learning self-monitoring.

Teach generalization

Since generalization usually does not occur automatically, special attention must be directed to this cortical process in treatment. Activities for encouraging generalization should begin as soon as the client has completed the establishment phase of treatment. In fact generalization of the correct phoneme may occur earlier than that because the sound can generalize or transfer to different positions or contexts within words, to different words and utterances, to other sounds that have similar distinctive features, and to other speaking situations or environments quite early in treatment. Activities for facilitating generalization include periodic probing for the target sound in a variety of phonemic contexts and physical environments, practicing the sound in many different environments, developing a core vocabulary that contains the target phoneme, reducing the frequency of reinforcements, involving a variety of "helpers," and eliciting large numbers of repetitions in the treatment setting. Additional ideas are included in Chapter 8. To reemphasize, generalization should be taught—it does not always occur spontaneously.

Teach several sounds at a time

Only in special instances should one sound be taught at a time. Most children and adults are capable of learning several sounds at once (Van Riper, 1972). Capability should be determined on the basis of stimulability testing and cognitive or conceptual abilities of the client and in some cases after several weeks of trial or diagnostic therapy. Reasons for working on several sounds simultaneously are for (1) expediting the rate of progress, (2) improving intelligibility more readily, (3) maintaining motivation, (4) reducing the chances for overgeneralization, and (5) financial or economical purposes—the faster the progress, the less the cost to the taxpayer or whoever is responsible.

We have mentioned elsewhere that cognates may not always need to receive individual attention; that is, working on /s/ may not always require working on /z/ because there tends to be generalization across cognates in some clients. We have found it to be expeditious to spend some time on cognates as well, since not all children show cognate generalization. Besides cognates, the clinician may elect to work on entire sound classes such as all of the stops or on a major feature that is lacking, such as sibilancy. In this manner the therapeutic process can be made more efficient.

Allow for clients who enter treatment at different levels

Heretofore we have not mentioned the possibility of different clients entering the treatment program at different levels. Not all clients are functioning on the same level insofar as articulation is concerned. Some children may be at the isolation level, and some may be at the sentence level. Since it is of utmost importance to start where the client is, the clinician must determine the level for each individual and begin treatment at that level. Appendix I includes a hierarchy of treatment levels. A particular client may enter treatment at any of these levels, once again emphasizing the importance of assuming an individualistic philosophy in treatment.

Follow-up of treatment

Any experienced clinician will admit that he or she has had "clinical failures." This is normal. However, some of these failures might have been prevented if a rigorous follow-up procedure had been practiced. There seems to be an unknown point in treatment beyond which maintenance will continue but before which maintenance will experience a relapse or regression. An analogy might be that of the cross-country skier trudging up a hill. Once beyond the crest or peak of the hill, skiing is easily accomplished as momentum and confidence are gained by traversing the downhill slope, but until that point is reached, there is always the possibility of losing footing and tumbling back down the slope, thereby losing confidence, patience, and interest. Since we do not know the point of the maintenance hill in each client, it would appear to be a prudent measure to follow up all clients 3 to 6 months posttreatment. In this way maintenance would be ensured.

Treatment must be realistic

An important aspect of the clinician's philosophy is to plan treatment strategies that are realistic. As used here, realistic treatment refers to activities that encourage meaningful and appropriate articulation. Examples of unrealistic expectations and activities follow. The client is asked the question, "How are you?" If the expected response is, "I am fine, thank you," this expectation would be unrealistic because this is not how we talk in real-life situations. The more acceptable answer would be, "Fine," "OK," "Great," or "Super." If the client is working on /s/ and is producing it acceptably but the clinician expects /s/ to be produced with greater sibilancy, the expectation is again unrealistic. If the clinician is working on transfer by drilling on reading word lists, the activity is inappropriate or unrealistic because it does not foster transfer of a specific phoneme to contextual speech. Unlike reading word lists, realistic treatment for achieving transfer must incorporate "functional" or "experiential" activities that are closely related to articulation behavior outside the clinic room, such as talking while playing or while building or cooking something. Realistic treatment is purposeful, interactive treatment. The client interacts with another client in a meaningful manner in the clinic and outside the clinic in order to achieve transfer and maintenance. Client-client and client-clinician interaction have been shown to be a very effective approach during these latter phases of treatment. Thus realistic treatment includes appropriate activities, interactions, responses, and expectations.

Use different articulation treatment approaches with different clients

In other words the same approach should not be used with every client. This guideline, like the previous one, is predicated on a thorough, accurate assessment of the client in which the speech-language pathologist becomes familiar with the individual and the exact nature of the patterns of articulation and misarticulations and related factors, including those that are maintaining the problem. During the assessment procedures the speech-language pathologist should be alert to any indication of a positive response to a particular learning procedure (Dickson, 1974). Such responses are hints at potentially effective treatment approaches for a particular client (see Appendix P).

One of Byrne and Shervanian's (1977) general treatment principles is that the uniqueness and individuality of each client must be recognized and considered in planning management programs. Similarly Powers (1971) contends that treatment cannot be the same for all clients but must be adapted to fit individual needs and deficiencies. For some clients it may not be essential to go through the entire treatment sequence if probing shows that the client already has the skills for certain steps of the program; perhaps only certain steps need to be emphasized (Winitz, 1975). This is one way of individualizing articulation approaches for particular clients. Additionally different clinical approaches may be better suited to different clients (Gerber, 1977). If this is true, the assessment procedures should differentiate among various clinical groups such as those displaying deviant articulation patterns versus delayed articulation, phonemic errors versus phonetic errors, and organic versus nonorganic cases. Diagnosis should also reveal whether a client is deficient in auditory perceptual or oral tactile and kinesthetic skills. Such deficiencies have implications for selecting an appropriate remedial approach. A period of trial treatment is often helpful in finding an effective approach.

Have available a large repertoire of treatment approaches and specific techniques

This principle is really a corollary to the preceding one since it is not possible to use different treatment approaches if the speech-language pathologist is competent in only one method of treatment. There is no recommended number of treatment approaches that should be mastered by a speech-language pathologist since little research has been done to compare various methods (Sommers and Kane, 1974). We do highly recommend utilizing an individualistic approach to diagnosis and treatment. Certainly competent articulation clinicians will not be limited to two or three approaches and will continue expanding their repertoire through reading professional literature, consulting with other clinicians, and attending classes, short courses, and seminars. The clinician should not be reluctant to change a planned remedial program if the client is not responding as expected or if new information indicates that a different approach might be more effective.

We have been discussing general treatment approaches such as those that will be described in the following chapter. A speech-language pathologist also must have a number of different techniques for eliciting sounds in isolation and for incorporating sounds into nonsense syllables and words. For example, a certain technique for eliciting correct /s/ from persons with a lateral lisp will not work for all who have a lateral lisp; therefore, the clinician must be ready with an armamentarium of techniques for the face-to-face situation with the client. The same is true for eliciting /r/, /l/, /f/, and, as a matter of fact, all sounds. Similarly a client does not often automatically produce sounds correctly in nonsense syllables or words even if production is correct in isolation. The clinician must be prepared with several techniques for accomplishing this task. Thus an effective articulation clinician will use various articulation treatment approaches and specific techniques with various clients.

Begin at the level of the client's articulation

One of Powers' (1971) principles for effective articulation treatment is to begin where the articulation level of the client is so that eventually new articulation patterns will replace incorrect ones. In other words the clinician should begin with what the client can already do and gradually build on new skills. If a client has multiple articulation errors, it usually is advisable to begin remediation with a sound or sounds that can most easily be produced correctly and are likely to result in early success for the client and a positive client attitude toward the clinical process. Later the persons probably will be more amenable to producing the more difficult phonemes. Easily produced sounds include those that are most stimulable, visible, and earlier developing. Certainly beginning with a sound that is stimulable, if there is one, is to begin where the client is, since correct production is already possible. Production of the error sound in nonmeaningful material, such as sounds in isolation, nonsense syllables, and nonsense words, tends to be easier than production in meaningful material because the client has habitually used misarticulations in meaningful contexts, but not in unfamiliar contexts. Therefore, it is suggested that the error sound be produced first in nonmeaningful material and later in meaningful contexts (Gerber, 1977; Johnson and associates, 1967; Winitz, 1969).

The clinician does not need to begin the treatment program at the beginning stage if the client is beyond that level. For example, if the client already can discriminate the correct sound from the error sound, it is not necessary to begin with discrimination training. Or, if the individual can produce a sound in words with stimulation, it probably is not necessary to begin with production of that sound at the isolation level. If the clinician begins where the client is and logically builds on more difficult tasks until the final objective is attained, the articulation treatment program should be effective.

Expect less than "perfect" articulation from some clients

This guideline refers to both organic and nonorganic cases. If an organic deficit, such as may result from cleft palate, cerebral palsy, and other dysarthrias, dyspraxia, and mental retardation, is not correctable, the speech-language pathologist needs to formulate treatment objectives that are within the client's potential (DiCarlo, 1974; Skinner and Shelton, 1978). This does not mean that such goals cannot be changed during the management process since the client may perform better or poorer than expected. Nevertheless the articulation goals must be realistic in terms of the physical, mental, or emotional capabilities of the client. It is also the clinician's responsibility to assist the client and family in acknowledging, accepting, and adjusting to the speech limitations.

In instances of nonorganic cases, the client also may not achieve "perfect" articulation even though the necessary physical and mental capacities seem to be present. There may be unknown organic deficits, or the client simply may not have the need or desire to achieve the goal set by the clinician. In this instance the speech-language pathologist should employ all feasible techniques for attaining the terminal objective of correct articulation but should not become frustrated or feel dejected because of failure to achieve the present goal. Not ev-ery person in the clinician's potential case-load will achieve perfect or even acceptable articulation.

Use a modified programmed behavioral treatment plan

Experience of the authors indicates that a modified programmed behavioral treatment plan is efficient and effective and that most approaches to treatment can be adapted to it. For example, even though McDonald (1964) and Van Riper (1972) did not formally develop behavioral programs, their approaches are easily adaptable to the method, as are others. Our treatment plan also includes meaningful experiential interaction. This type of interaction is especially helpful during the transfer and maintenance stages of treatment because the responses of the client are elicited in relation to meaningful interaction.

The modified programmed treatment plan does not eliminate a humanistic component or some other modifications since the clinical sessions involve interaction between two or more people. The clinician can be, and in most cases should be, warm, that is, "human," in carrying out the behavioral program. Gerber (1977) also contends that using programming principles greatly increases both the efficiency and effectiveness. The articulation treatment must encourage success by building on what the client can do and introducing new skills gradually while providing positive reinforcement and pleasant, meaningful experiences for the client. Below are some requirements of a programmed behavioral treatment plan (Collins and Cunningham, 1976):

1. Make sure the client has prerequisite behaviors before initiating the program. Examples are: demonstrating the concepts of "same" and "different," maintaining eye contact, and attending to the clinician.
2. Write the objectives in behavioral terms, i.e., they must be observable and measurable. An objective should specify exactly what the client is to do, under what circumstances, and how well (criterion for performance).
3. Specify small, logically-sequenced steps

which eventually lead to a final objective. A criterion level should be set for each step. Do not move on to the next step until the current one is completed. If the current step seems unachievable, add a branching or intermediate step to the program.

4. Specify the type of positive reinforcement and schedule for providing reinforcement for correct responses. Types of reinforcement include food, drink, tokens, social, e.g., "good," smile, pat on the hand, and ringing a bell. A clinician may choose to ignore or punish incorrect responses by saying "no" or "that's not right," taking away a token, or giving a

"black" mark. This is a way of providing feedback to the client.*

Use a minimum of motivational devices

At one time speech-language pathologists spent a great deal of time devising "games" and other motivational devices to make speech fun. Unfortunately this sometimes

---

*Adapted from Collins, P., and Cunningham, G.: Writing individualized programs, a workbook for speech pathologists, Gladstone, Oreg., 1978, C. C. Publications.

Name _____

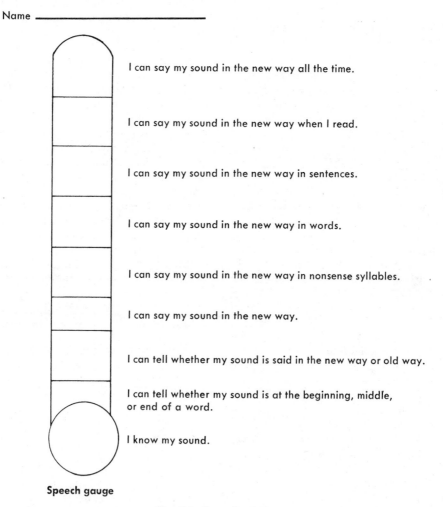

I can say my sound in the new way all the time.

I can say my sound in the new way when I read.

I can say my sound in the new way in sentences.

I can say my sound in the new way in words.

I can say my sound in the new way in nonsense syllables.

I can say my sound in the new way.

I can tell whether my sound is said in the new way or old way.

I can tell whether my sound is at the beginning, middle, or end of a word.

I know my sound.

Speech gauge

Fig. 7-1. Speech gauge.

results in inefficiency as the number of responses per unit time was minimal and often the game became more important than the speech. It now seems unnecessary to use so many of these devices to motivate clients to learn. This does not mean that clinical sessions should be drudgery; they should still be enjoyable, but not solely through the use of games. After all, the basic objective is using good articulation, which should not be obscured by just playing games. However, it is easier to "play" with a child than to "work" with a child, so this attitude of "play" might be preserved in treatment sessions that stress meaningful interaction. Effective reinforcement can be used to maintain the desire to improve articulation skills, and hopefully the client will become intrinsically motivated to work on articulation. It often is helpful to explain the sequential steps so that the client understands the need for the drill work at the various stages. There are ways of illustrating the sequence to even young children (Fig. 7-1). Having the client record daily progress on a chart also involves the person in the articulation program and provides a way of following self-progress. As a colleague of ours once said, the ultimate goal is "speech for speech sake" rather than "games for speech sake." "Motivation should be harnessed to good speech, not irrelevant to it" (Powers, 1971).

Elicit sounds in the simplest way

When teaching a client to produce a particular phoneme, use few and simple directions. Obviously the easiest way is to instruct the client to imitate the clinician's model. If this procedure is not successful after a few trials and if the phoneme is a visible one, a technique such as having the client look in the mirror and imitating the clinician's oral movements should be used. Other fairly simple procedures are to manipulate the client's tongue with a tongue blade, move the articulators from a sound the client can produce to the target sound, show pictures illustrating placement of the articulators, and with a tongue depressor, touch the points of two articulators that should contact one another when the sound is produced. Providing verbal directions for placement of the articulators may be effective if they are not too complex. Unfortunately often such directions are unclear, lengthy, and confusing. The rationale for this principle is that the motor movements must eventually become automatic, but if the elicitation procedure is too complex, the automatization process will be more difficult, if not impossible. A person who had received articulation treatment for an /r/ distortion reported that after 30 years it was still necessary to consciously place the articulators for /r/ because of having been taught to produce the sound through complex directions.

Elicit as many client responses as possible per unit of time

The purpose of a clinical session is to provide maximum opportunity for speech practice. A modified programmed approach helps meet this guideline. Clinical activities should be preplanned and the materials should be organized and ready for use so that clinical time is not devoted to deciding what to do and to gathering materials. If equipment is used, it should be in working order and checked prior to the session. Clinical activities should be simple to explain and to understand; otherwise valuable time will be spent answering questions and giving further explanations. Fairly rapid presentation of stimuli and provision of reinforcement results in eliciting more responses. It also keeps the client alert and attentive to the task, providing little opportunity to engage in off-task behavior. It is helpful to provide reinforcements that consume little time. For example, coloring a picture or working a puzzle can be quite time-consuming, whereas licking a sticker or taking a drink of juice is not. Setting time limits for reinforcement activities can alleviate the time problem. These are but a few suggestions for helping the client practice articulation skills as often as possible during the session.

Continuously assess the client's articulation problem and progress

Assessment of the client's articulation should extend throughout the treatment process, allowing for appraisal of the client's progress (Skinner and Shelton, 1978). This ongoing assessment provides a basis for changing the treatment procedures if progress is not commensurate with clinician expectations or if client responses indicate that a different approach would be more effective. The speech-language pathologist needs to be flexible and to modify methods when necessary in relation to the client's progress. This does not mean that treatment should be changed at the "whim" of the clinician, but occasionally plans do need to be changed when indicated by continuing reevaluation of the client. Progress should be measured in reference to the obtained baseline.

Include work on transfer and maintenance

Transfer refers to using the newly learned behavior in situations different from those in which it was learned. Maintenance refers to continuing use of the learned behavior. These two processes are commonly called carry-over. In articulation programming, carry-over refers to using the correct sound in other settings with other people for the rest of the client's life. After correct sound production is acquired, carry-over must occur for the treatment program to be considered successful. However, sometimes the latter stages of transfer and maintenance are ignored by the clinician. This wastes previous treatment time for both client and clinician.

The client must be an active participant in the treatment process

With the possible exception of very young children or of persons with extremely limited intellectual capacity, the client must be actively involved in the treatment process in order for it to be successful. The clinician must know how the client perceives the problem (Eisenson and Ogilvie, 1977). There should be a cooperative interaction between the client and the speech-language pathologist such that the former is active and informed, aware of the nature of the speech problem, the steps involved in the learning process, and the progress being made. Active participation can be aided through a fairly rapid pace of stimuli presentation, by varying the rhythm or flow of the sessions, and by making the treatment interesting and pleasant. The clinician needs to present the material and provide reinforcement enthusiastically rather than in a bored, routine manner. Such attitudes may be transferred to the client.

The tasks the client is to perform should not be too difficult or too easy. The overall correct responding rate should probably be somewhere in the range of 80% to 95%. The client can be aware of the progress rate by counting the number of correct and incorrect responses, charting the percentage of correct responses, and checking off treatment steps as they are accomplished. The clinician can require the client to self-evaluate responses rather than relying on the clinician's judgments. Gerber (1977) believes that evaluation of responses by the client is more effective than the outside assessment by the clinician. Group sessions may also encourage active involvement. The clinician can and should manipulate the clinical sessions to include the client actively in the treatment process.

Involve parents, siblings, teacher, and spouse in treatment process

As indicated in Chapter 4, inappropriate attitudes and reactions of important persons toward the client's speech may cause articulation disorders. Therefore, counseling these people becomes an important part of the management of the client's articulation problem. Additionally this will likely aid in the carry-over process. The articulation clinician should inform concerned persons about the nature of the disorder and frequently provide guidelines as to what they can do to aid in remediation (Skinner and Shelton, 1978). Every effort should be made to guide them to be supportive and encouraging of the client's efforts, that is, to be constructive in their interest and activity. The counseling can be done on an occasional basis or can be quite intensive, depending on the individual case (see Chapter 9). The amount of involvement of other persons in the treatment varies with such factors as severity of the problem, stage of treatment, quality of the client-person relationship, and motivation and intelligence of the concerned person. In many cases a parent or other concerned persons can become very much a part of the treatment program by observing the clinician at work with the child, preferably through a one-way mirror. A parent or other person in the room with the child and clinician often will distract the child, but in some instances and at selected times this can be done. Often there is a tendency to keep parents away from the treatment, but the opposite should be the case as often as possible (Lillywhite, 1948).

The clinician must be a humanist and artist as well as a scientist

Since the treatment process involves two or more people, the clinician needs to establish a relationship that will facilitate changes in the client's speech. Generally this is spoken of as "rapport building," which means development of an understanding, accepting, and warm relationship. Since what is known about disordered articulation is incomplete and imprecise and since no two problems are alike, clinicians must be creative in dealing with individual clients. Such creativity should be based on scientific information and certainly will be influenced by the clinician's educational and training background, as well as past experiences (Bloodstein, 1979). Perhaps someday research will identify, with greater certainty, which treatment procedures are most effective with which types of clients; however, until that time the speech-language pathologist must make creative use of clinical impressions, judgments, and intuition to strengthen those treatment procedures that have been most productive in the

past. In order to be an effective and efficient clinician, one must be a scientist, humanist, and artist.

SPECIAL CONSIDERATIONS

Some diagnostic categories may determine which treatment approach is selected by the speech-language pathologist. One such differentiation is phonetic versus phonemic errors. For example, a phonetic error is one in which there is an inability to produce motorically such a sound. This is likely to happen in dysarthrias, dyspraxias, facial and oral structural deviancies, oral sensory deficits, and possibly some nonorganic cases. Phonemic errors are those in which the individual motorically can produce the correct sounds but has not mastered the sound system of the language, that is, the phonologic or cognitive rules (Perkins, 1978; Winitz, 1969). These errors may be present in auditory perceptual deficits and in many nonorganic cases. It is difficult to state generalities about causes of phonetic and phonemic errors since each client must be evaluated on an individual basis and since a particular client can display both phonetic and phonemic errors. Certain treatment approaches seem best suited for phonetic errors, whereas others are more helpful for phonemic errors, as will be pointed out in Chapter 9.

A second diagnostic differentiation relates to delayed versus deviant articulation. Leonard (1973) has described the difference between the two types. Delayed articulation refers to following the normal sequence of development, but at a slower rate. The system used is less mature than the adult system. Examples of "normal" misarticulations are [w/r], [θ/s], [b/v], and [f/θ]. Children in this category with normal intelligence and without other deficits usually will acquire normal articulation without intervention, but not always. Deviant articulation cases are those in which a normal pattern of development is not followed; that is, the misarticulations are different from those of children in the normal process of articulation development. Commonly deviant articulation errors involve frequent omission of the distinctive features of [+strident], [−anterior], and [+continuant] and inappropriate use of a feature. In other words the 10-year-old child does not correctly produce sounds that are produced in the back of the mouth. Examples are omissions of sounds, lateralized sibilants, and [t/s]. Individuals who show such disordered articulation usually will not spontaneously correct their errors. Leonard (1973) urges that individuals with deviant articulation patterns be given priority for treatment over persons with delayed articulation. The opposite may be indicated in certain cases, however.

Third the speech-language pathologist needs to differentiate developmental dyspraxia* from dysarthria, language disorder, and nonorganic misarticulation, although this is a difficult task. In developmental dyspraxia articulation treatment can be an arduous process. It seems that an inordinate amount of treatment time is required, often with little improvement; progress is especially slow when moving from isolated words or monosyllabic words to the more complex sequencing tasks of phrases, sentences, and conversation (Yoss and Darley, 1974). "Even with intense stimulation by the clinician the children experience persistent difficulty repeating phonemes and words" (Chappell, 1973). Traditional articulation treatment does not seem to be effective with dyspraxic children. Some general principles and treatment techniques have appeared in the literature; they are presented in the following chapter. It is sufficient to say here that it is critical to diagnose differentially developmental dyspraxia in order to plan effective treatment.

TREATMENT OPTIONS

After making the diagnosis of articulation disorder and after determining a need for

*Here we are referring to dyspraxia in children rather than acquired apraxia in adults. (See Chapter 4 for a listing of the diagnostic characteristics of developmental dyspraxia.)

articulation treatment, the speech-language pathologist must select a treatment approach and design a program to implement it with a consideration of the principles identified in the preceding paragraphs. Three decisions need to be made at this point: (1) How many sounds will be taught at a time? (2) Which sound(s) will be taught first? and (3) Will specific auditory training be done? Usually treatment is begun with work on two phonemes if they are cognates of one another, for example, /s/ and /z/ or /t/ and /d/. When carry-over on the first sound is occurring, work can begin on a second one while continuing with the transfer stage of the first. One possible exception to the recommendation of working with only one sound at a time is with adults or older children who may be more motivated and better able to handle three or more sounds at a time (Johnson and associates, 1967). More than one sound may also be worked on at a time when the treatment approach specifies so, for example, motokinesthetic (Young and Hawk, 1938) and multiple-sound (McCabe and Bradley, 1975) articulation approaches, which are described later.

There are several criteria to aid in selection of phonemes. We previously mentioned that it is advisable to begin with a phonemic pair that is relatively easy for clients to produce. Some of the following criteria are related to that guideline, but others are concerned with client desires and the contribution of phonemes to improving communication.

Error phoneme that is the earliest to develop

Phonemes appearing earliest in speech development are often presumed to be the easiest to produce. This is not always the case among children.

Error phoneme that is the most stimulable

If a phoneme can be produced correctly with auditory stimulation and possibly some instruction, it probably is not difficult for the client to learn and would be a good place to begin. Occasionally a phoneme is quite stimulable, such as /s/ in a person who has tongue thrust, but carry-over can be very difficult if the abnormal swallowing is not simultaneously corrected.

Error phoneme that is produced correctly in a key word

Van Riper (1972) suggests that the diagnostician listen to the client speak spontaneously and note any words in which the misarticulated sound is produced correctly. Such words are called key words. Elicitation of the sound then can begin with a key word. McDonald (1964) developed a similar approach in which work on the error sound begins in a phonetic context (two words) in which the sound was produced correctly as determined by A Deep Test of Articulation (p. 121) (McDonald, 1968).

Error phoneme that occurs most frequently in speech

Certain sounds occur often in the English language, whereas others seldom are used. The Weiss Comprehensive Articulation Test (W-CAT) lists the relative frequency of English phonemes. Those that are used frequently usually contribute more to intelligibility and therefore are more important to communication. It is advisable to select an error sound that if corrected will improve intelligibility most. For example, correction of /s/, relative frequency of 5.04%, is more critical to intelligibility than /ʃ/, which has a relative frequency of 0.88%. However, the type of misarticulation is also an important variable in deciding with which sound to begin.

Error phoneme that is most consistent

It is generally assumed that those sounds that are most consistently misarticulated are the ones in greatest need of treatment. Those error sounds that are inconsistently produced are more frequently corrected through maturation. For this reason the error sound that is most consistently misarticulated should be considered a high priority for selection in treatment.

Error phoneme that is visible

The production of some phonemes can be easily seen by watching the speaker's mouth, whereas the production of others cannot. Examples of the former are bilabials, labiodentals, linguadentals, and lingua-alveolars. Examples of sound types that are not visible are glides and linguavelars. It is usually easier to teach the visible sounds first because visual as well as auditory stimulation can be used.

Error phoneme for which the client has been most criticized or penalized

Many clients have received negative reactions for misarticulating particular sounds because of the conspicuousness of the errors. A frontal lisp, nasalized production of /s/ and /z/, and a [w/r] substitution, along with facial contortions, are examples of articulation and associated errors that may be conspicuous to listeners and result in teasing, frowning, or other undesirable listener reactions. If a client corrects such errors, self-concept and attitudes toward speech should be enhanced.

Error phoneme that the client most desires to correct

Sometimes a client has a preference for beginning with a particular phoneme. This may be a sound that occurs in the client's name or address and therefore is used frequently, or it may be an error sound that has brought the most negative reactions. There are a number of other reasons for such client desires, and the speech-language pathologist should certainly consider them when deciding where to start.

Error phoneme whose production is least affected by physical deviations

There are many instances in which articulation skills are complicated by organic factors. Again, ease of production is important in deciding where to start; therefore, physical complications must be considered. For example, it often is easier for clients with cleft palate to produce nonpressure sounds than pressure sounds. Children whose upper central incisors are missing will probably experience less difficulty with sounds other than /s/ and /z/.

Error phoneme that is the same for a group of clients

In some clinical settings, especially schools, articulation treatment may be administered to a small group of clients. The selection of a sound that is misarticulated by all members of a group has some advantages in that all would work on the same sound at the same time.

Much has been written about the relationship between speech sound discrimination and articulation skills. Various opinions are held regarding whether or not to include discrimination training as part of the treatment for articulation disorders. Van Riper (1972) generally recommends it for all "functional" articulation cases; Winitz (1975) advocates it for many clients, but not all; and McDonald (1964) does not recommend it for any. The rationale for auditory training for better discrimination is that, according to feedback theory, speech is learned through the ear. A person has to hear a sound several times before all its features are perceived. In other words the client must be able to detect not only the error but also the correct sound before attempting to produce it. On the other hand the rationale for not using auditory training is that individuals usually can learn to produce correct sounds without it. In fact discrimination between correct and incorrect productions is probably learned during production training when the clinician provides feedback as to the correctness of the sound produced. Also, proceeding directly to production training seems to be more efficient. Perhaps the question should be one of providing specific auditory training or the typical auditory training that automatically accompanies all sound production training.

Before deciding whether or not to use auditory training, research results should be studied. Studies on the relationship between speech sound discrimination and articulation have been conflicting and inconclusive, but individuals with deviant articulation seem to have poorer speech discrimination ability (Johnson and associates, 1967; Powers, 1971; Winitz, 1977). Winitz (1977) and McReynolds, Kohn and Williams (1975) reported that some studies have shown that children have difficulty discriminating only the phonemes they misarticulate. Winitz (1975) recommends that discrimination be tested only for error sounds, not for those already produced correctly. Monnin and Huntington (1974) found that their kindergarten subjects who misarticulated /r/ did not accurately identify /r/ and /w/, whereas normal kindergartners did. Wolfe and Irwin (1973) found that children who misarticulated /r/ have difficulty discriminating their own misarticulations from the correct sound as produced by another speaker; however, they have no difficulty with the task when comparing their own tape-recorded misarticulations with correct productions of other speakers. Therefore, these authors recommend that children learn to compare accurately their own errors with correct sound production rather than receiving training in discriminating errors produced by other speakers. In contrast McReynolds, Kohn, and Williams (1975) found that children with multiple articulation errors discriminated their error sounds fairly accurately and thus question the use of discrimination training for articulation-defective children.

Some research has been done to determine if discrimination training has any effect on misarticulations and if production training has any effect on discrimination ability. Shelton and associates (1978) found that there was no difference in articulation skills between preschool children trained by their parents in speech sound discrimination and children who received no such training. Williams and McReynolds (1975) found that discrimination training improved discrimination ability but not production of sounds. Conversely production training improved both articulation and discrimination skills. They hypothesized that during production training discrimination work is simultaneously occurring because the client receives feedback on both the acoustic and articulatory aspects of productions. Also the client is hearing a model of correct sounds and compares his own production with that model; therefore, production training may be sufficient to train discrimination. However, Winitz (1975) contends that discrimination training will improve articulation if the distinctive features of the misarticulated sound are in the repertoire of the individual and if the training is extensive and carefully carried out.

Each speech-language pathologist must consider the preceding information in view of the fact that testing self-discrimination is extremely difficult and then decide whether or not to incorporate specific auditory training in articulation treatment. It would not seem to be efficient to spend much time on auditory training with individuals who can already discriminate their misarticulation from the correct sound, especially if self-monitoring skills are good. Testing must be done to determine this. It is probably more expedient to teach the client to discriminate between the error sound and the correct sound than to teach general discrimination skills. If discrimination work is done, the sounds should be presented in sentences in addition to isolation and individual words. It also seems feasible to incorporate auditory training with production work, that is, clients should be asked to evaluate their own productions during the latter stages of treatment. Whether or not specific auditory training is done and how it is done will be determined by the treatment approach selected and the needs of the client.

GENERAL PHASES OF ARTICULATION TREATMENT

Even though there are different treatment approaches, some general stages exist. A discussion of these stages follows.

Elimination of or minimizing causative factors

This stage is applicable to some clients in whom changes can be made to allow for ar-

ticulation skills to develop. This step usually precedes clinical intervention, but it may also be done concurrently.

Discrimination training

This stage is not a part of all treatment approaches, but when specific auditory training is done, it precedes production training. It may also occur concurrently with treatment.

Acquisition or production

At this stage of treatment the client learns to produce the sound correctly in a variety of contexts. It may begin with production of the phoneme in isolation and proceed to nonsense syllables, words, phrases, sentences, and conversation. This stage is generally conducted in the clinical setting. The client should achieve automatic, rather than deliberate, production at each level before moving to the next higher level.

Transfer or generalization

After production is strengthened, transfer should occur. This stage involves using the sound in connected speech in the clinical setting, outside the clinical setting, with the clinician, and with others. Here the client transfers correct articulation to everyday speaking situations.

Maintenance or habituation

This is the last stage of treatment in which the client habitually uses correct articulation patterns in all situations over a long period of time. Whether or not the treatment program is successful depends on retention or automatization of the responses learned in the clinical setting. The clinician periodically should recheck the client's speech to ensure that the new behaviors are retained and that carry-over has in fact occurred. If articulation skills do not become automatic, they tend to revert back to earlier error patterns.

These stages are not separate and distinct; they are overlapping. How each stage is accomplished varies with the particular treatment approach used and the individual clients and clinicians involved.

SUMMARY

Articulation is a subsystem of language and occurs concurrently with the use of other language systems. Thus articulation treatment involves all categories of language but emphasizes phonology. It is also a part of the communication process that contributes greatly to the intelligibility of a message. There is a wide range of articulation patterns that are within the normal limits of acceptability depending on the dialect, the speaking situation, and the age of the individual. Not every person who has misarticulations needs articulation treatment. Need is dependent on the social, cultural, ethnic, and occupational environment of the individual, family attitudes toward the speech problem, and the nature of the articulation deficiency.

There are some general principles to be followed in articulation treatment that help to plan for each client on an individual basis that use a modified programmed approach. We recommend that treatment be planned by taking into special consideration the diagnostic categories of phonemic versus phonetic errors, delayed versus deviant articulation, and organic versus nonorganic causes. Before implementing a treatment plan, the speech-language pathologist needs to decide how many sounds or features to work on at a time, which sound(s) or rules to work on, and whether or not to incorporate specific auditory training into the treatment program. There are five general stages of articulation treatment: (1) elimination of or minimizing causative factors, (2) discrimination training, (3) acquisition or production, (4) transfer or generalization, and (5) maintenance or habituation. Methods of providing treatment will be discussed in Chapter 9.

STUDY SUGGESTIONS

1. Discuss and compare ways in which treatment of articulation disorders relates to treatment of language disorders.
2. Describe and evaluate the relative importance of factors that determine whether or not misarticulations need treatment.
3. In what ways do the preceding factors influence treatment procedures and prognosis?
4. Relate normal articulation and deviant articulation to "other aspects of communication," as discussed in this chapter and to treatment procedures and anticipated results.
5. List and defend the most important treatment options.
6. Explain and give a rationale for the statement, "The clinician must be a humanist and artist as well as scientist."

REFERENCES

Bloodstein, O.: Speech pathology: an introduction, Boston, 1979, Houghton Mifflin Co.

Byrne, M., and Shervanian, C.: Introduction to communicative disorders, New York, 1977, Harper & Row, Publishers.

Chappell, G.: Childhood verbal apraxia and its treatment, J. Speech Hear. Disord. 38:362-368, 1973.

Collins, P., and Cunningham, G.: Writing individualized programs, a workbook for speech pathologists, Gladstone, Oreg., 1978, C. C. Publications.

DiCarlo, L.: Communication therapy for problems associated with cerebral palsy. In Dickson, S., editor: Communication disorders, remedial principles and practices, Glenview, Ill., 1974, Scott, Foresman and Co.

Dickson, S., editor: Communication disorders, remedial principles and practices, Glenview, Ill., 1974, Scott, Foresman and Co.

Dickson, S., and Fann, G.: Diagnostic principles and procedures. In Dickson, S., editor: Communication disorders, remedial principles and practices, Glenview, Ill., 1974, Scott, Foresman and Co.

Eisenson, J., and Ogilvie, M.: Speech correction in the schools, ed. 4, New York, 1977, Macmillan Publishing Co., Inc.

Gerber, A.: Programming for articulation modification, J. Speech Hear. Disord. 42:29-43, 1977.

Johnson, W., and associates: Speech handicapped school children, ed. 3, New York, 1967, Harper & Row, Publishers.

Leonard, L.: The nature of deviant articulation, J. Speech Hear. Disord. 38:156-161, 1973.

Lillywhite, H.: Make mother a clinician, J. Speech Hear. Disord. 13:61-66, 1948.

Mager, R.: Preparing instructional objectives, Palo Alto, 1962, Fearon Publishers.

McCabe, R., and Bradley, D.: Systematic multiple phonemic approach to articulation therapy, Acta Symbolica 6:1-18, 1975.

McDonald, E.: Articulation testing and treatment, a sensory-motor approach, Pittsburgh, 1964, Stanwix House, Inc.

McDonald, E.: A Deep Test of Articulation, Pittsburgh, 1968, Stanwix House, Inc.

McReynolds, L., Kohn, J., and Williams, G.: Articulatory-defective children's discrimination of their production errors, J. Speech Hear. Disord. 40:327-338, 1975.

Monnin, L., and Huntington, D.: Relationship of articulatory defects to speech sound identification, J. Speech Hear. Disord. **17:**352-366, 1974.

Mowrer, D., Wahl, P., and Doolan, S.: Effect of lisping on audience evaluation of male speakers, J. Speech Hear. Disord. **43:**140-148, 1978.

Perkins, W.: Speech pathology: an applied behavioral science, ed. 2, St. Louis, 1977, The C. V. Mosby Co.

Perkins, W.: Human perspectives in speech and language disorders, St. Louis, 1978, The C. V. Mosby Co.

Powers, M.: Functional disorders of articulation: symptomatology and etiology. In Travis, L., editor: Handbook of speech pathology and audiology, New York, 1971, Appleton-Century-Crofts.

Shelton, R., and associates: Assessment of parent-administered listening training for preschool children with articulation and language deficits, J. Speech Hear. Disord. **43:**242-254, 1978.

Shewan, C.: Speech and language disorders, selected readings, New York, 1978, Harper & Row, Publishers.

Silverman, E.: Listeners' impressions of speakers with lateral lisps, J. Speech Hear. Disord. **41:**547-552, 1976.

Skinner, P., and Shelton, R.: Speech, language, and hearing: normal processes and disorders, Reading, Mass., 1978, Addison-Wesley Publishing Co., Inc.

Sommers, R., and Kane, A.: Nature and remediation of functional articulation disorders. In Dickson, S., editor: Communication disorders: remedial principles and practices, Glenview, Ill., 1974, Scott, Foresman and Co.

Van Riper, C.: Speech correction principles and methods, ed. 5, Englewood Cliffs, N.J., 1972, Prentice-Hall, Inc.

Weiner, F.: Phonological process analysis, Baltimore, 1979, University Park Press.

Williams, G., and McReynolds, L.: The relationship between discrimination and articulation training in children with misarticulations, J. Speech Hear. Disord. **18:**401-412, 1975.

Winitz, H.: Articulatory acquisition and behavior, New York, 1969, Appleton-Century-Crofts.

Winitz, H.: From syllable to conversation, Baltimore, 1975, University Park Press.

Winitz, H.: Articulation disorders: from prescription to description, J. Speech Hear. Disord. **42:**143-147, 1977.

Wolfe, V., and Irwin, R.: Sound discrimination ability of children with misarticulation of the /r/ sound, Percept. Mot. Skills **37:**415-420, 1973.

Yoss, K., and Darley, F.: Therapy in developmental apraxia of speech, Lang. Speech Hear. Serv. Schools **5:**23-31, 1974.

Young, E., and Hawk, S.: Moto-kinesthetic speech training, Stanford, Calif., 1938, Stanford University Press.

GLOSSARY

acquisition Used here to refer to a client's first use of a target sound in the process of treatment or, more broadly, to a child's first use (acquisition) of developing sounds.

auditory stimulation Motivation (stimulation) of a client through auditory channels to try to learn and reproduce target sounds.

auditory training Teaching of specific sounds or of broader sound patterns through auditory channels.

developmental dyspraxia A condition in which a developmental deficiency in the central nervous system seems to result in inaccurate, uncontrolled voluntary movements of the articulatory organs. (*See also* Dyspraxia.)

discrimination A process in articulation training in which the client is helped to discriminate one sound from another and among several sounds.

labiodental Lips and teeth acting in conjunction to produce sounds. Sometimes a label given to specific sounds produced largely by lips and teeth in contact, such as /f/ and /v/.

lingua-alveolar Tongue and alveolar ridge acting in conjunction to produce sounds. Sometimes a label given to specific sounds produced by tongue and alveolar ridge functioning together, such as /t/ and /d/.

linguadental Tongue and teeth acting in conjunction to produce sounds. Sometimes a label given to specific sounds produced by tongue and teeth functioning together, such as /t/ and /s/.

maintaining causative factors Conditions (factors) that continue to cause or maintain articulatory problems, such as severe malocclusion.

maintenance Carry-over and continuing use of corrected sounds.

motokinesthetic A specific approach to articulatory training utilizing manipulation of motor and kinesthetic functions of the articulators in the treatment of error phonemes.

CHAPTER EIGHT

Types of articulation treatment

"Nothing is more useful than to speak clearly."
PHAEDRUS

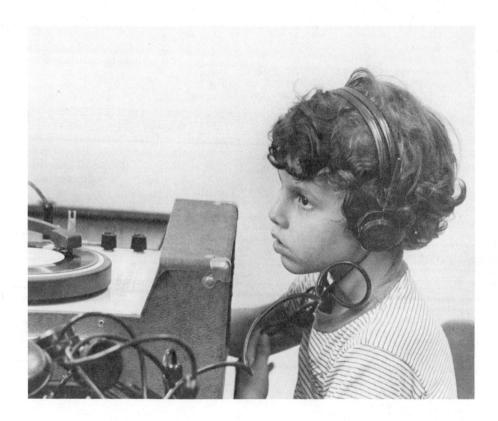

Various treatment approaches for articulation treatment have been used over the years, beginning with the phonetic placement approach of the 1920s and continuing to those currently being developed in terms of phonologic processes. All of the approaches imply the existence of a treatment sequence: planning, establishment or learning the sound, transfer or generalization, and maintenance or stabilization. Although these common elements exist, different rationales and philosophies relative to the nature and causes of articulation disorders have influenced the specific procedures and techniques that were devised for each approach.

The treatment methods described are generally presented in a chronologic order according to the time period when each was developed. They have been divided into (1) early approaches and (2) recent approaches. The more recent approaches clearly outline what the client is to do in treatment, under what conditions, and how well (Mager, 1962). More concise behavioral goals, objectives, and procedures have been developed to facilitate observing, counting, measuring, charting, and reporting progress. Some approaches specify the type of reinforcement, baseline data, and rationale underlying treatment procedures.

Descriptions of each of the following approaches include the developer's rationale or philosophy, actual goals and procedures utilized, and additional comments. Most of the methods have been described in terms of administering treatment to children, although certainly in most instances adaptations can easily be made for adults. Preferences have heretofore been an individualistic matter; however, we would like to suggest the possibility of some approaches being more effective for some clients than for others.

EARLY APPROACHES

Perhaps the first treatment approach was the phonetic placement approach developed by Scripture (1923) and Scripture and Jackson (1927). In this method the client is given general speech exercises to perform and is instructed in the specific placement of the articulators to produce various speech sounds.

Rationale

According to Scripture (1923), in order to move the speech organs correctly, a person must feel the movements and hear the sounds while producing them. An individual with an articulation deviancy must develop the ability to place the articulators in whatever position necessary for speech purposes and, consequently, must have complete control over them. The client, then, must attend to and consciously position the articulation structures and control articulation movements. An implicit assumption of this approach is that each sound is always produced in the same way using the same placement (Powers, 1971). Thus the role of the clinician is to teach the client "to carefully correct his faults" (Scripture, 1923). Tongue exercises are especially recommended for generally indistinct speech, and breathing and relaxation exercises are recommended for those who appear to be tense. Tongue and lip exercises and procedures for strengthening the velar musculature are to be used with "organic" disorders. Scripture emphasizes that correction of articulation deficits is important to a person's social and mental development and well-being; thus an individual with articulation deviancies should receive training in articulation skills.

Goals and procedures

The implicit goal of the phonetic placement approach is correct articulation of all sounds. Production of the sound begins in isolation and progresses through syllables, words, sentences, and prepared dialogue (Sommers and Kane, 1974). General relaxation, breathing, tongue, and lip exercises are performed by the client. Various techniques and devices, including the following, are utilized to demonstrate to the client where to place the articulators and how to direct the breath stream.

1. Tongue blades and sticks to manipulate or hold articulators in place
2. Manipulation of articulators with clinician's fingers
3. Verbal description and instruction
4. Breath indicator for mouth and nose
5. Graphic records, for example, spectrogram
6. Feeling breath stream with hand or seeing effects of breath stream on a tissue
7. Observing clinician and self in mirror while producing sounds
8. Feeling laryngeal vibration
9. Observing diagrams, pictures, or drawings of articulators while producing certain sounds
10. Observing palatograms of articulators while producing certain sounds

Scripture (1923) suggested using a "velar hook" (a sticklike device that is bent on one end to form a hook) to strengthen soft palate muscles in persons with too much nasal emission of air. There are probably other techniques that have been devised by speech-language pathologists, but the preceding list gives an indication of the sorts of procedures that are used. Van Riper (1978) states that when using the phonetic placement approach the client should understand exactly which tongue, lip, and jaw positions should be assumed before attempting the target sound. When produced correctly, the sound should be strengthened (that is, repeated) immediately many times with no distractions.

Comment

The phonetic placement approach can be implemented on either an individual or group basis and with either children or adults, although Scripture (1923) encourages early intervention. Specific instructions and techniques need to be adapted to fit the level and needs of a particular client. Scripture indicates that the approach can be used with any articulation-disordered client. Van Riper (1978) suggests that the approach is especially useful for hearing-impaired individuals and for cases in which

other sound elicitation procedures are unsuccessful.

Advantages of this approach are that it is faster than other methods in eliciting sounds in some clients and that it is useful in teaching compensatory articulation movements (Johnson and associates, 1967). Disadvantages are that it is a less direct procedure for producing sounds than others, sounds are less stable at first, and articulation placement of a sound varies with the phonemes that precede or follow it (Johnson and associates, 1967; Powers, 1971). Also the mechanics of phonetic placement require so much attention from the client that a sound taught in this way cannot be produced quickly or unconsciously in conversational speech (Van Riper, 1978).

MOTOKINESTHETIC APPROACH

Motokinesthetic articulation treatment was developed by Young and Hawk (1938) in the 1930s. It is an approach in which parts of the client's speech mechanism, especially the articulators, are directly manipulated externally (outside the mouth, jaw, and neck regions) by the speech-language pathologist.

Rationale

Young and Hawk (1938) emphasize that the air current from the lungs is the source of speech production and that this air current is acted on by muscles to produce sounds. The sounds are not produced in isolation, but in a sequence. In normal speakers the muscles of the speech mechanism produce an easy flow of movements proceeding from one sound to the next. Articulation learning requires coordination of muscular activities used in speech, control of the air current, and other facial expression. Individuals who have misarticulations need to learn the "feel" of articulation movements. Through the clinician's manipulations and productions of the sounds, the client associates the articulation movements with the auditory input and learns to articulate sounds. The client reproduces the articulation movements through the kinesthetic sense. It is assumed that positive kin-esthetic and tactile feedback is established by having the clinician manipulate the client's articulators (Sommers and Kane, 1974).

Goals and procedures

Young and Hawk's (1938) stated objectives are to prevent incorrect articulation learning and to aid in the correction of mis-articulations. Manipulations by the clinician set the patterns for the location, direction, and form of articulation movements; that is, they indicate where the movement is to occur, in which direction the articulators are to move, and the manner in which the sounds are to be produced. There is a standard stimulation for each sound, and the clinician uses that stimulation each time the sound is to be produced. Thus the speech-language pathologist guides the muscular actions that act on the air current. The sounds so stimulated are produced sequentially, without pausing between sounds. No procedures are given for transferring the client from passive to active sound production and then on to carry-over.

The clinician says the syllables while manipulating the client's articulators; therefore, the client receives kinesthetic, tactile, and auditory stimulations simultaneously. By having the client watch the clinician's face, the visual sense is also utilized. The "feel" of movements is "learned" and becomes associated with auditory input of the clinician. In other words, after the client feels the movements, they can be reproduced through the kinesthetic sense.

Young and Hawk caution that the whole client needs to be considered and that manipulation rarely begins during the first meeting with the client. When using this approach, the client is placed in a supine position so as to facilitate relaxation. The clinician then manipulates the articulators with the "skill of a typist." Sometimes when initially teaching a sound a tongue depressor is used inside the mouth if the standard manipulation is ineffective. The use of the tongue depressor is discontinued

as soon as possible. No auditory discrimination training is done, and sounds are not produced in isolation, but rather in syllables, words, phrases, sentences, and paragraphs. The motokinesthetic stimulations for this method appear in Appendix I.

Comment

The motokinesthetic approach can be used only with individuals, not with groups. It is appropriate for both children and adults. Young and Hawk recommend the approach for the categories of sound substitutions, delayed speech, speechlessness, cleft palate, hard of hearing, deaf, blind, deaf-blind, cerebral palsy, and aphasia and for the development of infant speech. Young and Hawk (1938) give more detailed information about adaptations of the method for various types of clients. Sommers and Kane (1974) indicate that the approach is likely to be most effective with neurologic and motor deficits, for example, cerebral palsy, other dysarthrias, and dyspraxia. We have found manipulations for individual sounds to be useful in comparing and contrasting a target sound with a substitute sound when a client is confused as to when to use each.

Probably the best way for a speech-language pathologist to learn this method is to be trained by one who has skill in using the approach. It would be extremely difficult, if not impossible, to learn to use motokinesthetics by reading the textbook. This is perhaps the primary disadvantage of the approach.

STIMULUS APPROACH

In 1939 Van Riper first formulated what now is generally considered to be the traditional approach to articulation treatment, the stimulus approach. Since then the approach has been revised five times. The last published revision of this approach appeared in 1978, which we will use as the reference here. The stimulus approach emphasizes auditory training, which precedes sound production. After the sound is elicited in isolation, it is produced at various levels by the client through the use of auditory stimulation. The client generally is "bombarded" with auditory stimulation.

Rationale

Van Riper (1978) contends that the basic error in an articulation disorder consists of a misarticulated sound or sounds and that the individual error sound should become the focus of treatment. It is especially difficult for the client to identify and isolate the error sound because production of a sound is brief, varies with the phonetic context, and involves different sensory modalities in the discrimination process. Characteristics of the sound must be made vivid enough to be mastered. Therefore, ear training is emphasized and sound production begins in isolation rather than in more complex articulation movements involved in syllable, word, and sentence production. Van Riper indicates that if the client learns to produce the sound in isolation, syllables, and some words, the tools are there for the client to articulate correctly the error sound in all words in which it occurs.

The treatment process should begin where the client is so that progression through each phase of the recommended program is not necessary; that is, work can begin at any level appropriate to the client's pretreatment skills. The clinician must design a treatment plan but should be flexible enough to make revisions as new information about the client's skills and progress presents itself. Van Riper further indicates that the approach can be programmed according to operant conditioning principles and methods. As a matter of fact, many articulation programs written by others follow Van Riper's principles and techniques.

Goals and procedures

1. To become aware of characteristics of the standard phoneme
2. To recognize characteristics of misarticulations and how they differ from the target sound
3. To produce the standard sounds at will and use them in isolation, syllables, words, phrases, and sentences

4. To use standard sounds in spontaneous speech of all kinds and under all conditions, that is, achieve carry-over

Generally one sound or one pair of cognates is worked on at a time so as not to confuse the client. Characteristics of sounds that are selected for treatment include those that are correct in some phonetic contexts, that require simple coordinations, that are most stimulable, that are earlier-developing, and that the client is motivated to work on. The first two phases of treatment involve auditory training. The first phase deals with identification of the standard sound produced by the clinician; at this time the client does not attempt to produce the "new" sound. From the clinician's productions the client is to locate and isolate the sound and to discriminate it from others. In the second phase of treatment the client listens to himself; that is, it is a "self-hearing" process. The standard sound is discriminated from its error through scanning the client's own speech and comparing it with the standard phoneme production. Initially the clinician signals when errors occur. Progressively the client identifies the error after, during, and before it occurs; that is, progress goes from recalling to perceiving to predicting misarticulations. This phase is to be continued throughout the treatment process since it is critical that the client continuously evaluate his own productions.

The third phase of treatment involves elicitation of the target sound through the process of varying and correcting the client's attempted productions. This phase must be accomplished at all successive phonetic levels and may begin at whichever level is appropriate for the client's skills. Generally production begins at the isolation level. Van Riper describes five alternate methods for evoking the sound:

1. *Progressive approximation,* or shaping, which consists of a series of sounds that progressively, more closely resemble the target sound until it is produced correctly, that is, a gradual shift from a sound the client can produce to the standard sound (Shriberg [1975]

outlined a progressive approximation program for /r/)

2. *Auditory stimulation,* in which the clinician produces the sound several times and instructs the client to imitate

3. *Phonetic placement,* in which various procedures are used to teach the client where to place the articulators and how to direct the breath stream

4. *Modification of other sounds,* in which the client makes a sound and then moves the articulators while continuing to produce the first sound

5. *Key word,* in which work begins on a word where the target sound is correctly articulated

The progressive approximation method seems to be preferred most by Van Riper, whereas phonetic placement is the least preferred.

The fourth phase of treatment is stabilizing the target sound. The "new" sound must be strengthened before it will be produced correctly in conversation. Various techniques for strengthening are suggested, including repetition, prolongation, increasing intensity, whispering, and simultaneous talking and writing. The sound is then evoked and stabilized in successive phonetic levels, that is, syllables, words, phrases, and sentences. This phase includes transfer or carry-over. At this point in treatment the client must develop a feedback system that will scan utterances and automatically identify and correct any errors that occur. Van Riper (1978) gives further information on numerous techniques for achieving the objectives for each phase of the auditory stimulus treatment approach. Some of these techniques include creating key words, slow motion speech, echo speech, unison speech, correcting clinician's production, and role-playing.

Comment

The stimulus approach, or variations of it, seems to be used widely. Carrell (1968), Johnson and associates (1967), and Powers (1971), among others, have described it in their books as the preferred approach to use; however, it has not been particularly effective with dyspraxic children. Although Van Riper's descriptions of treatment sessions imply that it is to be used for individual sessions, it can be easily adapted for group sessions. This approach can also be adapted for use with adults. Advantages seem to be ease and simplicity of use, directness, and absence of distracting or irrelevant cues (Johnson and associates, 1967).

INTEGRAL STIMULATION APPROACH

In 1954 Milisen and associates devised and reported on an articulation treatment program called integral stimulation. In it a client must use all relevant stimuli, including auditory, visual, and perhaps kinesthetic, in order to produce speech sounds correctly. Treatment begins with production rather than with auditory training.

Rationale

Milisen and associates' (1954) basic premise is that deviant articulation results from a disruption in the normal learning process and that it can be corrected if training is appropriate, initiated early enough, and continued long enough. Treatment is based on learning principles appropriate for the skill level of the client. The approach should be positive, rather than negative, that is, it should focus on producing correct responses rather than "unlearning" incorrect responses.

Milisen and associates enumerated four criteria of a good treatment program that they believe their program meets:

1. Should handle all types of articulation deviancies, all age levels, and all environmental and physical limitations

2. Should involve methods, based on learning theory, which are easy to understand and teach, enable successful performance, and challenge the client

3. Should present material in a whole or complete speech response that enables the client to produce it correctly

4. Should not conflict with psychotherapy

According to Milisen and associates (1954), "A speech movement skill cannot be learned until it is produced." Thus the stimulus complex must elicit correct production. In order to elicit a correct response, the stimulus must be vivid for the client. Use of all available sensory stimuli aids in obtaining correct responses. Other techniques such as phonetic placement and tongue and lip exercises fractionalize or "break up" the speech process. One study showed visual-auditory stimulation to be more effective than either visual or auditory stimulation alone. Further, the results of another study showed that large amounts of stimulation resulted in better ability to produce sounds after a time lapse.

This approach is based on the assumption that clients are most strongly motivated if they can see and hear themselves producing the whole sound. Finally features learned while producing easily stimulable sounds are transferred to sounds that were not stimulable at first but later become stimulable because of the success in producing other sounds.

Goals and procedures

Milisen and associates (1954) do not specifically identify goals and procedures. They describe a rather elaborate system for sound selection. Basically, misarticulated sounds are listed in the order of stimulability and in terms of level of distractibility to listeners. Visibility of the sounds, auditory acuity and discrimination abilities, general speech environment (others in child's environment displaying similar misarticulations), organic conditions, and motivational influences are secondary factors to be considered. The treatment process begins with sounds that are more stimulable and progresses to sounds that are less stimulable. If any phonemes remain unstimulable after intensive stimulation, ear training procedures are used or, as a last resort, fractionalizing methods are utilized.

Once a sound is selected, the clinician uses integral stimulation, which includes clinician production of the sound such that the client hears, sees, and perhaps feels it; the client's response, which the clinician sees, hears, and feels; and evaluation of the response by both the clinician and client. The clinician uses every device to make the sound heard and seen. All points of articulation should be made as visible as possible to the client.

Throughout the treatment process the clinician manipulates three variables so that the client is challenged but does not completely fail. Generally two variables are held constant while the third one is being manipulated. The first variable is the amount of assistance needed for the client to produce the speech unit. In other words the clinician varies the amount of stimulation and help given to the client depending on how much is needed to elicit a correct response at a particular stage of treatment. A second variable is the complexity of the speech unit. Treatment begins with easier speech units such as an isolated consonant and proceeds to more complex configurations such as sentences and conversation. The third variable is audience or listener reaction. "Friendly" listeners tend to facilitate more accurate responses, whereas an "unfriendly" audience may cause a client to regress to incorrect speech patterns. At the later stages of treatment the three variables should be at the most adverse level with the client using correct productions. Milisen and associates (1954) believe that success of articulation treatment frequently is dependent on the amount of success experienced with the first sounds worked on since improved speech positively changes the attitudes of the client and persons in the environment. Success with the first sounds provides a model learning pattern and motivation for the client.

Comment

Powers (1971) also recommends a multisensory approach rather than relying only on the auditory modality; however, Powers emphasizes the need for discrimination training, which Milisen and associates (1954) do not. The approach seems adaptable to both group and individual sessions. Milisen contends that his treatment approach is effective with all types of articulation deviancies, age levels, and physical and environmental limitations since the speech-language pathologist can emphasize whatever aspect is appropriate for an individual client.

GROUP APPROACH

Backus (1957) and Backus and Beasley (1951) have devised a method of working with all types of speech deviancies in a group setting. Speech skills are taught through developing interpersonal relationships and group interactions. The clients begin with a speech pattern in a context or situation. The pattern is then "broken down" and finally put back into context. In other words the sequence of working on speech patterns proceeds from whole to part to whole.

Rationale

Backus and Beasley (1951) developed the group approach because their observations showed that speech behavior changes are more dependent on variables of interpersonal relationships between the client and clinician and among a group of clients than on speech drills and ear training. Additional observations revealed that the ability to produce correct speech patterns in structured drill situations does not necessarily carry over to social situations (Backus, 1957). Backus further notes that persons with different types of speech disorders showed some similar behaviors and that persons with the same disorder displayed basic differences; therefore, the use of speech-disordered labels becomes meaningless as does development of special treatment procedures for specific speech disorders. These observations led to development of a group interactive approach rather than an individual drill-type approach. Speech is therefore viewed as an aspect of the total behavior of an individual rather than merely as a motor skill.

Backus and Beasley (1951) made the following assumptions about learning, which apply to speech development as well as to other areas of human development:

1. Learning proceeds from the whole to parts by a process of progressive differentiation
2. Learning involves a process of organization in which the individual must perceive the whole or a patterning of the parts
3. The whole person does the learning

With a consideration of these assumptions, treatment procedures deal with the functional organization, social skills, and speech patterns, thus going from the whole person (functional organization) to parts (social skills) and finally to subparts (speech patterns). The functional organization of a person is comprised of perceptions of self, perceptions of the environment, basic needs, which include a feeling of belongingness and safety, value standards, and techniques for adjusting to the environment. The social skills are adjustive techniques that allow the individual to develop positive interpersonal relationships and that facilitate learning.

The clinician's role in the group approach is based on three assumptions of interpersonal theory (Backus, 1957):

1. Each person does his or her own growing, changing, and learning.
2. An individual will grow and learn unless barriers block the growth.
3. Critical learning variables are contained in interpersonal relationships.

Backus thus defines treatment as "a particular kind of interpersonal process in which at least one of the participants seeks consciously to keep creating the sort of environment in which the other participant can develop his own potentialities to the greatest extent possible at successive points in time." It is not the speech-language pathologist's role to provide psychotherapy, although the two fields interrelate and use some of the same techniques. However, the speech-language pathologist is primarily concerned with speech and language usage and the mechanics of speech production, whereas the psychotherapist deals with other behaviors.

In summary Backus and Beasley's approach (1951) adheres to four treatment principles that evolved from these viewpoints. The first principle is that group instruction should be the core of management. In this way a variety of interpersonal situations and real speaking situations can be structured. The value lies in an optimum situation for meeting individual needs. Second group membership should not be segregated by types of disorders of symptoms. Individual group members are exposed to a range of problems to be solved. The positive aspects of speech are stressed. Third treatment should provide a corrective "emotional" experience. This is not to be construed as psychotherapy. Instead speech is used as a means to create significant interpersonal relationships. Last, treatment should be structured in terms of interpersonal relationships involving conversational speech. The interpersonal relationship comprises the whole, the speech behavior is a functional part of the whole, and the subpart is sound production mechanics.

Goals and procedures

The goal of the speech-language pathologist in this approach is to help individual clients change behavior in interpersonal relationships in order to function more adequately in terms of satisfaction and security. Backus and Beasley (1951) explain that speech is one of the behaviors to be changed in order for speech to be used adequately in social situations.

Goals of the individual client are different at different stages of treatment and are different for each person within a group. The goals revolve around changing the functional organization, social skills, and speech patterns of the clients. The first goal, improving the functional organization of individuals, is achieved by developing a positive psychologic climate by interacting warmly, being relaxed, developing a group structure in which each client is encouraged to participate and will experience acceptance and success, being permissive, accepting feelings, helping clients succeed,

keeping the situation speech-oriented, and setting rational limits. Individual group members contribute to verbal interaction, serve as a model for others, and reinforce others (Sommers and Kane, 1974). Social skills that are to be developed include the ability to follow conventional social patterns, win acceptance and support from others, share attitudes, and develop flexibility in role-taking.

The final goal is speech development. As stated previously, a speech pattern is introduced in context and patterned language is utilized. All group members respond with the same pattern and evaluate one another while the clinician gives directions to aid in production. The correct aspects of speech production are reinforced, and the incorrect aspects are described as needed improvement for the whole group. No techniques for eliciting individual sounds are provided, but repeated experience with selected sounds is provided by using the same response in a variety of situations. The response is one that is used frequently in real-life situations. Sounds are selected on the bases of ease of learning, needs of the group, and frequency of occurrence but not on the basis of developmental order. They often begin with /θ/ and /v/ and later add /s/.

Seven types of interpersonal situations provide the means for achieving the objectives:

1. Experiences in human relatedness occurring in everyday life, for example, greetings, introductions, invitations, asking favors, sharing, and apologizing
2. Specialized experiences in analyzing use of speech by enacting everyday situations and discussing them
3. Specialized experiences in observation of part functions in which speech patterns are observed through the senses and motor patterns and evaluated in terms of the difference between what a person did and what is usually done
4. Specialized experiences in using the method of science in behavior by mak-

ing available tools for observing, evaluating, and solving problems using general semantic principles

5. Specialized experiences in communicating about feelings
6. Experiences in acquiring specific information (applied in skills), for example, telling time, colors, calendar, and arithmetic
7. Experiences in developing certain abilities for pleasure, for example, sewing, singing, card tricks, and sports

A sample lesson is presented in Appendix J to aid in understanding the group approach. Additional samples appear in Backus and Beasley (1951).

Comment

The number of clients per group varies, but Backus and Beasley indicate that eight to ten is an effective number. Subgroup sessions can be scheduled to meet individual needs, or the larger group can be divided into smaller groups during regular sessions. The approach can be used with all age levels, including adults, and with all types of speech disorders. Backus (1957) recommends that levels of locomotion ability, age, and interest levels are important considerations in grouping. She further suggests that at least two members of the same sex should be included in a group rather than only one member of a sex. Short-term intensive management, utilizing fairly long sessions, is preferable to shorter sessions meeting over a longer period of time.

Advantages of the approach are that it tends to provide motivation for success and to facilitate carry-over (Sommers and Kane, 1974). A disadvantage is that it requires clinical skills that many speech-language pathologists do not possess. Backus (1957) cautions that a person needs to become acquainted thoroughly with the rationale and procedures she recommends before implementing them.

SENSORY-MOTOR APPROACH

The sensory-motor approach was devised by McDonald (1964). Production begins at the syllable level, which is considered to be the basic unit of speech. Sounds that the client already produces correctly are practiced in the context of bisyllables and trisyllables. After production of each bisyllable the client describes the movements of the articulators, that is, which two articulators touched and in what direction the tongue moved. Stress patterns are varied during this bisyllabic and trisyllabic drill, and the client identifies the stressed syllable. Actual training of a misarticulated phoneme begins in a phonetic context in which it was produced correctly, that is, in a two-word combination either in releasing or arresting position as determined by the McDonald Deep Test of Articulation (p. 121).

Rationale

The sensory-motor articulation treatment method emphasizes all the sensory and motor processes involved in speech production, since speech results from the interaction of certain sensory and motor processes. These processes evolve from simple to complex skills as a child matures from birth through 8 years of age. The integration of auditory, proprioceptive, and tactile sensations results in the use of precise, intricate articulation movements that normal speakers learn.

McDonald describes the movements of articulation as ballistic and overlapping. Ballistic movements occur as a result of rapid contraction of a muscle group followed by a short period of no contraction with the involved structure continuing to move because of momentum. The movement is subsequently stopped by contraction of the antagonist muscle group. According to McDonald, all skilled movements, including articulation, are ballistic. Articulation movements also are overlapping; that is, articulation of a particular phoneme is influenced by the sounds that precede and follow it. As McDonald (1964) stated, ". . . when a group of movements typical of an isolated consonant is combined with another consonant or vowel, the result is not the sum of the two movements, but a new group." Thus the exact articulation of any sound depends on its phonetic environment or context; each different context means that a different movement pattern must be used. For example, /s/ followed by /t/ is produced somewhat differently than /s/ followed by /k/. There are three types of overlapping movements:

1. Overlapping of different parts of the same structure, for example, in the articulation of "oaks," two different parts of the tongue are used
2. Overlapping of different structures adjacent to one another, for example, in the articulation of "spool," the lips and tongue tip are involved
3. Overlapping of different structures remote from one another, for example, in the articulation of "something," the lips, soft palate, and laryngeal muscles are used

From his viewpoint, then, McDonald (1964) defines articulation as a "process consisting of a series of overlapping, ballistic movements which place varying degrees of obstruction in the way of the outgoing air stream and simultaneously modify the size, shape, and coupling of resonating cavities."

These overlapping, skilled articulation movements are superimposed on the syllable, which McDonald considers to be the basic unit of speech, both physiologically and morphologically. A syllable has three components: (1) release, which may be through a consonant or by chest muscles, (2) vowel shaping, and (3) arrest, which may be through a consonant or by chest muscles. McDonald contends that sounds do not occur normally in isolation or even in the initial, medial, or final positions of words. Instead sounds are parts of the movement sequences of syllables. Consonants function to release or arrest syllables. Words are not physiologic units in running speech but sequences of syllables. The syllables are produced with differing rates and stress patterns. McDonald identifies three types of consonants as they occur in syllables: (1) simple, that is, a single consonant

that arrests or releases a syllable, as illustrated by /se/, (2) compound, that is, two or more consonants that function as a single consonant, as in /ste/, and (3) abutting, that is, adjacent consonants with one arresting the first syllable and the other releasing the second syllable, such as /istɚ/.

McDonald criticizes more traditional articulation approaches for several reasons. He contends that testing sounds in the initial, medial, and final positions of words is haphazard sampling rather than a representative sample of the client's articulation skills. Sounds should not be taught in isolation because they do not occur naturally in isolation; the syllable is the basic unit of speech. Ear training emphasizes only one sensory channel and utilizes analysis of another person's production rather than attending to all sensory input channels. Finally commercially prepared or clinician-prepared materials do not place responsibility for learning on the client and likely do not utilize the client's own vocabulary. Thus McDonald devised a treatment approach with a consideration of these factors and of his viewpoint of the articulation process.

Goals and procedures

The goal of this approach is to increase the number of phonetic contexts in which the target phoneme is produced correctly rather than to teach a "new" sound. McDonald (1964) points out that defective articulation is not always consistent, some phonemes may never be produced correctly, others are sometimes produced correctly, and still others are always produced correctly in certain contexts. This variability is because articulation develops from simple to complex skills as the sensory and motor processes mature over time.

There are three general goals to be reached in the sensory-motor approach. The first is "heightening responsiveness to patterns of auditory, proprioceptive, and tactile sensations associated with overlapping ballistic movements of articulation." In this first phase of training the client imitates the clinician's auditory stimuli and describes tactile and kinesthetic sensations by indicating which two articulators touched, in which direction the tongue moved, and which syllable was stressed. The stimuli progress from simple to complex movements, using varying stress patterns. On the bisyllabic drills, only correctly articulated consonants, as shown by testing, are used. The following stimulus sequence is presented for bisyllables:

1. CVCV (consonant-vowel-consonant-vowel) with the same consonant and vowel and with equal stress, for example, /bibi/
2. 'CVCV with the same consonant and vowel and with trochaic stress patterns, for example, /'bibi/
3. CV'CV with the same consonant and vowel and with iambic stress patterns, for example, /bi'bi/
4. CVCV with different vowels and various stress patterns, for example, /'bibu/
5. CVCV with different consonants and various stress patterns, for example, /bi'ki/
6. CVCV with different vowels and consonants and various stress patterns, for example, /'biku/

Following bisyllabic drills, trisyllables are presented with various vowels, consonants, and stress patterns. Different movement sequences are practiced beginning with larger changes of movement so that diverse parts of the articulators are used, for example, /po ki te/, in which the movement shifts from the front of the mouth at the lips to the back of the tongue and finally to the tongue tip. Progressively smaller articulation movement shifts are used as in /ti se mo/, in which the tongue tip is used twice in succession followed by a front of the mouth bilabial consonant. At this point in the program phonemes that were incorrectly produced on the articulation test are presented since McDonald believes that the bisyllabic practice and descriptions of various movement sequences may result in correct production of these error phonemes. However, if the client continues to misarticulate them, no attempt is made to teach correct production at this trisyllabic drill stage of treatment.

The second general goal is "to reinforce correct articulation of the error sound." McDonald (1964) recommends allowing the client to select the sound. Additionally a sound should be selected that can quickly be habituated, that is earlier developing, and that is not correct in a high percentage of phonetic contexts but is correct in at least one phonetic context. The correct phonetic context is the starting point for production of the error sound. Procedures for practicing the correct articulation in the phonetic context include "slow motion" speech, equal stress on both syllables, prolongation, and practice in short sentences.

The third goal is "to facilitate the correct articulation of the sound in systematically varied phonetic contexts." This phase of treatment begins by changing the vowel following the target sound. The phonetic context is then further modified in additional word combinations and sentences. At this stage the client makes a list of words beginning and ending with the target sounds. These words are used in various combinations, stress patterns, and rate patterns. Sentences with these words are constructed and practiced with different stress and rate patterns.

Comment

McDonald (1964) recommends this approach for children whose articulation errors seem to be the result of arrested or retarded articulation development and for those who correctly articulate the sound in at least one phonetic context. It seems to us that this approach is especially appropriate for clients who have multiple errors; the approach seems a bit tedious for those with only one or two errors. Rosenbek and associates (1974) recommend a variation of this method for dyspraxic children. The approach can be adapted to group treatment, to individual work, and to adults, although it was designed for children.

Sommers and Kane (1974) criticize the

approach on the bases that the drill, imitation, and description of articulation sequence movements seem tedious and the client is given no feedback as to how to change incorrect production attempts. Giving the client responsibility for treatment material and using the client's vocabulary may facilitate carry-over. Incorporating the concept of "overlapping movements" in articulation treatment, more commonly referred to as coarticulation, may also expedite management.

RECENT APPROACHES
Programmed instruction approach

The programmed instruction approach to articulation treatment could be accurately referred to as operant conditioning, behavior modification, behavior therapy, or as learning theory since it is based on principles formulated in these areas. Programmed instruction is an approach in which the stimuli and client responses are behaviorally specified prior to initiation of treatment. Stimuli are arranged in small, sequential steps leading to the desired terminal objective. The client is given immediate feedback about the adequacy of responses in the form of positive reinforcement for correct responses and sometimes in the form of negative reinforcement or punishment for incorrect responses. Progress is continuously monitored through tracking and recording procedures. Many people in the field of speech-language pathology have contributed to the development of the programmed approach, but Mowrer (1977) is the primary source for the information presented in the following paragraphs.

Rationale

Mowrer (1977) points out that in the 1960s and 1970s there has been a rapid increase in the use of behaviorism in which operant conditioning techniques play a major role and from which programmed instruction has developed. Operant conditioning has been quite influential in the methods currently being used by speech-language pathologists. Treatment is directed toward

modifying observable problem behaviors or symptoms rather than toward the underlying causes. A specified behavior is modified by manipulating stimuli that both precede (antecedent event) and follow (consequent event) the client's responses. Behavior modification procedures are characterized by specification of behavioral objectives in quantifiable terminology, precise measurement of behaviors, systematic use of reinforcement schedules, and use of programmed instruction. These features, among others, will be discussed.

An important component of programmed instruction is observing, assessing, and recording speech behaviors in an objective way. Appropriate and accurate observation helps the clinician assess the effect of treatment. In order to assess objectively a behavior, the behavior must be clearly stated and defined so that anyone observing would see the same behavior. Subjective estimates of progress merely provide a "feel" for the effectiveness of treatment, but knowing the exact increase or decrease in the frequency of correct or incorrect responses allows the clinician to evaluate accurately the effectiveness of treatment procedures.

Another critical component is stating the objectives behaviorally, that is, identifying objectives that can be observed and measured. A behavioral objective describes what the learner will be able to do as a result of a learning experience; the objective specifies what the learner is to do, under what conditions, and how well. Behavioral objectives are hypothesized to have three functions, although research has not supported these hypotheses:

1. Provide direction in the form of concise goals of teaching and curriculum development
2. Provide guidance in evaluation of goals
3. Facilitate student's learning (Mowrer, 1977)

As mentioned previously, behaviorists control behaviors through the stimuli presented in order to elicit a response. The learning principle to which this is related is referred to by Mowrer as the S-R laws, which can be written as R=f (S) under c. This formula refers to the relationship between stimulus events (S) and response events (R) under certain environmental conditions (c). It is reasoned that if a specified response always varies directly as the stimulus is manipulated, the stimulus causes the response. Thus one can control the response by manipulating the stimulus that precedes it, that is, by controlling the antecedent event. Of course 100% control never occurs when dealing with human behavior. However, if speech-language pathologists desire to change speech behaviors, the use of the functional relationship between stimuli and responses can result in such a change.

In addition to manipulating antecedent events, behavior is controlled by the consequence that follows a response to increase or decrease the frequency of a specified client response. This process has been called contingency management, which seems to be a term analogous to behavior therapy and behavior modification. There are three basic procedures for increasing and decreasing responses by manipulating consequent events (Mowrer, 1977). The first procedure is reinforcement, which may be either positive or negative. Positive reinforcement is a "pleasant" consequence that increases a particular response. If the frequency of a response does not increase, the consequent stimulus is not a positive reinforcer. The effect of positive reinforcement is influenced by the amount of reinforcement, the number of trials that are reinforced, and the schedule of reinforcement. The reinforcement schedule refers to how often a response is reinforced. Negative reinforcement also increases the frequency of a response, but it does so through the removal of an aversive stimulus. Unlike punishment, the unpleasant stimulus is presented before the response and is removed as a consequence of a desired response.

A second procedure used to control behavior is the use of punishment, in which an aversive stimulus is presented following a response in order to decrease the frequency of occurrence of the response. Time-out is a specialized form of punishment in which positive reinforcement is removed. The client must be removed from a pleasant situation, or the removal is not punishing. Another form of punishment is response cost, in which only one positive reinforcer is removed at a time, such as taking away a token, a "good mark," or a penny.

A third procedure of manipulating consequent events is the combining of positive reinforcement and extinction. Such a procedure is used in shaping behavior, that is, progressive approximation as described by Van Riper (1978). Behaviorists sometimes call the procedure response differentiation. A certain response is reinforced initially in the treatment process but later is not reinforced because the client is now using a behavior that is closer to the terminal behavior. This process of reinforcement and extinction continues until only the terminal behavior is reinforced. Thus the initial response becomes extinguished while another response is rewarded. A second way in which a combination of positive reinforcement and extinction is used is in discrimination training, in which a response is used in the presence of one stimulus but extinguished in the presence of another stimulus. For example, /s/ is to be used when a picture of a "sink" is shown but not when a picture of a "drink" is shown. This also may be what occurs when a client produces /s/ correctly when talking to the clinician but not when talking to the teacher. The clinician is a discriminative stimulus for /s/, but the teacher is not.

We have been discussing procedures for acquisition of behaviors. Now we will turn to principles of transferring behaviors to other situations. Positive transfer of training refers to the process by which the learning of one behavior facilitates learning of another behavior. According to Mowrer (1977), there are two forms of transfer. The first is stimulus generalization, in which a response is elicited by a stimulus that is similar to the original stimulus. Because of this process, clinicians do not need to teach a sound in every possible word in which it occurs; instead the correct response generalizes to words not taught. The second form of positive transfer is response generalization, in which one stimulus elicits several different responses. This process seems not to be applicable to articulation treatment. Negative transfer of learning also occurs. In this phenomenon the learning of a second behavior is more difficult because of what was learned during an earlier event, which results in more time needed to learn the second response. This may be what is happening when attempting to teach new articulation responses. The misarticulation has been learned and consequently interferes with the learning of a different, correct response. Use of unfamiliar stimuli may facilitate teaching a "new" sound in that the misarticulation has never been used in the nonmeaningful speech unit.

After presenting a background for programming, Mowrer (1977) cautions that "unless these concepts and procedures can be unified into a plan for executing instruction, their haphazard use may have only minimal effect on increasing the effectiveness of learning." Costello (1977) identifies the behavioral principles and characteristics of programmed instruction:

1. *Successive approximations.* The program begins with a response that the learner already has and gradually changes in small, logically sequenced steps to terminate with the target behavior.
2. *Active participation.* The learner responds overtly and frequently.
3. *Immediate knowledge of results.* Immediate feedback is provided to the learner.
4. *Mastery learning and self-pacing.* Correct responding on each step is a prerequisite to moving on to the next step so that the client proceeds at his own pace.
5. *Fading stimulus support.* The models, prompts, and cues are gradually faded

so that the stimulus becomes less supportive.
6. *Concept learning through varied repetition.* Many examples of a rule or principle are presented so that the concept or rule will be learned.

Goals and procedures

The goals of treatment of a programmed instruction approach are determined by the clinician. Whatever the objective, it is to be behaviorally stated, that is, the behavior to be achieved must be observable and countable. The objective should specify what the client is to do, under what conditions, and how well. Each program generally has a terminal objective, that is, the goal of the entire program and subobjectives or transitional objectives. Mowrer (1977) indicates that the intent of the objective should be specified if it is not the same as the behavior that indicates the intent. Following is such a statement: "To discriminate between /s/ and /θ/ by pointing to a red card when the clinician says /s/ and pointing to a blue card when the clinician says /θ/ in nineteen out of twenty trials." To rephrase this objective as "to point to a red card when the clinician says /s/ and to point to a blue card when the clinician says /θ/ in nineteen out of twenty trials" would not accurately reflect the intention of the objective, although it accurately reflects what the client is to do. An example of behaviorally stated goals, objectives, and procedures is included in Appendix N.

Collins and Cunningham (1975) have clearly outlined a method for speech-language pathologists to use when writing their own programs. The first step is to *identify a target behavior* that the client needs to attain. Examples are "articulation of /f/" and "discrimination of /s/ from other sounds." Second a *terminal objective is formulated,* as described previously. Third a *pretest and posttest are constructed* that test for the behavior identified in the terminal objective. Next a *task sequence is developed,* that is, the steps of the program are delineated. A *task analysis* follows, in which prerequisite behaviors for each task are listed. Last the *task sequence is put into a delivery system* that specifies stimuli, cues, client responses, reinforcement schedule, reinforcers, criteria for passage and failure for each step, and a procedure for recording progress.

Costello (1977) describes the components of a program that are similar to those used by Collins and Cunningham. Each component is to be specified for each step. The function of the stimulus is to elicit a response. It is modified throughout the program, from providing very supportive conditions to providing minimal cues. The client response begins with a behavior in the client's repertoire and progresses toward the terminal objective. Effective reinforcement must be determined for each client. Initially reinforcement is usually administered for every correct response; however, it should become more natural and intermittent as the program progresses. Both pass and fail criteria should be specified. Determining whether or not a criterion is met is dependent on tracking and recording the client's correct and incorrect responses.

Many articulation programs have been developed and published and thus are readily available for clinician use. Gerber (1977) and Mowrer (1977) give brief descriptions and critiques of available programs. Sommers and Kane (1974) and Winitz (1961) also present relevant discussions on the use of teaching machines. Appendix K includes a bibliography of articulation programs.

Comment

The programmed approach is used with both children and adults. It probably is easier to implement on an individual basis but is certainly adaptable to group situations.

This approach has been quite controversial in the field of speech-language pathology, as well as in other fields. Critics contend that humans are free to do as they choose and that their behavior should not be controlled, that it is dehumanizing to reduce behavior to S-R laws, that the approach deals with specific behaviors only

and not with the whole person, and that the clinician may develop into a mechanistic and inflexible technician (Mowrer, 1977). Shelton (1978) believes that the client is relatively passive, although others indicate that the client must actively respond. After analyzing several articulation programs, Gerber (1977) concluded that the greatest shortcoming of the approach is reliance on a prewritten approach that restricts flexibility. She continues that ideally each clinician should apply principles of programming, but with knowledge, skills, and sensitivity, so that each individual client is optimally served.

Costello (1977) enumerates several advantages of the approach. Treatment is effective in that terminal behaviors are usually learned thoroughly and quickly at a high success rate. Procedures can be replicated, since they are standardized, and often can be used by paraprofessionals. The method is economic in that the time required for learning is often short, it is applicable to several students, and it reduces the time needed for lesson planning and preparation. A good client-clinician relationship is fostered because of the reinforcement. Last, a clinician gains a better understanding of the communication process and learning principles. Sommers and Kane (1974) point out the advantage that the client progresses at his own pace. Mowrer (1977) believes that clinicians will continue to develop and use such programs because they facilitate accountability, which is being demanded by federal, state, and local agencies. Certainly most other articulation approaches are adaptable to using programmed instruction principles and procedures.

NONSENSE MATERIAL APPROACH

The nonsense material approach to articulation treatment was developed by Gerber (1973). In this method the client achieves correct articulation of error sounds in nonsense syllables and words used with the characteristics of conversational speech before proceeding to "real-word" production.

In other words, nonmeaningful words are produced automatically, rapidly, and effortlessly with normal stress, juncture, and intonational patterns. Only then does the client produce the error sound in meaningful words.

Rationale

Gerber (1973) developed the nonsense material approach because of the frustration over clients not achieving carry-over. She observed, as have many clinicians, that when a newly acquired sound is used in conversational speech, it is deliberately and carefully produced, but when the client's attention changes to the content of the message, misarticulations often recur. Initially the sound must be produced with careful and deliberate attention because the former articulation response (misarticulation) interferes with the correct response, because the person is focusing on the sound instead of on the meaningful word as a whole, or perhaps because of other reasons. Whatever the reason, this deliberate speech production interferes with carry-over to spontaneous speech, which is not deliberate.

Gerber (1973) hypothesizes that there are two different levels of speech: *deliberate* and *spontaneous*. Table 11 compares the characteristics of the two modes of speech. The overriding principle of the nonsense material approach is to "bridge the gap" between these two levels. Using nonsense syllables and words with the characteristics of spontaneous speech aids in "bridging the gap" or in facilitating carry-over. In other words sound production occurs effortlessly in sentences and stories with normal prosody before meaningful words are introduced. According to Gerber, after this objective is achieved the client will likely produce the sound in meaningful material without undue effort and exaggerated articulation. The client, then, is free to focus more attention on content because of the prior practice on nonsense material. The nonsense material is programmed with a consideration of phonetic complexity in that stimuli using easier articulation movements are introduced before more difficult ones.

Accuracy in evaluating and monitoring the client's own speech is critical, in most instances, for achieving carry-over. In Gerber's method this skill is systematically trained in order to develop a more effective means of monitoring speech by detecting and correcting misarticulations. Generally auditory perception is stressed, but some clients may need training in visual, tactile, or kinesthetic perception or any combination of these.

Gerber recommends using an approach midway between a "game" approach and operant conditioning. In this way the client responds at a rapid rate to material designed to arouse interest. Active client participation is required while focusing on the quality of speech production, not on the game. A "game" approach is not effective because games tend to distract attention away from speech and because the response rate is re-

Table 11. Contrastive analysis of the attributes of spontaneous and structured speech

Spontaneous speech	Structured speech
Articulatory movements are rapidly overlapping and effortless	Articulatory movements are frequently artificially prolonged and strenuous
Articulation is subordinated in consciousness to the content of the message; therefore, production is relatively automatic	Attention is focused on the mechanics of sound production; therefore, production is deliberate, frequently emitted from a preparatory set
Segmental sounds are modified by natural patterns of stress, juncture, and intonation related to meaning	Stress patterns are frequently distorted through exaggerated production; rhythm and melody are often stilted and artificial

From Gerber, A.: Goal carryover: an articulation manual and program, Philadelphia, 1973, Temple University Press.

duced. On the other hand an operant conditioning approach tends to be uninteresting because of straight drill work. Therefore, a combination of the two approaches is used.

Goals and procedures

The goal of the nonsense material approach is automatic production of the target sound in spontaneous speech with the criterion specified as "90 to 100 percent correct production of the target sound in a communicative situation wherein the client's attention is focused on the content of the message and not on the deliberate control of the mechanics of speech production" (Gerber, 1973). No procedures for acquisition of sounds are provided except for /r/; other sources can be consulted for sound-acquisition techniques.

The nonsense material is presented in levels of increasing complexity:

1. CV, VCV, and VC syllables
2. More complex syllables, for example, CCV, VCCV, and VCC
3. Simple nonsense words, for example, CVC
4. Multisyllabic nonsense words, for example, /ˈkakɪ/
5. Phrases comprised of nonsense words, for example, /ˈkakɪ pʌnəd fæk/
6. Conversations in nonsense words
7. Using nonsense words in meaningful contexts, for example, "I say a /sot/."

Each level of nonsense material is programmed to be produced eventually with the characteristics of spontaneous speech, that is, consistently correct with normal juncture, with rapidness, in stressed and unstressed syllables, in varying levels of phonetic complexity, and in natural syntactic structures. After the highest level of nonsense material is produced as if it were conversational speech, real words are introduced. The client's own vocabulary is used and the words are eventually produced in sentences and connected speech. Gerber (1973) provides several techniques for the previously described treatment process, including "sound hopscotch," "sound hurdles," riddles, word-building blocks, "follow the beat," "model sentence drills," and

stories. The procedures emphasize speed of production and natural prosody.

Simultaneously with the production training, self-monitoring training is incorporated. This is programmed in the following six steps to be used at each level of production work:

1. Evaluate clinician's live speech productions
2. Evaluate clinician's taped speech productions
3. Evaluate taped samples of clinician and client productions with each producing one sound unit
4. Evaluate taped samples of clinician and client productions with each producing three sound units
5. Evaluate taped client productions without clinician model
6. Evaluate client productions without clinician model prior to playing back the taped utterances

The client strives to produce the sound consistently and to evaluate productions accurately at increasing levels of speed.

Comment

The nonsense material approach is designed for older children who have passed the stage of articulation development through maturation, that is, children who are 7 or 8 years of age and adolescents. The material can be adapted for adults, although it has not been widely used with adults. Less direct approaches are recommended for children under age 7 years. The approach can be used on an individual or group basis. Gerber indicates that not all clients need to perform all activities at all levels. The advantages of Gerber's approach are that the client develops strong internal motivation, the material is highly organized, and carryover is facilitated (Sommers and Kane, 1974).

AUDITORY CONCEPTUALIZATION APPROACH

The auditory conceptualization approach was devised by Winitz (1975) and further developed by Weiner (1979). Treatment begins with auditory discrimination training.

General discrimination work is not provided, but training on the difference between the error and standard sound is emphasized. Production training begins with nonsense syllables and nonsense words; nonsense words are practiced in sentences and conversation. Later treatment involves production of the target sound in words, phrases, sentences, and conversation.

Rationale

Winitz (1975) believes that articulation errors represent learned behavior in nonorganic cases. He further notes, as have others, that misarticulations are often variable, that is, a particular phoneme is not always produced incorrectly and the error is not always the same. During developmental stages a word may be produced incorrectly because a child has had only limited exposure to the words and children tend to say words before all phonetic elements are produced correctly. Habitually producing a sound incorrectly hides perceptual differences; that is, a child is not able to discriminate between the error sound and the target sound. Winitz's review of the literature supported this assumption in that the literature showed a fairly high relationship between discrimination and articulation skills. Winitz believes that a child who does not detect differences between sounds cannot be expected to produce them correctly and that the ability to discriminate between the error sound and standard sound is an important prerequisite to correct articulation. Therefore, this articulation treatment program begins with discrimination training.

Winitz recommends that target sounds be practiced first in nonsense words. This usually results in more rapid acquisition since the sound has not been learned and practiced incorrectly in such contexts, resulting in minimal interference. The error sound does not interfere with correct production in nonsense words, as is the case with meaningful words.

Prior to treatment a client's articulation skills need to be thoroughly evaluated since the speech-language pathologist needs to know where the articulation breaks down.

Assessment begins with examination of misarticulations in conversation and in isolated words. The consistency of the errors should be noted as well as words in which the error sound is produced correctly. Stimulability is examined. If errors are not stimulable, a distinctive feature analysis is done to determine which features are in error. Such an evaluation aids in determining where to begin treatment, since not all clients must proceed through the entire sequence of treatment.

Winitz contends that developmental articulation tests should not be used to exclude a child from treatment. Even if a child has articulation skills commensurate with developmental norms, the child should be treated if the parents are concerned. In this way the parents can be shown how to handle their child's speech patterns.

Articulation treatment is characterized by Winitz as a complex process dealing with training in articulation production skills and in generalization of these skills to other situations. He believes that controlled experimentation is important in developing effective treatment procedures so that relevant variables can be identified and manipulated in the treatment process. He seems to advocate a behavioral modification approach as a way to functionalize or manipulate the treatment environment for those who have previously experienced failure. Further, in order for intervention to be effective, Winitz insists that the client be actively involved rather than being a passive participant. Conceptualization training also includes teaching of contrasting features.

Goals and procedures

There are four processes in Winitz's (1975) articulation treatment approach: (1) discrimination training, (2) production practice, (3) transfer of training, and (4) retention. Fig. 8-1 is a flow chart of these four processes.

Discrimination training begins with assessment of a client's discrimination skills. The clinician examines for specific discrimination errors rather than for general auditory discrimination abilities and for specific

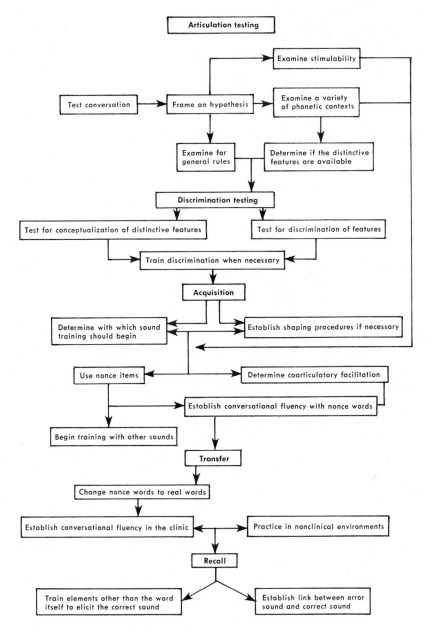

Fig. 8-1. Block diagram of clinical process of articulatory training. (From Winitz, H.: From syllable to conversation, Baltimore, 1975, University Park Press.)

linguistic contexts in which the errors occur. For example, if a client substitutes /w/ for /r/, the clinician tests for the ability to discriminate between /w/ and /r/ in syllables and meaningful words. If the client discriminates accurately between the two sounds or if the target sound is stimulable, auditory discrimination training may be eliminated. In this phase of treatment the client is trained to distinguish between the error and target sounds. Training is implemented by presenting contrasting pairs in which the phonetic differences are carefully sequenced beginning with large differences and progressing to smaller differences until the error and target sounds are contrasted. Initially the error sound is compared with other sounds and only later in the sequence is the standard sound presented. For example, in a /w/ for /r/ substitution error, /w/ could be contrasted with /s/, /θ/, /j/, etc. before comparing it with /r/. Discrimination training progresses through conversational speech. Winitz emphasizes that interesting materials should be used so that the client will become actively involved in the process. During this stage of treatment, when the child uses misarticulations the clinician responds inappropriately. For example, if the child says /wɪŋ/ when requesting a /rɪŋ/, the clinician could say something such as, "I don't have a wing." Sound production should not begin until auditory discriminations are easily made in sentences. Sometimes auditory discrimination training results in correct production with no need of continuing with the subsequent three levels of treatment. This potentially can occur when the distinctive features in the target sound are produced correctly in nonerrored sounds.

The second phase of training is production practice. If the target sound is stimulable, the clinician indicates to the client when it is produced correctly. If such key words are found, production treatment proceeds to the transfer phase of training. If the sound is never produced correctly, the clinician looks for the production of distinctive features that comprise the error sound and generalizes the missing feature to the target sound. If a feature is not used by the client, production training begins with a verbal response that contains the missing feature. This sound is eventually transferred to the target sound through the process of shaping. Coarticulation factors are to be considered when programming for production training. The clinician begins with phonetic contexts that facilitate correct production. An example might be to begin with words in which the preceding consonant has features similar to that of the target sound and unlike the error substitution, such as a word that begins with /n/ for a client who substitutes /w/ for /l/. The sound is then used in nonsense syllables and words that are subsequently practiced in sentences and conversational speech. The nonsense words are then transformed into real words. Throughout production training, immediate positive reinforcement is provided to the client for correct productions.

The third stage of articulation treatment is transfer of training, or transfer of the newly acquired sound from one context to another. A procedure for doing this is to vary the syllabic divisions. For example, if the client can say /'aste/, the syllables should be changed to /a 'ste/. Winitz (1975) indicates that transfer of a sound to words occurs more rapidly when first used in nonsense words. The sequence of training proceeds from nonsense words to nonsense words in conversation to English words to phrases to sentences to conversational speech. At this stage the client's articulation skills are probed (tested) to determine if the features in the target sound are now used in other error sounds. If so, production and transfer training should be implemented for those sounds.

The final stage of treatment, retention, is of great concern to speech-language pathologists. This stage refers to carry-over or automatization of the target sound, that is, correct habitual production of the sound in all speech contexts and environments. Retention involves training in nonclinical situations. Training in spontaneous speech is begun with the client and clinician in environments similar to and near the regular clinical setting. Later a second clinician, unknown to the client, converses with the client in these same settings.

Winitz (1975) reviews methods for achieving carry-over but contends that recall of the target sound is what is needed because the client may be able to produce the sound but not be able to retrieve it. Intensive ear training facilitates recall. He also suggests incorporating a procedure to strengthen the association between correct and incorrect sounds by listening to the clinician produce the incorrect sound and responding with the correct one. Winitz concludes by emphasizing that his program need not be followed without deviation since it is always subject to revision.

Comment

Winitz describes his program as used individually with children, although it could be adapted for adults and for group settings. The program was primarily developed for nonorganic cases. Winitz is not always clear in describing exactly what the clinician is to do, but his examples clearly explain the treatment principles proposed.

MULTIPLE PHONEMIC APPROACH

The multiple phonemic approach was developed by McCabe and Bradley (1975). In this approach all misarticulated sounds are treated at the same time. Each sound is produced at the client's proficiency level, that is, isolation, syllables, monosyllabic words, etc. Sounds are elicited in isolation with whatever techniques are appropriate for the client. No auditory discrimination training is done. An essential part of the program is that the client's performance be recorded for each session.

Rationale

McCabe and Bradley indicate that their approach is quite similar to traditional approaches except that several sounds are worked on at the same time. The client can proceed at an appropriate pace for each error sound. The rate of progress for each sound varies depending on the difficulty for the client. In the first phase of treatment the client produces all consonants, including those produced correctly, as well as those produced incorrectly. This is done to provide success from the beginning of treatment and to train the client to attend to several phonemes at a time rather than only to those that are misarticulated. In the final stages of treatment the objective is to articulate whole words correctly instead of only the target sound. The client then is responsible for correct production of several pho-

nemes at once. In phrases the client must attend to articulation of more than one phoneme, to word sequences, and to semantic aspects of the utterance. According to McCabe and Bradley (1975), if this is accomplished by the client, progress through the remaining steps will be relatively easy.

Throughout treatment the *client's own vocabulary* is used rather than words that happen to contain target phonemes but that may not be useful to the client. The client should experience success throughout the treatment process. Each session begins and ends with an activity that the client can achieve. Additionally if the correct responding percentage for all tasks falls below 80% during one session, the tasks are modified to allow for a higher success rate. McCabe and Bradley use a programmed approach and emphasize the necessity for tracking all client responses so that the clinician can determine when to proceed to the next step for each sound, when to modify tasks to accommodate the client's skill level, and when to branch.

Goals and procedures

There are three phases of articulation treatment in the multiple phonemic approach: (1) establishment, (2) transfer, and (3) maintenance. Each phase is composed of steps, each of which has a specific stimulus, client response, reinforcement schedule, and criterion level. The purpose of the establishment phase is to achieve correct production of all error sounds in isolation using only visual stimulation; for example, the client is presented the grapheme of a sound printed on a card and asked to say it. If the client initially needs more than visual stimulation to achieve correct production, auditory and tactile stimulation are added. The second step of the establishment phase is considered to be a "holding" procedure for sounds that have reached the criterion level in the first step but for which there is insufficient time to work on in subsequent steps. In this step each phoneme is produced once in isolation with only visual stimulation. In this way the client practices all error sounds during each session.

Six steps comprise phase II, transfer of sounds into syllables, words, phrases, reading, and conversation. *Step 1* is characterized as a "word probe" or test of the sound in monosyllabic words. If the client does not produce the sound in six of ten words, *step 2*—practice of the sound in CV and VC syllables and in multisyllables—is implemented. If the client meets criterion on the word probe, treatment proceeds to *step 3*—production of the target sound in monosyllabic and multisyllabic words. Words used are selected on the basis of the client's age and vocabulary and include nouns, verbs, adjectives, and other parts of speech. *Step 4* consists of practice of the target sound in phrases and sentences. At this stage the objective may change from correct production of the sound to correct articulation of the whole word. In *step 5* the client reads stories or paragraphs. Usually the objective is correct articulation of whole words rather than only of a specific sound. Error words are practiced after the reading. Last, *step 6* involves spontaneous speech with the objective of whole-word accuracy.

The last phase of training is maintenance of correct articulation in various speaking situations. In *step 1* the client engages in conversational speech in the clinical setting with minimal cues. *Step 2* involves maintenance of articulation skills over time without direct intervention. The client is evaluated 3 and 6 months after treatment is terminated.

Each misarticulated phoneme progresses through all three phases at a pace that is appropriate for the client. For example, three sounds may be in phase I, four sounds in phase II, and two sounds in phase III. Thus all error sounds are worked on at the same time.

Comment

The multiple phonemic approach has been used with children who have repaired cleft palates and other corrected orofacial anomalies as well as with those who have functional articulation problems. The age range has been 5 to 14 years, although it certainly is an approach appropriate for older individuals. The approach seems to be more usable with individuals than with groups since it would be difficult to record client responses for more than one person at a time.

The advantage of working on more than one sound at a time is that intelligibility is improved more rapidly. The approach also seems to be more efficient than traditional approaches. A possible disadvantage is that working on several sounds at a time may be confusing to the client.

Sommers and Kane (1974) also recommend work on more than one sound at a time, but in a more selective way. This approach is called the *"wedge" approach*. It is based on the assumption that not all error sounds need direct treatment since learning to produce one sound may generalize to other sounds with similar distinctive features. The clinician selects two or more misarticulated sounds that are phonetically dissimilar, for example, /ʃ/, /k/, and /r/, to work on at first. These sounds are "wedges" in that they "open up" the incorrect articulation pattern. The features of the selected sounds then transfer to other error sounds, often without direct intervention.

DISTINCTIVE FEATURE APPROACH

The distinctive feature approach for articulation treatment originally was developed by McReynolds and Bennet (1972). In this approach distinctive features of phonemes are taught, such as voicing, rather than individual phonemes. This is done by the client producing two sounds, one of which contains the feature to be taught and one of which does not. The contrasting phonemes are produced in isolation and nonsense syllables. In some programs the sounds are also contrasted in words, sentences, and conversational speech.

Rationale

The distinctive feature approach is based on the premise that distinctive features are the basic elements of sounds, that is, sounds are composed of a bundle of features (McReynolds and Engmann, 1975). They are the elements that distinguish one sound from another. When developing articulation skills, a child systematically acquires features rather than phonemes. As more features are added, more phonemes are articulated correctly. Distinctive feature theorists contend that articulation errors are systematic. A child with articulation errors often has a phonemic rule system that is different from the adult system (Costello, 1975). Misuse or omission of a distinctive feature may result in the misarticulation of several sounds. The intent of the distinctive feature approach is to aid the client in learning the rules of the adult phonology system (Van Riper, 1978). The client learns distinctive features rather than specific sounds (Drexler, 1976). If a feature is acquired, it may transfer to other sounds that contain the feature. More than one sound thus may be changed by teaching a particular feature. If this is true, using a distinctive feature approach would appear to be more efficient than traditional approaches.

How are distinctive features taught? Distinctive features do not appear in isolation; therefore, they are taught in the context of sounds. Both positive and negative aspects of a feature are taught through two or more phonemes that ideally are minimal pairs, that is, the two phonemes contain the same features except that one contains the feature to be taught and the other does not. For example, /k/ and /g/ could be used to teach voicing, and /t/ and /s/ could be used to teach stridency. Often the clinician selects the target sound and the substituted error for contrast. Such a procedure enhances the feature contrast the client needs to learn.

Various feature systems have been developed and used to analyze and treat articulation disorders. McReynolds and Engmann (1975) use Chomsky and Halle's (1968) system but indicate that any system may be used. Costello and Onstine (1976) prefer the system devised by Singh and Polen (1972). Drexler (1976) developed a simplified system using terminology familiar to speech-language pathologists, for example, vowel, nasal, glide, fricative, and alveolar (see Appendix L).

Costello and Onstine (1976) and McReynolds and Engmann (1975) advocate an indepth feature analysis of a client's articulation system. This is necessary in order to know where to begin treatment and on which sounds. To implement feature analysis treatment, the clinician needs to determine the patterns of feature errors, that is, the phonologic system the client is using. Conversely Drexler (1976) does not recommend such a thorough evaluation because clinical time limitations preclude it.

Goals and procedures

Three different distinctive feature programs will be described here, although there are certainly similarities among them. The general goals of the programs are to teach the client how to produce a specified distinctive feature in the context of phonemes and where to use the feature; that is, the client is to learn the rules for correctly using a particular distinctive feature.

We will begin by describing McReynolds and Engmann's (1975) approach, which was developed for research purposes. They indicate that the approach may need to be modified for clinical purposes, but the treatment principles are useful nonetheless. From the analysis the clinician determines the percentage of incorrect usage of the positive and negative aspects of each of thirteen features. If a feature error occurs in less than 25% of the trials, it is not necessary to deal with it in treatment. If a feature is used incorrectly 40% to 50% of the time, it is inconsistently produced and may need to be modified. If a feature is incorrect 65% of the time, it should be considered in treatment. Finally, if the percentage of errors for a feature is above 80%, it has a high priority for being included in training. After analyzing the evaluation results, a feature is selected for training and two sounds are used for teaching the feature contrast. One sound contains the feature to be taught and the other does not.

The client produces both consonants throughout the treatment process; no auditory training is done. A programmed instructional approach is used. Stimuli consist of nonsense pictures and verbal stimuli using the two contrasting consonants and the vowels /a/, /i/, /æ/, and /u/. The responses are initially imitative and progress to spontaneous productions. Reinforcement schedules and criterion levels are specified. Production training begins with the production of the phoneme containing the feature to be learned, imitatively and spontaneously. In the feature contrast training the two sounds are produced in CV syllables with the vowels, imitatively and spontaneously. The two sounds are then produced in VC syllables with the vowels, imitatively and spontaneously. Generalization of the feature to other sounds is tested. If generalization has not occurred, the same treatment process is administered again using two other phonemes as a contrasting pair for the same feature.

Although Drexler (1976) does not utilize a distinctive feature analysis as thorough as that of McReynolds and Engmann (1975), she expands on their treatment program. The contrasting phonemes ideally are the same in all features except the one being taught; however, sometimes it is necessary that they vary in two features. There are five phases in Drexler's program: (1) initial position, which includes the phonemes in isolation and CV syllables; (2) final position in VC syllables; (3) words; (4) phrases; and (5) sentences. The first two phases follow McReynolds and Engmann's format. At the word level minimal word pairs are produced, for example, "suit/toot" and "pass/pat." At the phrase and sentence levels words containing the contrasting phonemes are produced in meaningful, short phrases and sentences.

Costello and Onstine (1976) advocate a thorough distinctive feature analysis. Features are selected for training on the following bases: (1) developmental order of feature acquisition, (2) whether the feature is completely omitted or misused, and (3) number of phonemes affected by the feature. Costello and Onstine also implement a programmed instruction approach. In contrast to the two programs described previously, they select for training two sounds that contain the feature to be taught and one that does not contain the feature. They use two sounds with the feature on the assumption that the client can more easily conceptualize the feature than if only one sound is used. The three sounds are each produced by the client in the following sequential levels:

1. Isolation
2. CV and VC syllables
3. Words in releasing and arresting positions
4. Phrases in releasing and arresting positions
5. Sentences in releasing and arresting positions
6. Stories
7. Conversation

A sample distinctive feature program appears in Appendix M.

Comment

The distinctive feature approach has primarily been implemented with children on an individual basis, although it seems feasible to adapt it for adults. Group treatment also would be possible. The approach is recommended for phonemic deviancies but not for phonetic deviancies. McReynolds and Engmann (1975) indicate that a distinctive feature analysis should be reserved for those who have four or more sound errors since it is probably not useful to analyze the articulation pattern of those with fewer errors.

The approach seems to be quite efficient in that once a feature is acquired the feature seems to generalize to other sounds. Two studies have shown that such generalization occurs (Costello and Onstine, 1976; McReynolds and Bennet, 1972). Overgeneralization does not tend to occur as it does in more traditional approaches, and the client tends to substitute the "new" sound for previously incorrectly articulated sounds. A disadvantage is that most distinctive feature analyses are quite time-consuming. McReynolds and Engmann indicate that the time required for analysis must be compared with the hours spent in treatment when such an analysis is not done.

PHONOLOGIC PROCESSES APPROACH

Phonologic methodologies have evolved from psycholinguistic research (Ingram, 1976; Jakobson, 1968; Compton, 1970; Morehead and Morehead, 1976). This approach has been helpful in identifying the processes that underlie certain articulation problems. Once these detrimental processes have been identified, the clinician can proceed toward their alleviation.

Rationale

The phonologic processes approach is based on the theory that misarticulations may be phonetic problems, phonemic problems, or a combination thereof. If the errors are phonemic, then a conceptual, cognitive, or linguistic approach should be considered. Phonologic concepts can best be taught by emphasizing rules and contrasts. Once a particular concept is taught, such as an addition or elimination of a phonologic process, that concept or rule will generalize to other contexts, thereby expediting the treatment process. However, there is some concern whether or not generalization occurs consistently or pervasively (McReynolds and Bennet, 1972).

Goals and procedures

As with other approaches, the phonologic approach considers the individual child's needs. Training should not focus on isolated phonemes but rather on the general processes of phonologic acquisition (Ingram, 1976). This approach attempts to eliminate the client's tendency to simplify speech while establishing a new, more appropriate behavior. Emphasis is placed on teaching contrasts, provided of course that they are lacking in the client's articulation system. Acquisition of phonology is concerned with

acquiring the ability to use sounds contrastively. Three deficiences in the use of contrasts have been reported in the psycholinguistic literature: (1) unstable use of speech, (2) use of a large number of homonyms, and (3) a small inventory of contrastive elements (Ingram, 1976). Treatment then is to stabilize phonetic variations by first stabilizing the client's own contrastive form of a word either by eliciting it or by accepting it when pronounced, but rejecting other alternatives. Reducing the large number of homonyms (a word meaning many different things) in the client's repertoire is another therapeutic necessity. This can be most efficiently accomplished by first selecting the homonyms with the most different meanings for treatment—those that are the most contrastive. The last aspect of treatment deals with increasing the client's inventory of contrastive elements. Establishing new contrasts considers the client's entire phonologic system. This third goal is accomplished through the use of a wide variety of words.

Selection of contrasts is provided by Jakobson (1968), such as beginning with the basic vowel contrasts between /a/ and /i/ or /u/. Ingram (1976) suggests two guidelines for teaching contrasts: (1) establish contrasts that result in a system comparable to that used by young children, and (2) proceed in a way that contrasts are established by eliminating processes in their most general form. Contrasts should be taught gradually. The use of discrimination training in phonologic treatment is not clearly defined at this time. It may be beneficial in regard to some sound classes such as fricatives.

Comment

The phonologic processes approach appears to be more effective in diagnosis than in treatment at this time. This approach would seem to be useful with clients having multiple misarticulations or lacking several contrastive features. Teaching concepts and processes may eventually expedite articulation treatment; however, at this time the phonologic processes approach lacks specificity, refinement, and subjection to scientific investigation. Nevertheless it appears to have significant potential in remediating articulation disorders, especially if generalization of these phonologic processes would occur in treatment.

OTHER ARTICULATION TREATMENT APPROACHES

It is not possible to discuss all articulation treatment approaches that have been developed. However, we think it is useful to comment briefly on a few additional approaches.

Nondirective approach

Hahn (1961) indicates that not all children with speech disorders will respond optimally to direct treatment approaches. Some need a nondirective approach because they have formed barriers against changing their communication patterns. Indications of need for a nondirective approach include such client behaviors as not responding favorably to directions or suggestions, displaying extreme tensions, destroying materials, and retreating from people. Hejna (1960) suggests that this approach is applicable to clients in whom emotional factors or fear responses precipitate or maintain speech disorders, that is, clients in whom personality differences or behavioral characteristics preclude success with direct approaches. According to Hahn (1961), in a nondirective approach the client supposedly needs to solve problems in adapting to the environment before attending to speech skills. The client develops a desire to communicate and experiences pleasure from successful communication interactions. The role of the clinician is to be "a comfortable listener and observer who has provided a situation in which the child can act out and express freely." Hejna (1960) gives further information on how to apply nondirective treatment approaches to articulation intervention.

Paired-stimuli approach

Developed by Weston and Irwin (1971), the paired-stimuli approach seems to be a modification of Van Riper's key word approach to articulation treatment. A word in which the target sound is correctly produced is used as a frame of reference and as a starting point for transfer of that sound to other words. If no word exists in which the target sound is used correctly, one should be taught to the client. This approach should be used with one phoneme at a time.

The initial stage of this word approach requires selection of a target sound and key word, one that is correctly articulated 90% of the time in the key word. Then training words are selected in which the sound is misarticulated two out of three trials. Next the client is asked to produce the key word followed by each of the successive training words. Words, both key and training, are varied in regard to sound position. Once criterion is established, question and answer activities are used so that the training words are produced in simple phonemic contexts, followed by spontaneous conversation. This approach facilitates sound transfer at the word level and as such is not a complete treatment program.

Coarticulation approach

A coarticulation approach to articulation development is currently being developed by Schukers (1978) but is as of yet unpublished. Coarticulation refers to the phenomenon in which the articulators simultaneously move in the production of speech sounds that are perceived to occur sequentially. In other words the articulation movements of a sound are influenced by sounds that closely precede and follow it. McDonald (1964) considers this aspect in the sensory-motor approach when he refers to "overlapping" movements. It is believed that coarticulation needs to be considered when evaluating and treating articulation disorders. Coarticulation factors can be used to facilitate production of sounds (Eisenson and Ogilvie, 1977). For example, in order to help prevent lip-rounding of /r/, /r/ should be used in combination with a nonrounded vowel. To aid in the production of /k/, a back vowel rather than a front vowel should be used. A second application of this phenomenon is to practice the target sound in systematically varied phonetic contexts so that correct production is achieved no matter which sounds precede or follow it (Shelton, 1978). The client needs to learn to coarticulate a wide variety of phonemes. More information will likely be appearing in the literature relative to the application of coarticulation factors to articulation treatment.

PREVENTION OF ARTICULATION DISORDERS

The foregoing treatment approaches have been used quite effectively with several different kinds of articulation disorders, but what approaches are available to the clinician for preventing articulation disorders from occurring? Should not also the clinician be equally concerned with preventing articulation disorders from developing? Concern for prevention is well justified when it is realized that articulation problems may be easier to prevent than to "cure." It would seem to us that if as much attention had been placed on prevention as has been given to treatment, a number of effective preventive approaches might now be broadly employed. The result would be articulation problems becoming less commonplace. Be that as it may, clinicians should strive toward developing more and better preventive approaches. Some attempts have been made in preventing speech disorders (Schoolfield, 1973; Van Riper, 1950; Weiss and Lillywhite, 1976).

Factors that may assist in preventing articulation problems include (1) parent education, (2) increased awareness among other professional persons, (3) greater availability of helpful suggestions, and (4) special courses or greater emphasis on prevention in training programs. Each area will be briefly discussed.

Parent education

The value of involving parents in treatment programs has been recognized for many years (Lillywhite, 1948; Lassers, 1954; Stoddard, 1940), but only recently have parents been encouraged to assist in preventing communication disorders from developing. Reasons for the delay in utilizing parents may include a number of factors, such as the following: parents are too busy; they do not know how to help; they are not always effective; and sometimes they may actually interfere with articulation development. Some of these reasons may be valid. We certainly know that not all parents can or should be involved in an active program of prevention. We also have observed effective parental intervention, especially when parents were appropriately educated and trained.

Education should provide normative data on articulation development. Knowing this, parents will be in a better position to know where and when to begin an intensified program of stimulation. Education should include ideas for ways of stimulating articulation. Activities such as modeling, echoing, ear training, placing articulators for different sounds, and reinforcing speech efforts must be explained to, demonstrated for, and learned by the parent. Finally education should include recording, charting, and reporting articulation behavior. Parents must become good listeners so that they can readily learn to recognize and record good or bad speech productions. The recordings may be as simple as number of correct productions of /l/. Charting need not utilize a six-cycle graph but rather a simple graph that illustrates the total number of responses of a specific sound and the percentage of time those responses were correct. Hopefully the graph will be meaningful to the child as well as to the parent. Reporting should also be simple and concise. In fact the data recorded on the graph or chart may be sufficient for the supervising speech-language pathologist. This information can be supplemented with a tape recorded sample of the child's speech and given to or sent to the clinician (Weiss and Lillywhite, 1976). After analysis of the progress, the clinician can decide if the parent should move on to another sound or continue working on the present sound. In some instances parents might be asked to determine for themselves when a new task or target sound should be initiated. Careful instruction should precede such parental independence. For example, after the child uses the /f/ and /v/ sounds correctly 80% of the time in 5-minute sessions of conversation 3 days in a row, work should be begun on a new pair of sounds. If carefully selected and instructed, many parents can be helpful in preventing articulation disorders.

Increased awareness among other professional persons

Some articulation problems could be prevented if persons in disciplines other than speech-language pathology would become increasingly aware of these problems. Workshops and courses should be taught to professional persons who are intimately involved in the welfare and management of children. Some of these disciplines include medicine, dentistry, psychology, special education, general education, nursing, occupational therapy, physical therapy, social work, and early childhood specialists.

Awareness can be increased through various educational processes. However, education should relate the importance of prevention to the potential contributions of these disciplines, showing how they can help the child develop articulation competence. Once persons in these disciplines are more aware of the potential problem and some ways of preventing it from developing, their assistance will be forthcoming. By assistance we are not implying intensive daily stimulation but praise, encouragement, interest, concern, and love. The effectiveness of prevention can be greatly enhanced by increasing the awareness among other professional persons.

Greater availability of helpful suggestions

All persons interested in the welfare of children should be provided with helpful suggestions. Good intentions are useless if unaccompanied by appropriate knowledge. In the past decade we have seen a proliferation of information aimed at helping parents and others to assist children's communication development. These suggestions range from where to get materials to how to provide speech stimulation and measure its effectiveness. Many of these materials are commercially available and are advertised in catalogs. Other materials are now available at meetings, in bookstores and libraries, in children's stores, and occasionally at training centers. We will reserve judgment on the quality of some of these "helpful" materials for now.

Special courses

Until students in training are given more formal instruction on ways of preventing articulation disorders, only minimal inroads will be made in this area. Courses should include some developmental landmarks of articulation, a review of the various causes of defective articulation, and some commonsense ideas on how to help a child with delayed articulation development. As more information is obtained on how to stimulate articulation development, prevention will assume a more scientific quality that will improve its effectiveness and efficiency. Courses that improve one's listening and other observational skills, such as phonetics and diagnostic testing, might also be helpful for persons interested in preventing articulation problems. A course on behavioral management would likewise be beneficial. The general courses that are now offered to a variety of students including non–speech-language pathology majors include courses such as introduction to speech-language pathology and phonetics. These courses should include more suggestions for detecting and helping persons with articulation disorders and a range of ideas for preventing these disorders from happening. In this way existing courses, as well as new courses, will provide more useful information on preventing communication disorders in general and articulation disorders in particular.

SUMMARY

Several widely used articulation treatment approaches have been described. These are phonetic placement; motokinesthetics; traditional stimulation; integral stimulation; sensory-motor, programmed instruction; nonsense material; auditory conceptualization; and multiple phonemic, distinctive feature, and phonologic processes. Each approach has been at least partially effective in managing articulation-disordered individuals. Speech-language pathologists need to be familiar with these approaches in order to plan and carry out treatment programs for individuals with articulation disorders.

STUDY SUGGESTIONS

1. Compare and contrast the preferred treatment approaches for dysarthria and dyspraxia.
2. Describe and compare articulation approaches that utilize auditory discrimination and discuss the factors that would indicate the use of this kind of training.
3. Describe and relate principles to be followed and components that need to be specified in a programmed instruction approach.
4. Describe "distinctive features" in articulation and relate these features to the diagnosis and treatment of articulation disorders.
5. Show how and where distinctive features can be used in various other approaches to treatment, including the phonologic processes approach.
6. What "other approaches" can be taken when a client does not respond to any direct treatment approach?

REFERENCES

Backus, O.: Group structure in speech therapy. In Travis, L., editor: Handbook of speech pathology and audiology, New York, 1957, Appleton-Century-Crofts.

Backus, O., and Beasley, J.: Speech therapy with children, Boston, 1951, Houghton Mifflin Co.

Bloodstein, O.: Speech pathology: an introduction, Boston, 1979, Houghton Mifflin Co.

Bzoch, K., editor: Communicative disorders related to cleft lip and palate, Boston, 1972, Little, Brown and Co.

Carrell, J.: Disorders of articulation, Englewood Cliffs, N.J., 1968, Prentice-Hall, Inc.

Chomsky, N., and Halle, M.: The sound pattern of English, New York, 1968, Harper & Row, Publishers.

Collins, P., and Cunningham, G.: Writing individualized programs: a workbook for speech pathologists, Gladstone, Oreg., 1975, C.C. Publications.

Compton, A.: Generative studies of children's phono-

logical disorders, J. Speech Hear. Disord. **35:**315-339, 1970.

Costello, J.: Articulation instruction based on distinctive features theory, Lang. Speech Hear. Serv. Schools **6:**61-71, 1975.

Costello, J.: Programmed instruction, J. Speech Hear. Disord. **42:**3-28, 1977.

Costello, J., and Onstine, J.: The modification of multiple articulation errors based on distinctive feature therapy, J. Speech Hear. Disord. **41:**199-215, 1976.

Crickmay, M.: Speech therapy and the Bobath approach to cerebral palsy, Springfield, Ill., 1966, Charles C Thomas, Publisher.

Darley, F., Aronson, A., and Brown, J.: Motor speech disorders, Philadelphia, 1975, W. B. Saunders Co.

Drexler, H.: A simplified application of distinctive feature analysis to articulation therapy, J. Oreg. Speech Hear. Assoc. **15:**2-5, 1976.

Eisenson, J., and Ogilvie, M.: Speech correction in the schools, ed. 4, New York, 1977, Macmillan Publishing Co., Inc.

Finnie, N.: Handling the young cerebral palsied child at home, New York, 1975, E. P. Dutton & Co., Inc.

Gerber, A.: Goal: carryover an articulation manual and program, Philadelphia, 1973, Temple University Press.

Gerber, A.: Programming for articulation modification, J. Speech Hear. Disord. **42:**29-43, 1977.

Hahn, E.: Indications for direct, nondirect, and indirect methods in speech correction, J. Speech Hear. Disord. **26:**230-236, 1961.

Hartbauer, R., editor: Counseling in communicative disorders, Springfield, Ill., 1978, Charles C Thomas, Publisher.

Hejna, R.: Speech disorders and non-directive therapy: client-centered counseling and play therapy, New York, 1960, The Ronald Press Co.

Ingram, D.: Phonological disability in children, New York, 1976, Elsevier North-Holland, Inc.

Jakobson, R.: Child language, aphasia, and phonological universals, The Hague, 1968, Mouton.

Johnson, W., and associates: Speech handicapped school children, ed. 3, New York, 1967, Harper & Row, Publishers.

Lassers, L.: Fun and play with sounds and speech, Salem, Oreg., 1954, State Department of Education.

Lillywhite, H.: Make mother a clinician, J. Speech Hear. Disord. **13:**61-66, 1948.

Ling, D.: Speech and the hearing-impaired child: theory and practice, Washington, D.C., 1976, Alexander Graham Bell Association for the Deaf.

Lowell, E., and Stoner, M.: Play it by ear, Los Angeles, 1960, John Tracy Clinic.

Mager, R.: Preparing instructional objectives, Palo Alto, 1962, Fearon Publishers.

McCabe, R., and Bradley, D.: Systematic multiple phonemic approach to articulation therapy, Acta Symbol. **6:**1-18, 1975.

McDonald, E.: Articulation testing and treatment: a sensory-motor approach, Pittsburgh, 1964, Stanwix House, Inc.

McDonald, E., and Chance, B.: Cerebral palsy, Englewood Cliffs, N.J., 1964, Prentice-Hall, Inc.

McReynolds, L., and Bennet, S.: Distinctive feature generalization in articulation training, J. Speech Hear. Disord. **37**:462-470, 1972.

McReynolds, L., and Engmann, D.: Distinctive feature analysis of misarticulations, Baltimore, 1975, University Park Press.

Milisen, R., and associates: The disorder of articulation: a systematic clinical and experimental approach, J. Speech Hear. Disord., Monogr. Suppl. **4**:1954.

Morehead, D., and Morehead, A., editors: Normal and deficient child language, Baltimore, 1976, University Park Press.

Morley, M.: Cleft palate and speech, Edinburgh, England, 1970, E. & S. Livingstone.

Mowrer, D.: Methods of modifying speech behaviors, Columbus, Ohio, 1977, Charles E. Merrill Publishing Co.

Newby, H.: Audiology, New York, 1972, Appleton-Century-Crofts.

Oyer, H., and Frankmann, J.: The aural rehabilitation process, New York, 1975, Holt, Rinehart and Winston, Inc.

Powers, G.: Cleft palate, Indianapolis, 1973, The Bobbs-Merrill Co., Inc.

Powers, M.: Clinical and educational procedures in functional disorders of articulation. In Travis, L., editor: Handbook of speech pathology and audiology, New York, 1971, Appleton-Century-Crofts.

Rosenbek, R., and associates: Treatment of developmental apraxia of speech: a case study, Lang. Speech Hear. Serv. Schools **5**:13-22, 1974.

Sanders, D.: Aural rehabilitation, Englewood Cliffs, N.J., 1971, Prentice-Hall, Inc.

Schiefelbusch, R., editor: Language of the mentally retarded, Baltimore, 1972, University Park Press.

Schlanger, B.: Speech measurements of institutionalized mentally handicapped children, J. Speech Hear. Disord. **19**:339-343, 1954.

Schoolfield, L.: Better speech and better reading, a practice book, Boston, 1973, Expression.

Scripture, E.: Stuttering, lisping and correction of the speech of the deaf, New York, 1923, Macmillan Publishing Co., Inc.

Scripture, M., and Jackson, E.: A manual of exercises for the correction of speech disorders, Philadelphia, 1927, F. A. Davis Co.

Shelton, R.: Disorders of articulation. In Skinner, P., and Shelton, R.: Speech, language, and hearing, Reading, Mass., 1978, Addison-Wesley Publishing Co., Inc.

Shriberg, L.: A response evocation program for /ɜ˞/, J. Speech Hear. Disord. **40**:92-105, 1975.

Singh, S., and Polen, S.: Use of a distinctive feature model in speech pathology, Acta Symbol. **3**:17-25, 1972.

Skinner, P., and Shelton, R.: Speech, language, and hearing: normal processes and disorders, Reading, Mass., 1978, Addison-Wesley Publishing Co., Inc.

Sommers, R., and Kane, A.: Nature and remediation of functional articulation disorders. In Dickson, S., editor: Communication disorders: remedial principles and practices, Glenview, Ill., 1974, Scott, Foresman and Co.

Spriestersbach, D., and Sherman, D., editors: Cleft palate and communication, New York, 1968, Academic Press, Inc.

Stoddard, C.: Sounds for little folks, Magnolia, Mass., 1940, Expression Co.

Turnbull, A., and Schulz, J.: Mainstreaming handicapped students, Boston, 1979, Allyn & Bacon, Inc.

Van Riper, C.: Teaching your child to talk, New York, 1950, Harper & Row, Publishers.

Van Riper, C.: Speech correction principles and methods, ed. 6, Englewood Cliffs, N.J., 1978, Prentice-Hall, Inc.

Weiner, F.: Phonological process analysis, Baltimore, 1979, University Park Press.

Weiss, C., and Lillywhite, H.: Communicative disorders: a handbook for prevention and early intervention, St. Louis, 1976, The C. V. Mosby Co.

Wells, C.: Cleft palate and its associated speech disorders, New York, 1971, McGraw-Hill Book Co.

Westlake, H., and Rutherford, D.: Speech therapy for the cerebral palsied, Chicago, 1961, National Society for Crippled Children and Adults, Inc.

Weston, A., and Irwin, J.: The use of paired-stimuli in the modification of articulation, J. Percept. Mot. Skills **32**:947-957, 1971.

Winitz, H.: Articulatory acquisition and behavior, New York, 1961, Appleton-Century-Crofts.

Winitz, H.: From syllable to conversation, Baltimore, 1975, University Park Press.

Young, E., and Hawk, S.: Moto-kinesthetic speech training, Stanford, Calif., 1938, Stanford University Press.

GLOSSARY

auditory conceptualization Grasping, understanding, and framing concepts from incoming information via auditory channels.

ballistic movements Rapid contraction of a muscle group followed by short periods of no contraction, but the involved structures continue to move because of the momentum.

behavior modification A system for modifying, shaping, or changing behavior based on principles of positive and negative reinforcement. Improving or modifying speech or any segment of speech can be considered behavior in this context.

behaviorism A doctrine that observed behavior provides the only valid base for constructing a plan to change behavior. Behaviorism largely rejects the mind and psychologic processes as factors in behavior change.

bombardment Refers to a process in treating articulatory disorders in which the client is subjected to many repetitions (bombardment) of a target sound in one or many situations.

contingency management Analogous to behavior therapy and behavior modification. The management or manipulation of antecedent and subsequent events to bring about a specific response in an individual and reinforcement of that response.

directive Used here to designate a direct rather than a nondirect approach to treatment of articulatory disorders.

echo speech A technique in which the clinician repeats (echoes) specific utterances of the client in order to stimulate the client to continue verbalizing and to provide auditory training.

extinction A technique in behavior modification applying to discontinuing (extinguishing) a stimulus or response of the client in a structured sequence of treatment.

fractionalizing Separating or "breaking up" verbalizations into separate segments to facilitate the treatment process.

iambic stress A stress pattern of two syllables in which the first syllable is unstressed and the second stressed, usually a consonant-vowel-consonant-vowel (CVCV) combination, used as stimulus in articulatory training.

isolation Used here to refer to a single phone isolated from a phoneme, syllable, or word.

morphologic Refers to the structure of words as opposed to that of phones, phonemes, or syllables.

nondirective Indirect treatment techniques, such as role-playing, games, counseling, etc.

operant conditioning Analogous to behavior modification, behavior therapy, programmed instruction, and sometimes learning theory. Essentially stimuli and responses are specified prior to initiation of a particular treatment procedure and the client is given immediate feedback after the response in the form of positive or negative reinforcement.

overlapping movements Certain movements of the articulators overlap other movements preceding or following the production of a particular phoneme, often influencing or modifying that phoneme.

phonetic rule system Theoretically a child unconsciously develops phonetic rules or patterns that form an individual system for evolving speech. If speech is disordered it may be that the child's rule system is different from the expected norm.

programmed instruction Analogous to operant conditioning, behavior modification, behavior therapy, and sometimes learning theory. (*See* Operant conditioning.)

reinforcement A procedure in programmed instruction for providing a client with feedback and motivation immediately after a response by means of positive or negative reinforcement.

stabilizing Used here to refer to making a newly learned sound stable by incorporating it into the client's speech outside the clinic.

stimulability The ability of a client to reproduce sounds when given the vocal-visual model (stimulated) by the clinician.

stimulation The act of motivating a client to make a specific desired response, such as a clinician's saying a target sound to stimulate a similar response from the client. Stimulation may be given by vocal, visual, tactile, or kinesthetic methods and may be direct or indirect.

strengthening *See* Stabilizing. Refers to the same process.

stridency High-frequency or high-friction sound such as in /s/ and /z/. Stridency is sometimes used to refer to a shrill, coarse voice quality.

successive approximation A procedure in which the client starts with a sound already learned correctly and progresses by stimulus and response through a series of sounds gradually more closely approximating the target sound.

tactile The sense of touch. Skin or mucous (surface) sensitivity of the organism.

target sound A specific error sound of the client that becomes the "target" of procedures taken to correct it.

task sequence A programmed instruction procedure in which a specific objective is attempted through a carefully programmed sequence of tasks.

transfer The process by which the learning of one behavior (sound or other aspect of communication) facilitates learning of another related behavior.

trochaic A stress pattern in which an accented syllable is followed by an unaccented syllable, vowel-consonant-vowel-consonant (VCVC).

CHAPTER NINE

Techniques for treatment of special problems

"Speech and reason distinguish men from beasts."

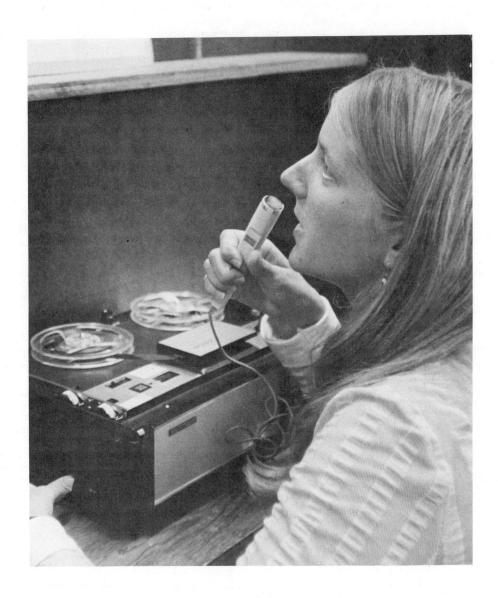

In the previous chapter discussion centered around the different types of articulation treatment. These methods have been quite successful with articulation problems in the mainstream. However, because they have a wide, general application, they may not be as efficient and effective with certain special aspects of articulation management. For this reason the following information will include techniques for treating special problems.

Certain aspects of articulation treatment and types of articulation disorders pose specific problems for speech-language pathologists. Unhealthy or erroneous parental attitudes toward the child and the child's speech can be a deterrent to successful articulation management (Hartbauer, 1978). Throughout this chapter when we speak of parents we are including any others who might be most responsible for a child's care, such as foster parents or guardians. A primary approach for coping with this problem of unfavorable attitudes is counseling.

A second problem area is failure to achieve carry-over in treatment. It is understandable that carry-over commonly poses problems for the clinician because it requires the client to acquire new phonologic rules, habitually produce different distinctive features, and achieve cognitive competence in articulation. In treatment, criterion levels are usually systematically and easily achieved until the client must transfer the consciously produced sounds into subconscious utterances in settings other than a structured clinic room. At this point the rate of progress begins to falter. To aid in alleviating the problem of achieving carry-over, helpful suggestions are provided.

Previous reference has been made to articulation disorders caused or accompanied by dyspraxia, mental retardation, cerebral palsy, cleft palate, hearing impairment, and multiple educational handicaps. Because these special problems are not always effectively managed with general, traditional approaches, we have included some special techniques.

With the advent of the federal mandate for providing appropriate, minimally restricting education for all handicapped children, public school speech-language pathologists more and more will be dealing with clients who have multiple problems. Along with these multiple handicaps will be a wide range of articulation disorders. Special techniques will need to be devised for members of this population who have special needs. This chapter will share some ideas for these special children.

Last, an important problem area for any kind of treatment but especially for articulation disorders because they are so common, is that of insufficient time to accommodate all individuals needing treatment. Group treatment, block scheduling, and the employment of communication aides, parents, and other professionals or team members provide partial solutions for this problem area. Information will be included to assist with the problem of limited available time.

COUNSELING

Most success in articulation improvement occurs when the person being counseled has a healthy and constructive attitude toward the client and the client's speech; therefore, all parents of children with deviant articulation and other key persons in the child's environment should be provided with information and guidance relative to the child's development (Powers, 1971). Counseling is an approach through which such information can be given, but counseling can also accomplish much more than just giving information and guidance. Parents can become effective participants in the management program, especially when special and difficult problems are involved, but also when general and less severe problems are present. Usually the more information parents and other key members in the child's environment have, the more effective will be their participation.

The very important step of counseling in articulation management can occur several times: after the diagnostic workup, periodically during treatment (particularly if counselee behavior is to be modified), at the time treatment is terminated, and during the carry-over period. The direction and emphasis vary with the purpose of the counseling session, the person being counseled, the client being discussed, the duration and number of counseling sessions anticipated, and the philosophy of the counselor— whether counseling is viewed as an educational experience, a psychotherapeutic process, or both.

Counseling requires a number of skills, some of which are discussed below. We know that an effective counselor must possess interpersonal relationship skills, know about the articulation disorder in particular and about communication development and its disorders in general; give and receive information, establish a basic contract or understanding between counselor and counselee, and know mechanics of beginning and ending counseling sessions; have integrity; provide ways of establishing rapport and freedom to explore feelings and facts; clarify attitudes about oneself and others; be aware of the pragmatics and nonverbal aspects of communication; respect the private world of each person; and have an acute sense of perception and judgment in relation to the person being counseled (Webster, 1977). Another quality important to counseling, but one that is not teachable, is common sense. It is defined as sound practical judgment independent of specialized knowledge. Without it, even though all the aforementioned characteristics are present, one probably could not become an entirely effective counselor. Hopefully persons engaged in counseling will have common sense. Unfortunately common sense is not common.

Students continually express concerns and anxieties about how to counsel. These concerns are justified partly because of the paucity of training available in counseling communication disorders and partly because of the complexity involved in effective counseling (Patton and Griffin, 1974). For example, how does one best respond to a crisis during a counseling session? What is the most appropriate response of the counselor when a counselee begins to cry or becomes enraged? Where, in the typical university curriculum, is this taught?

What can be done to improve one's counseling skills? Webster (1977) and Hartbauer (1978) suggest a number of activities and principles that can improve counseling skills. We will mention some of them and refer to the sections on interviewing in Chapter 5 and reporting in Chapter 10 for providing a helpful supplement to the following suggestions.

Gain knowledge

Since counselors in communication disorders receive information, give information, help clarify ideas, attitudes, and emotions, and assist parents in learning new behaviors, an ample amount of knowledge is imperative. This knowledge should include all facets of articulation problems, child growth and development, and interpersonal communication skills. This is knowledge that can be gained through a course of study, observation of exemplary counseling, observation of children's behavior, and experience in counseling. Like many activities of the "helping" or health professions, counseling skills are not developed through studying and reading alone but through experience in counseling as well.

Question attitudes and assumptions

To question one's own attitudes and assumptions is to understand better the attitudes and assumptions about parents or others being counseled (Webster, 1977). Such questioning increases levels of awareness about our attitudes and assumptions. This guards against making hasty value judgments and imparting inappropriate information. As Rogers (1951) so aptly stated, "It is unlikely that a counselor can accept others unless he is also in the process of accepting himself." This lifelong process of self-acceptance requires considerable effort in self-analysis, critically viewing oneself, and asking others to help interpret one's attitudes and assumptions. Coursework in psychology and sociology can also be helpful in this regard.

Improve interpersonal communication skills

Since interpersonal relations are dependent on communication, any improvement in communication skills might also improve counseling. These communication skills involve conveying and receiving messages through verbal and nonverbal means. They require adherence to semantic rigor and careful monitoring of voice, inflection patterns, rate, stress, and other prosodic features of speech. Here again, improvement dictates practice in attending to and using these skills, increasing levels of awareness, and improving self-analysis abilities. One way of improving interpersonal communication skills is through conscious efforts of practicing better communication and interaction. Courses in this area and in general semantics are also helpful.

Remember that information can be conveyed in different ways

As mentioned earlier, information can be conveyed verbally and nonverbally, orally or in writing, clearly or ambiguously. However it is conveyed, information should be checked with receivers of the information for accuracy of interpretation. These probes for understanding will provide information about the counselor's effectiveness. Another way to improve this aspect of communication is by perfecting communication skills through practice in organized group discussions, increased knowledge, and defining and refining methods of assessing the accuracy of the counselee's interpretations.

Become a better listener

The art of listening is integrally related to interpersonal communication and counseling. It is a skill that can always be improved but is often neglected. Better listening leads to better understanding, which in turn, leads to better counseling (Barbara, 1958). Practice in listening should be done actively and intensely (Nichols, 1955). At first listening might be assisted by making more elaborate notes of what is being said or by tape-recording the session. By listening to the tape several times and reanalyzing it, the counselor should improve listening skills. The counselor should be prepared to listen to a range of experiences from crisis to happiness. Also the counselor must resist the great temptation to start talking too soon or to talk too much. As Weiss and Lillywhite (1976) stated, "The professional person is especially vulnerable with respect to the temptation to ververbalize because there is a captive audience and much to say. The client is in trouble and needs to be told what to do." The task of the counselor is not to tell the client what to do but to help the client find what to do on the client's own initiative.

Structuring the session

Webster (1977) recommends structuring the session by placing certain limitations on the counseling session. These limitations provide a sense of order and security and clarify the ground rules from the outset. Structuring should improve efficiency, particularly when counseling includes several sessions. Improving this aspect of counseling usually occurs with practice and with a mutual understanding of the goals to be accomplished.

Respect the rights and abilities of counselees

In some area of life nearly everyone is superior to others. Regardless of your role as counselor, the counselee may have abilities and knowledge superior to yours. Be aware of them, acknowledge them, and utilize them, even if it means relinquishing your leadership role at times. This is especially important if counseling occurs in a group setting. Counselees also have a right to express themselves, a right that must be granted if counseling is to be truly a feedback process. Improvement in this area usually comes with increased awareness and practice.

Use simple, descriptive language

This point is discussed in Chapters 5 and 10 dealing with interviewing and reporting. Many misunderstandings could be avoided if the counselor would only remember to talk simply and descriptively. Avoid becoming "intoxicated by the exuberance of one's own verbosity," "technical jargon," fancy labels, unnecessary polysyllabic words, and long, elaborate sentences. Constantly strive to monitor the counseling session in regard to every concept being conveyed. Remember, the purpose of the session is to communicate, which can usually be accomplished through skillful listening and by using simple, descriptive language. Listening to a tape recording of the counseling session can be very revealing and helpful.

End the session on a positive theme

This attribute of effective counseling combines common sense and basic psychologic principles. We suggest positive termination in regard to each counseling session. Ending on a pleasant note is a matter of awareness and planning. The counselor must plan how to end the session positively. It is important to end on time and without making unwarranted statements or impossible promises. Experience in counseling should improve this area.

Teach counselees how to change behaviors

If counseling is for the purpose of changing behavior rather than of merely informing the parent or others about the child's condition or progress, then several ideas should be presented. These ideas should provide options on what to do and how to do it. Skill in this area presupposes knowledge and experience in behavior modification on the part of the counselor.

These are some areas that should be improved if counseling skills are to become more effective. Improvement requires knowledge of communication disorders, communication development, counseling skills, and considerable practical experience. Improvement in these skills should enhance the overall treatment process in the habilitation or rehabilitation of persons with articulation and other communication disorders.

Now we shall discuss some of the special problems in the management of articulation disorders that not only involve extensive counseling but also require special techniques of treatment and other phases of management.

CARRY-OVER

Possibly the most perplexing and frustrating aspect of articulation treatment is carry-over. This is well illustrated by the results of a survey in which public school speech-language clinicians ranked lack of carry-over as their most difficult problem (Sommers, 1969). Many clinicians have had the discouraging experience of hearing a client misarticulate a sound outside the clinic room after hearing the client produce the sound correctly in conversational speech during several clinic sessions. Just what is meant by the term "carry-over"? *Carry-over* can be defined as the habitual use of a target sound in all speaking situations, including conversational speech in and out of the clinic. It also involves articulation of the target sound without deliberate or conscious effort (Gerber, 1973; Sommers and Kane, 1974). Various other terms are used when describing the carry-over process: transfer, generalization, maintenance, retention, automatization, and habituation. *Transfer* refers to using the same response to stimuli not used in the training process, for example, using the sound correctly in different words, using the sound in sentences when only words have been trained, and using the sound when talking with persons other than the clinician (Mowrer, 1971). *Generalization* also occurs when the newly acquired sound is used in the presence of stimulus conditions not present during the training process and in the absence of reinforcement (Costello and Bosler, 1976). *Maintenance* and *retention* refer to continued use of the target sound in all speaking situations over time (Mowrer, 1977). *Automatization* and *habituation* indicate correct production of the sound that occurs without conscious or deliberate effort (Manning, Keappock, and Stick, 1976; Sommers and Kane, 1974).

Carry-over occurs at different rates for different individuals and sometimes is never achieved. Occasionally a client is dismissed from treatment only to be reentered at a later time because carry-over did not occur. We really do not know what variables account for success in this phenomenon or for differences in the learning rate, but some of these variables may be client characteristics, such as stimulability, consistency of error production, history of reinforcement, and intelligibility in addition to variables in articulation programming (Costello and Bosler, 1976; Mowrer, 1971). Winitz (1975) hypothesizes that the reason a client produces a sound correctly during word and phrase practice but not in conversational speech is that the error response interferes with the newly acquired sound. In other words, what a person has learned previously interferes with retaining and using the new behavior as a substitute for the "old" behavior; the years of practice a child or adult has had in using the misarticulation (habit strength) intervenes in the ability to remember the newly learned sound (Mowrer, 1977).

Some clinicians apparently assume that carry-over occurs automatically during the treatment process with little attention given to it; however, often this is not the case (Costello and Bosler, 1976; Powers, 1971). Carry-over does seem to take a certain period of time and considerable planning and incorporation in treatment for correct articulation of target sounds to transfer or generalize to conversation in all speaking situations. Actually the carry-over process begins at the initiation of treatment, but in the later stages specific procedures need to be incorporated to facilitate generalization and habituation. Many suggest that carry-over activities can be initiated when the client easily and unhesitatingly produces the sounds in words (Eisenson and Ogilvie, 1977; Johnson and associates, 1967; Pow-

ers, 1971). Carry-over may be facilitated if treatment includes four general principles of positive transfer (Mowrer, 1971):

1. *Stimulus similarity*—the more similar the stimuli in training and in test activities, the greater the transfer
2. *Amount of training*—the more training on a task, the greater the transfer, up to a point
3. *Reinforcement variability*—when correct responses are reinforced immediately, the greater the transfer; intermittent reinforcement results in greater transfer than constant reinforcement
4. *Punishment*—punishment of incorrect responses may lead to greater transfer of the correct response

Several techniques and programs have been suggested and devised for achievement of carry-over. Some of these procedures have been researched, but many have not. Some involve only in-clinic activities, whereas others require out-of-clinic (extra-clinic) activities and the assistance of people other than the clinician and client. In-clinic procedures will be described first.

In-clinic activities

Gerber (1973) devised the *nonsense material approach* to articulation treatment primarily for the purpose of effecting carry-over. She hypothesized that individuals with deviant articulation disorders need to learn to produce target sounds effortlessly and consistently. Use of nonmeaningful verbal material facilitates achievement of this objective in that the old articulation habit patterns do not interfere with the motor patterns necessary to produce the newly learned sound. Old learning does not interfere with new learning. Only after the target sound is produced automatically in nonmeaningful contexts is meaning introduced. At this point "real" words are easily produced by the client, who can then concentrate on the content of the message while attending minimally to the mechanics of articulation. According to Gerber, if meaningful material is introduced too early in the treatment process, articulation of the sound in these words will be deliberately and laboriously produced. Many treatment approaches certainly involve practice of the target phonemes in nonsense material, but not to the extent that Gerber suggests.

A study conducted by Leonard (1973) investigated the effectiveness of using nonsense drill material. Leonard divided eight subjects with [θ/s] substitutions into a "nonsense" group and a "meaningful" group. The former group was taught to produce /s/ in words with nonsense definitions, and the latter group was taught to produce the same /s/ words in meaningful contexts. The "nonsense" group learned the correct production more effectively; however, the "meaningful" group had better generalization. Leonard suggests that nonsense contexts may facilitate acquisition of the target sound but may not be as effective for generalization so that possibly one should begin with nonmeaningful words and move to meaningful ones. Gerber's approach (1973) does proceed from nonsense to meaningful material, and the approach is reported to be effective in achieving carry-over.

After reviewing research results, Winitz (1975) also recommended the *use of nonsense words* (alone and in conversation) prior to practicing the target sounds in meaningful material. Mowrer (1977) points out that meaningful words usually are retained longer than nonsense words and cautions that some practice materials used by speech-language pathologists, for example, rhymes, tongue twisters, and poems, are really not meaningful for a client and thus may not contribute much to carry-over of the target sound into spontaneous speech. It seems to us that the use of nonsense materials emphasizes the motor or mechanical aspects of articulation, that is, production without the competition of meaning and former negative habit patterns. Later, during carry-over phases, meaning is added to the motor component of articulation.

Another "motor" approach to articulation treatment was proposed by Bankson and Byrne (1972), although they utilized meaningful words. They experimented with a carry-over approach, the purpose of which was to develop articulation motor skills so that phonemes could be produced easily and rapidly. They hypothesize that carry-over may not occur because of inadequate practice of the motor skills used in production of the target sound; therefore, *"overpractice"* may be important in maintaining correct production of the target sound rather than reverting to habitual error patterns. Caution should be practiced, however, since overpractice can result in overgeneralization. Byrne and Shervanian (1977) also suggest that overlearning may foster carry-over. In the program of Bankson and Byrne the client reads a sixty-word list twenty-five times per session in a given time limit. The time limit is reduced by 2 seconds each time the list is read with 100% accuracy. Ten seconds are added to the time limit at the beginning of each succeeding session, providing a "warm-up" period, and 2 seconds are taken off with each successful reading. If misarticulations occur, the time limit is expanded by 2 seconds for five trials. The goal is correct, effortless, automatic articulation. Using this procedure over a 10-day period, five of five subjects showed improved performance in the training task and four of five achieved at least some carry-over to three different settings. Gerber (1973) also stresses rapid, effortless, and consistent production, suggesting that competition during clinical activities helps fast production. Activities requiring responses under a time limit are also recommended by Gerber.

Another component emphasized is *client self-evaluation,* for which auditory training forms the base (Gerber, 1973; Powers, 1971; Van Riper, 1978; Winitz, 1975). Training in self-monitoring occurs throughout the treatment process, primarily through the auditory modality, although the visual, tactile, and kinesthetic modes are sometimes also used in Gerber's approach. The rationale is that the clients need to detect their own errors. The client is trained to do this through a series of steps that are briefly described in Chapter 8 and through positive reinforcement of accurate self-evaluation. Winitz emphasizes training in distinguishing between the client's own misarticulations and the standard sounds in words, sentences, and conversation. According to Winitz (1975), sometimes discrimination training is enough to effect correct articulation without actual production training. Winitz further describes a rather unique technique for training self-monitoring skills. When a client misarticulates the target sound, the speech-language pathologist initially responds inappropriately and eventually responds appropriately by articulating the word correctly several times (see Chapter 8). Eventually as a result of this procedure the client will likely produce the sound correctly. Another self-monitoring procedure requires clients to evaluate their own productions (scanning and self-analysis) before being reinforced. If they produce the sound correctly and identify it as correct, they are reinforced. Engel and Groth (1976) also found this procedure to be helpful in achieving carry-over. Powers (1971) indicates that thorough auditory discrimination training is critical to the achievement of carry-over since persons need to be able to identify their own errors in order to use correct articulation in conversational speech. If generalization to spontaneous speech is not occurring, possibly the clinician should incorporate specific auditory training procedures into the treatment process, including training in connected speech.

For the purpose of generalization Winitz (1975) suggests using a procedure to develop and strengthen an *association between the error and correct sounds*. In the clinic session the clinician articulates words incorrectly and the client responds by producing the word correctly. The child never intentionally produces the word incorrectly; it is only heard incorrectly (a form of negative practice). In this way, it is hypothesized, the client associates the incorrect production with the correct production. Later, when misarticulating the sound, the clients may associate the error with the standard sound and correct themselves.

Irwin and Weston (1975) developed the *paired-stimuli approach* to articulation management to assist generalization. First the clinician locates words that contain the target sound and that the client articulates correctly, that is, key words as described by Van Riper (1978). If no key words are found, one is taught to the client. The client then pairs this correctly produced key word with the training words, that is, words that are misarticulated in two or three trials. Thus the key word serves as a model for the training words and for providing correct auditory and tactile feedback. All correct productions are reinforced by the clinician. The three steps of the paired-stimuli program for the client are:

1. Pair the correctly articulated key word with the misarticulated training words until eight or ten training words in each position are correct on two successive trials.
2. Answer structured clinician questions using the training words.
3. Use training words in spontaneous conversation.

A study (Irwin and Weston, 1975) was conducted with eighty experimental subjects who were administered the program and eighty control subjects who were not. The experimental group performed better on conversational posttests administered immediately following treatment and again 1 month later, suggesting that such an approach may facilitate carry-over.

Mowrer (1971) seems to prefer using a *systematic programmed approach* without manipulation of external stimuli. If the program is carefully and logically designed with an emphasis on techniques to facilitate positive transfer, it may not be necessary to plan extraclinic activities. Mowrer cited one study that showed a programmed approach to be more effective for carry-over than a nonprogrammed traditional approach. Regardless of the treatment approach used, carry-over activities must be incorporated into the overall design, both in-clinic and out-of-clinic.

Other specific techniques for in-clinic

carry-over activities have been suggested. It is beneficial to practice *nucleus words and phrases* (for example, greetings, courtesies, names, and frequent requests) in clinic sessions and to encourage the client to articulate correctly these expressions in everyday situations (Johnson and associates, 1967; Powers, 1971). Some time should be devoted to such practice every session. Along these same lines, words from classroom subject matter, vocabulary related to holidays and special events, and core vocabularies (words meaningfully related) can be practiced in and out of clinic sessions. Punishment of misarticulations calls the client's attention to the errors and thus should result in a decrease in their occurrence. Johnson and associates (1967) indicate that the client should use self-punishment, for example, track or note errors, write down error words, or tap a foot. Such a negative procedure should first be practiced in the clinic setting where the speech-language clinician can monitor the client's self-monitoring accuracy. Later the clients can track themselves outside the clinic.

Negative practice (deliberate production of the error) is occasionally suggested. The purpose is to make the client aware of errors; however, such a procedure may actually strengthen the error pattern. Therefore, caution should be exercised when employing negative practice. It may be helpful to place the responsibility for changed articulation behavior on the client since desire to improve is a "powerful force" in achieving carry-over (Engel and associates, 1966). It is often motivating for clients to follow progress of the treatment process so that they understand what has been accomplished and what the future goals are. Results can be shown objectively through graphs, charts, and other records. Time should be devoted to the client and clinician conversing with one another and engaging in other activities requiring the client to use connected speech, for example, role playing, storytelling, dramatizations, and puppetry. It is helpful to introduce games, competition, and similar activities in clinic sessions after

the target sound is produced in connected speech in ideal conditions in order to heighten a client's emotional level. Such activities tend to induce excitement and distraction. Such speech productions could be tape-recorded for later analysis by both the client and clinician. Masking noise can be used so that the client has to produce the standard sound without auditory feedback (Van Riper, 1978). Numerous other in-clinic techniques can be used to aid carry-over into conversational speech, but now extra-clinic techniques will be considered.

Out-of-clinic activities

Since the final goal is correct articulation of the standard sound in all speaking situations, several techniques have been devised to help generalization to extraclinic settings. Speech notebooks may "bridge the gap" between the clinic and outside environments. The client puts pictures or words containing the target sound in the notebook, which is used for home practice. New words are not added until the client demonstrates proficiency in producing them within the clinic session. The purpose is to increase the client's awareness of speech between sessions and to provide stimulus material for the client, teacher, parents, and other key persons. Powers (1971) suggests establishing a weekly quota of words to be produced correctly outside the clinic session. Other types of assignments can be given to aid in carry-over, but certain cautions should be taken. Assignments should be made for particular times or situations, not for all day everyday. Remember that clients cannot generalize to all words at once. For the assignments to be useful, the client must identify all misarticulations.

Winitz (1975) suggests that the child and clinician engage in *conversational speech* in the clinic setting and then in *outside environments* similar to and near the clinic room. Still later, an unfamiliar clinician or someone trained to detect misarticulations converses with the client in these same environments. Training in two or more different settings was also recommended by Griffiths and Craighead (1972), especially for trainable mentally retarded individuals. Creating discriminative stimuli or reminders in extraclinic environments should foster carry-over (Engel and associates, 1966; Gerber, 1973). Examples are signs placed in outside environments, books used during clinic sessions and read in other settings, word lists taped to the desk and bedroom door, and so forth.

Enlisting the assistance of interested persons, such as parents, teachers, siblings, classmates, and aides, facilitates carry-over. In most instances for such a procedure to be effective the speech-language pathologist must train the person aiding in the treatment process. In the public school setting classroom teachers are often asked to assist in the treatment process. They can help the client carry out speech assignments, monitor the client's speech during certain activities, provide classroom material to be used during clinic sessions, track the client's errors, and intermittently reinforce correct sound productions. Mowrer (1971) cautions that a classroom teacher should only be requested to perform activities that do not demand much time and that are compatible with normal classroom activities. Additionally instructions should be clear and specific, preferably in written form. Some teachers do not desire to assist or do not have the time; therefore, demands should not be made on them, but they should be asked if they would like to help.

Parent involvement is frequently solicited by the speech-language clinician for the purpose of facilitating carry-over. Remember that not all parents can work effectively with their child on articulation skills. The speech-language pathologist must first make a judgment about whether a parent will work positively with the client before embarking on a training program with the parent (Skinner and Shelton, 1978). Factors to be considered include the complexity of the problem, the nature of the parent-child relationship, amount of desire to help, and possibly the intelligence level. If it appears that parents will not be helpful in the treat-

ment process, siblings, classmates, or aides can be used instead. Most parents who are interested in assisting must be trained in some way (Eisenson and Ogilvie, 1977; Mowrer, 1971). Merely providing them with instructions is usually not sufficient since they do not have the background and skills needed to evaluate and reinforce their child for articulation proficiency. Parents need to learn to discriminate between their child's correct and incorrect sound productions in words, sentences, and conversation, to reinforce positively, to correct misarticulations, and possibly to track articulation performance. Ideally such training includes explanation by the clinician of the articulation treatment program, parent observation of clinic sessions with the client and clinician working together, verbal and written explanation of the parent role in treatment, and practice by the parent and child in the clinic setting with observation and critique by the clinician.

An articulation carry-over program implemented by parents was developed by Wing and Heimgartner (1973). They contend that the final phase of treatment, conversational speech, is too broad for both the clinician and client in that there are varying levels of difficulty in this last step of treatment. Therefore, a five-level carry-over program was devised:

1. Oral reading within a limited time span (10 minutes)
2. Oral reading and oral discussion of the reading with a limited time span (5 minutes of reading and 5 minutes of discussion)
3. Structured conversation about pre-selected topics within a limited time span (10 minutes)
4. Unstructured conversational speaking within an increased time span (10 minutes within a certain hour)
5. Unstructured conversational speaking within an expanded time span (10 minutes within a day)

Criterion for movement from one step to the next is zero errors for three consecutive practice sessions on at least 3 different days.

The five-step program is carried out by the parent and child with weekly clinician-parent telephone conferences. These telephone conferences serve to monitor progress, answer parent questions, maintain interest, and reinforce the child and parent. Training consists of familiarizing the parent with the child's treatment program, training the parent how to identify and record articulation errors, explaining the five-step carry-over program, and training the parent in how to maintain and record data for each home practice session. Results of a pilot study using the program with six subjects showed it to be effective in generalization of correct articulation patterns to other speaking situations as reported by parents, teachers, and speech-language clinicians. It is assumed that this program is effective because home assignments are clearly defined, length of home sessions is specifically prescribed for frequent intervals, realistic achievable objectives are specified, results are recorded daily, and periodic telephone contacts are used. For more specific information about the parent training procedures, selection of clients, home practice assignments, and recording procedures, refer to Wing and Heimgartner (1973). Similar programs could be used involving siblings, aides, classmates, older students, or other key persons in the client's environment. Again we must caution that the speech-language pathologist must be selective in instituting a client-parent or other person carry-over program since not all have the necessary time, desire, or skills to implement it effectively.

Another program has been devised to transfer correct articulation responses to the client's everyday environment after the clinician teaches the target sound in words (Shelton, Johnson, and Arndt, 1972; Shelton and associates, 1975). *Parents are trained to make auditory discriminations* between sounds. For 3 consecutive days the parent elicits ten different words from the child. Then thirty different words are elicited in conversational speech for a period of 4 weeks. Correct responses are positively reinforced, incorrect responses are punished, and all responses are tracked. The procedure was found to be somewhat but not totally effective with preschool and school-aged children.

Winitz (1975) believes that parents generally serve only to remind the client to produce the standard sound. Their role in the carry-over process is seen as relatively minor, especially if conversational proficiency has not occurred in the clinic setting. Many articulation clinicians do not agree with Winitz's contention, but it does seem logical not to expect the client to use the target sound in conversation outside the clinic setting until proficiency is achieved in the clinic. A good rule of thumb is never to assign a task for the client to perform outside the clinic until the task is achieved within the clinic setting.

Peers and older students have also been used to aid with carry-over. Marquardt (1959) was one of the first to report on the effectiveness of "speech pals." A classmate who has normal articulation is selected to be a client's "speech pal" and attends the speech sessions with the client once a week. After the clinician determines that the classmate can effectively assist the client and after a conference, the "speech pal" helps the client practice speech while reading and conversing outside the clinic 15 minutes per day. The parents of the client and of the speech pal, principal, and teachers should approve of the plan before it is implemented. The rationale of the procedure is that peers are powerful reinforcers. Marquardt reported that the procedure is quite effective in achieving carry-over.

In addition to classmates, older students in the school can serve as "speech pals." Mowrer (1971) also has suggested using peers but cautions that they must be trained by the speech-language pathologist in order for the procedure to be effective. The peer is trained to discriminate between correct and incorrect productions and to reinforce the client. Also it often is effective to reinforce and punish the peer for the client's performance, for example, to award the peer points for correct productions and take away points for incorrect productions. In this way the peer has a vested interest in the client's performance and progress. From their research Johnston and Johnston (1972) concluded that peers function well as discriminative stimuli for correct articulation. Two clients were taught to monitor correct and incorrect speech sounds of each other. This monitoring continued in the classroom even when reinforcement was not provided for doing so. It appears, then, that peers can be a valuable aid in the carry-over process.

Determining carry-over

An inherent problem with the final phase of articulation treatment is how to determine if carry-over has been achieved since it is not feasible for the speech-language pathologist to evaluate the client's articulation in all speaking situations (Irwin and Weston, 1975; Manning, Keappock, and Stick, 1976). Additionally the presence of the clinician in various outside speaking environments may serve as a stimulus for the client to use the target sound, whereas the client may use misarticulations when the clinician is not present. Thus speech observed by the clinician may not be representative. No universal systematic procedure for measuring carry-over has been developed. However, it might be helpful to clarify the client's progress by differentiating among three types of generalization and evaluating articulation performance for each type (Costello and Bosler, 1976):

1. *Intratherapy generalization,* which occurs within the treatment program in that correct articulation generalizes to different stimuli, for example, in different word positions, levels of production, different stimulus conditions, and different words
2. *Carry-over,* which is generalization from treatment to spontaneous speech in the clinic
3. *Extratherapy generalization,* which occurs outside the treatment setting in that correct articulation generalizes to different environments

Often articulation production is evaluated only in the clinic setting yet accurate evaluation of spontaneous speech within the clinic and outside the clinic is important in determining when to dismiss a client (Manning, Keappock, and Stick, 1976).

Manning, Keappock, and Stick (1976) suggest using an auditory masking procedure to determine if automatization of articulation production has been achieved. The rationale for this procedure is based on Van Riper's theory (1978), which indicates that if a person correctly produces words without auditory feedback, the articulation movements are relatively stable. It was thus hypothesized that if correct articulation occurs in the presence of auditory masking, articulation movements have become automatic, but if the masking disrupts correct production, automatization has not yet been achieved. Since auditory masking appears to result in making more accurate estimates of automatization than testing carry-over without masking noise, more research needs to be conducted.

Costello and Bosler (1976) took another approach. They trained mothers of children with articulation disorders to administer a home treatment program. Extratherapy generalization was measured in the clinic environment since treatment was conducted in the home. The clients were tested on twenty-five words (twenty used in training plus five new words) in four situations: (1) mother and client in a small clinic room, (2) experimenter and client in a small clinic room, (3) experimenter and client in a large classroom, and (4) a different experimenter and client in the waiting room on a couch. The results did not differ in these four situations, suggesting that the physical dimensions of the evaluation situation do not seem to influence the client's articulation performance. Although Costello and Bosler (1976) did evaluate extratherapy generalization, they did not assess carry-over of correct articulation into spontaneous speech.

Much more research needs to be done to determine how to evaluate efficiently and accurately articulation proficiency in spontaneous speech in all situations. In the meantime, in order to evaluate carry-over one would need to assess the client's articulation proficiencies in spontaneous speech both inside and outside the clinic setting. Winitz (1975) suggests weekly or biweekly probes of 5 to 10 minutes of conversational speech done when the client is achieving some success in words and phrases. This should be done inside and outside the clinic setting. The speech-language pathologist records the percentage of correct productions in order to track the progress for intratherapy generalization and carry-over. Sometimes parents, siblings, classroom teachers, and classmates can be trained to be accurate evaluators and to report progress to the clinician. Another way to evaluate articulation carry-over is for a clinician not known to the client to interact and assess the client's spontaneous speech in various settings. Additionally the clinician can unobtrusively observe the client in any of a variety of settings, for example, in the classroom, on the playground, in the lunchroom, with the mother in the clinic room, with friends outside the clinic room, and at home. It is important to be accurate in the assessment of carry-over in order to determine when to dismiss the client. The final test is consistently correct production of the target sound in rapid speech under somewhat stressful or emotional conditions when attention is directed to the meaning of what is being said rather than to the mechanics of articulation.

In addition to the special techniques discussed so far in this chapter, there are several special types of disorders that require unusual treatment procedures. Discussion of these follows.

Childhood dyspraxia

Traditional articulation management approaches generally are not effective with dyspraxia in children (Mitcham, 1975). Rosenbek and associates (1973) discuss principles of articulation treatment for dyspraxia in children. The objective is for the child to "acquire as near normal volitional speech as physiological limitations will allow." Auditory discrimination training and muscle strength exercises are not helpful procedures. Instead it is useful to teach the client to use even stress and pauses in polysyllabic words, to slow the speaking rate by prolonging vowels, and to use the intrusive schwa in blends (for example, /bəlu/ for /blu/). A second principle is that treatment should emphasize articulation movement sequences in CV and VC syllables rather than beginning production training in isolation. A third principle is to sequence tasks with a consideration of phonetic principles. Treatment should begin with visible, voiceless consonants and progress to nasal sounds and then to visible, voiced consonants. These sounds are used in reduplicating syllables (for example, /bibi/), and the client learns to use a slow rate, even stress, and careful self-monitoring. Later the vowels and consonants are changed similarly to McDonald's (1964) sensory-motor approach. The fourth principle is to use a limited amount of stimuli. Next an intensive, systematic drill that is spaced should be used. Much drill is needed since the progress is slow. The visual modality is to be stressed. Written stimuli are often helpful for older school-aged clients. Last, correct responses should be facilitated by using motor movements and patterns of rhythm, intonation, and stress. In essence a form of melodic intonation treatment is used. Singing, rhyming, using written accent marks, pausing between syllables, pairing a motor movement with speech, and "beating" time while speaking are helpful procedures.

Chappell (1973) also has suggestions for treating childhood dyspraxia. This treatment approach begins with production of four isolated vowels and five consonants that are easily distinguished (have markedly contrasting features) from one another, for example, /p/, /t/, /k/, /f/, and /s/. These selected sounds are used to teach articulation patterns by blending the sounds. Gradually the length of utterances is expanded. Each pattern is repeated several times in order to assist motor memory of how the words are to be articulated. While working on these basic patterns, Chappell recommends that the client be taught to produce a few meaningful monosyllabic words that will be useful to the child in the environment.

Adult dyspraxia

Rosenbek and associates (1973) developed a treatment program for adult clients with dyspraxia. They begin by stating principles for sequencing articulation responses:

1. Begin with the easiest sounds and systematically proceed to more difficult ones.
2. Select articulation sequences that gradually increase the distance between sounds in juxtaposition in regard to place.
3. Consider the initial sound when selecting stimuli.
4. Increase the length of stimuli systematically.
5. Select meaningful words that have a high frequency of occurrence.

An eight-step program was devised to implement treatment:

1. Client and clinician simultaneously produce utterance and client is instructed to attend to visual and auditory cues.
2. Client imitates clinician while clinician simultaneously "mouths" the utterance.
3. Client imitates clinician with no simultaneous cues.
4. Client imitates clinician and says the utterance several times without cues.
5. Client reads written stimuli.
6. Client reads written stimuli after the stimuli are removed.
7. Client answers clinician's question.
8. Client uses appropriate utterances in role-playing situations.

Deal and Florance (1978) have also found this sequential procedure to be effective.

Dabul and Bollier (1976) have devised a four-step process for training articulation skills in clients with dyspraxia. The program is designed to aid the client in stabilizing articulation postures and in sequencing phonemes. The first step is to master the production of isolated consonants. We prefer to bypass sound production in isolation and begin with syllables or words whenever possible. Second the client rapidly produces the acquired consonant with the vowel /a/. The third step involves rapid production of the consonant in various CVCV and CVC nonmeaningful combinations. Last, the client approaches words that are seemingly impossible to articulate by producing each sound in isolation and then blending them into syllables and eventually into words. Dabul and Bollier (1976) indicate that auditory stimuli are not helpful in teaching the production of phonemes. Instead they recommend using visual stimulation or phonetic placement procedures. Printed cues are also useful for clients who can read. We have found this approach effective with some of our clients.

Darley, Aronson, and Brown (1975) outline three principles for dealing with dyspraxic persons: (1) imitating speech activities, such as phonating on command and producing diphthongs and vowels while facing a mirror, (2) using automatic responses, such as familiar expressions, counting, reciting serial content (days of week and numbers), and even singing, and (3) phonemic drill in isolation rather than at the word level, again using a mirror, the "listen and watch me" approach, and progressing from easy sounds and contexts to more difficult sounds and contexts. They also mention a ten-step sequence for motor programming of consonant sounds. This approach, as well as the other mentioned, is not the ultimate answer to the complex problem of verbal dyspraxia, but it certainly appears to be a step in the right direction.

Mental retardation

Another special problem that speech-language pathologists often deal with is an articulation delay or disorder associated with mental retardation. An approach that has proved to be quite effective with this population is behavior modification or operant conditioning. Because this approach is relatively simple, highly structured and repetitive, carefully programmed, and easily followed, it has been useful with persons having impaired intellect. In this approach the client is asked to imitate a sound, usually beginning in isolation, and then is reinforced with some tangible reward when the sound is correctly imitated. Some form of punishment or aversive stimulus is presented to the client when the response is not acceptable. If the client has difficulty achieving success at a particular level, the clinician can go to the next easier level or use a system of progressive approximations, that is, moving the client's responses closer and closer to normal through systematic steps or increments, each of which is rewarded for being closer to the target sound. Following the accomplishment of criterion at one step, the client and clinician then move on to the next more difficult step, and so on.

The advent of operant conditioning has influenced the development of a number of programmed approaches to articulation treatment (Bloodstein, 1979). One such program for persons who are mentally retarded was developed by Raymore and McLean (1972). Their motivation for developing such a program was directly related to the fact that clinicians have not been productive in dealing with the speech and language disorders of the mentally retarded. They point out that the need for articulation treatment in this population is especially great because retarded persons generally also have deficient language systems. Because of their typically abnormal syntax, intelligibility is even more dependent on articulation proficiency. The stimulus shift program of behavior modification was developed by McLean (1970) to assist in generalization from one stimulus condition to another and in generalization to all word positions. The program consists of seven steps:

1. *Echoic stimulus condition*—client imitates the clinician's model of a word containing the target phoneme.

2. *Echoic stimulus condition paired with textual/picture stimulus condition*—client imitates the clinician in conjunction with presentation of a picture of the word.
3. *Picture stimulus condition*—client identifies the picture with no clinician model.
4. *Picture stimulus condition paired with textual/printed word stimulus condition*—client identifies the picture in conjunction with the presence of the written word.
5. *Printed word stimulus condition*—client identifies the printed word.
6. *Printed word stimulus condition paired with intraverbal stimulus condition*—client identifies the printed word in conjunction with completing a sentence presented by the clinician, for example, I put the shoe on my _____.
7. *Intraverbal stimulus condition*—client completes a sentence presented by the clinician.

The printed stimulus conditions are not used with those clients who cannot read. This program can be used only when the target sound is stimulable. If not stimulable, the response needs to be shaped until the sound is produced. Raymore and McLean (1972) found that mentally retarded individuals tend to overgeneralize, that is, inappropriately use the newly acquired sound for other sounds. In such cases one needs to implement a program to respond discriminatively with the two involved sounds.

Raymore and McLean (1972) hypothesize that it is not necessary to train the client to use the sound in various settings. However, two studies showed that this was not the case with trainable mentally retarded (TMR) subjects (Garcia, Bullet, and Rust, 1977; Griffiths and Craighead, 1972). These experimenters recommend that the client needs to be reinforced for correct productions in various settings. Other personnel or interested persons can provide such reinforcement.

An interesting approach to teaching articulation of final consonants was used with a trainable mentally retarded subject (Ferrier and Davis, 1973). The subject's receptive and expressive vocabulary was increased, which resulted in fewer omissions of final consonants. Minimal word pairs were initially taught receptively and then expressively. For example, "seat" and "seal" could be differentiated through the use of pictures. When the final consonants were critical to the meaning of the word, the client correctly produced them. Such a procedure might also be useful with other types of clients. Ingram (1976) uses a linguistic approach in correcting final sound position omissions.

Clinicians must learn to remediate articulation disorders of mentally retarded individuals in an effective and efficient way since articulation proficiency is critical to their being understood by others. However, in doing so clinicians must also remember that these persons have a reduced ability to learn, slower development, and more problems in adjustment and attention span than do intellectually normal persons (Schlanger, 1954). The clinician should be prepared to work at a slower pace, spend more time at each stage of treatment, present information more concretely, establish easier, more realistic goals, and expect less from these persons than might be expected from persons with functional articulation problems. Since traditional approaches as used in the schools have been of little value with rare exceptions (Sommers, 1969), other approaches need to be developed. At this time a programmed approach of behavior modification seems to be the most effective (Schiefelbusch, 1972; McLean, 1972).

Cerebral palsy

Articulation problems associated with cerebral palsy will vary with the type—spasticity, athetosis, rigidity, ataxia, or tremor—the degree of severity, and the age of the client (McDonald and Chance, 1964). Most articulation disorders related to cerebral palsy are described by the general term known as dysarthria, which has been previously differentiated from verbal dyspraxia.

Communication problems related to dysarthria usually are multiple in nature, involving, besides a motor speech disorder, respiration, phonation, ambulation, and not uncommonly vision, hearing, eating, posturing, education, and vocation. Treatment requires a team approach because speech, orthopedic, occupational, and physical therapy are typically needed. In addition the client may need braces, special shoes, counseling, employment, recreation, furniture, and education.

Crickmay (1966), who utilizes the Bobath approach, lists three general treatment principles: (1) inhibition of abnormal reflex behavior, (2) facilitation of more mature movements, and (3) performance of movements under the voluntary control of the patient. She goes on to outline eleven systematic manipulative procedures ranging from normalizing muscle tone to specific procedures for correct use of the articulators and phonation. She appears to prefer the motokinesthetic approach to articulation treatment. During the overall program, time is also spent on self-concept and psychologic desensitization.

Darley, Aronson, and Brown (1975) suggest working on:
1. Slowing the rate of speech
2. Using a syllable-by-syllable attack
3. Exaggerating consonant production in final and medial positions
4. Including difficult sounds in isolation, such as /l/, /t/, /d/, /n/, /s/, /z/, /ʃ/, and /tʃ/
5. In severe cases working directly on consonant production rather than on "strengthening the muscles" per se

Additional suggestions are provided for working on phonation, resonation, prosody, and respiration.

Westlake and Rutherford (1961) encourage the provision of early sensory information and the development of communication behavior. They outlined the following activities:
1. Working from relaxed conditions
2. Emphasizing perception of movements

3. Using stabilization
4. Posturing
5. Working from vegetative to voluntary movements
6. Using resistance
7. Progressing from gross to specific movements
8. Progressing from passive to resisted motion
9. Controlling primitive patterns
10. Working beyond minimum motor requirements
11. Developing tolerance
12. Doing negative practice
13. Using, using, using, and using (simply repeating activities)

Breathing, phonation, and gross tongue, lip, and jaw movements are also included along with attention to muscles of mastication and facial expression.

Finnie (1975) urges the inclusion of gestures during the first year of life. She also includes work on abnormal breathing and on sounds in isolation. Most of her other suggestions are similar to those already mentioned.

Articulation treatment of persons who have cerebral palsy can incorporate the aforementioned activities by using a number of treatment approaches: motokinesthetic, sensory-motor integration, progressive approximation, or visual. Whatever approach is used, it should be kept in mind that treatment must be an interdisciplinary team approach, compensatory in nature, and realistic in terms of client expectations.

Cleft palate

Children born with a cleft palate are children who also need to be managed by an interdisciplinary team of specialists because of the multiplicity of the problem. The range of services needed usually includes surgery, orthodontic and prosthodontic dentistry, otologic and audiologic intervention, and speech and language treatment. Genetic and nutritional counseling and psychologic and pediatric services are sometimes necessary. Coordination and timing of all these services are extremely important.

Powers (1973) indicates that communication treatment will depend on the type of client. He lists three types of individuals: (1) those with clearly inadequate closure, (2) those with clearly adequate closure, and (3) those with marginal closure. He obviously thinks that the important variable among persons born with a cleft palate is the velopharyngeal mechanism. Clients with inadequate closure should be considered for a speech appliance or for additional surgery because articulation and resonance treatment cannot be completely successful if the velopharyngeal mechanism is inadequate. In fact the speech-language clinician and the client will typically experience considerable frustration in treatment if the client does not have the physiologic potential for normal articulation and resonance.

Treatment for those clients with clearly adequate closure can be similar to that for clients with functional articulation problems except that attention must be given to residual problems commonly associated with cleft palate, such as glottal stops, pharyngeal and laryngeal fricatives, pharyngeal /l/, faulty habits with pressure consonants, and some possible hypernasality. Treatment for these clients is largely a matter of breaking down old habits that might have been related to the cleft and other faulty habits unrelated to the cleft and then replacing these incorrect habits with correct habits.

Clients with marginal closure might benefit from velopharyngeal exercises, an appliance that stimulates the palate or pharynx, or methods emphasizing compensation (Spriestersbach and Sherman, 1968). Compensatory training might include tongue placement variations, light tongue contacts, light velopharyngeal closure for pressure sounds, and other articulator adjustments. Wells (1971) includes a number of activities for stimulating velopharyngeal closure.

Whatever the individual characteristics of the client, the clinician must remember that management is a team effort, is long term, and must begin early, as with other organically caused articulation problems. Early treatment should (1) develop the child's confidence, (2) allay parental anxiety, (3) encourage development of communication skills, and (4) minimize or prevent the development of undesirable compensatory articulation (Philips, 1972). The treatment goals should be tentative and include (1) speech discrimination, (2) correct phonetic placement, and (3) automatic use of the newly acquired sounds (Spriestersbach and Sherman, 1968). In other words treatment should (1) inhibit learning of faulty patterns, (2) facilitate required normal movements, (3) associate, through experience, these movements of articulation, and (4) stabilize these movements (Morley, 1970).

To summarize, articulation treatment must alleviate glottal stops, pharyngeal and laryngeal fricatives, pharyngeal /l/, weak production of the sixteen pressure consonants, and hypernasality whenever any of these characteristics of faulty articulation and resonance are present. If the velopharyngeal mechanism is inadequate, a speech appliance or additional surgery should be considered because speech treatment by itself is usually ineffective in this situation. Although there does not appear to be a best method of treating this heterogeneous population, distinctive feature, multiple sound, motokinesthetic, and phonetic placement approaches have worked quite well.

Hearing impairment

Another group of persons presenting special treatment needs is the population with hearing impairment. The needs, like those of persons with cerebral palsy, will vary with the degree of hearing impairment from mild hearing loss to the legally deaf, with the age of the client, and with the age of onset of the hearing disorder. The three major communication problems among this population are articulation, language, and voice deviations.

Articulation training typically includes the sounds /s/, /r/, /l/, /ʃ/, and /tʃ/ (Newby,

1972). Other defective sounds include the high-frequency, low-intensity sounds /s/, /f/, /tʃ/, and /θ/, other later developing sounds, and the less visible sounds. Visual-tactile-kinesthetic and phonetic placement approaches have been effective with hearing impaired persons. These approaches can be coupled with an auditory training unit, illustrations of nonvisible sounds, feeling the differences on the larynx between voiced and nonvoiced sounds such as /t/ and /d/, feeling the breath flow for plosive and fricative sounds, and feeling the nose for nasal sounds. Ling (1976), Oyer and Frankmann (1975), Lowell and Stoner (1960), and Sanders (1971) provide ideas for the overall processes of aural rehabilitation—speech reading, auditory training, hearing aid orientation, articulation and language training, speech conservation, and counseling. Ling (1976) especially stresses the importance of order in teaching speech sounds. He states that sounds should be taught by order of natural acquisition: (1) undifferentiated vocalization, (2) nonsegmental voice patterns varied in pitch, intensity, and duration, (3) distinctly different vowel sounds, (4) simple consonants, and finally (5) consonant blends. High front vowels should be taught before low central vowels, and the remaining vowels should be taught last.

Hearing impaired persons present multiple problems in communication. In addition to having an understanding of these communication problems, the speech-language clinician must be familiar with different types of amplification, counseling needs in the area of child acceptance, education, and eventual vocation. Even though no generally accepted method of treatment has been developed, several methods emphasizing visual and motokinesthetic approaches have been quite successful. The crucial question for the clinician is, "Should perfection be expected or required of the severe hearing impaired person?" This question probably must be answered individually if the most effective treatment approach is to be utilized.

Multiple educational handicaps

Although persons with mental retardation, dyspraxia, cerebral palsy, cleft palate, and hearing impairment all have multiple problems, special mention should be made of learning disabled children. These children have problems in motor incoordination; cognitive disability; listening problems; communication problems; reading, writing, spelling, and arithmetic difficulties; perceptual problems; and motor activity or hyperactivity. Various state and federal laws fortunately have made it necessary to provide appropriate treatment for those multiply handicapped schoolchildren.

The special role of the speech-language pathologist is one of team member, resource person, supportive person, and primary clinician. Because these children are frequently mainstreamed (Turnbull and Schulz, 1979), the speech-language clinician must develop intervention strategies that will complement the philosophy of mainstreaming and the multiple learning problems of the children. Since specific articulation approaches have not been developed for this population and since treatment approaches should be determined on the basis of the child's overall problems and their etiologies, several of the approaches mentioned in Chapter 8 may be sufficient. It is important that the speech-language clinician become somewhat knowledgeable about educational principles, philosophies, and procedures for this population. An understanding of the special education needs of these children and how best to provide them using a team approach would also be valuable. Finally sharing of information and techniques and following the principles of team functioning are indispensable attributes for successful management of schoolchildren with multiple learning problems.

In addition to the foregoing discussion, three other special treatment situations merit consideration.

GROUP TREATMENT

A major management problem for many speech-language pathologists is insufficient time to treat all individuals with articulation deviancies. This is particularly true for public school clinicians. Therefore, alternative methods of administering treatment have been devised to result in more efficient intervention. One such method is treatment of clients in a group situation (Van Hattum, 1969). In some instances work with clients on an individual basis is necessary because of severity level, causal factors, and other complicating factors (Johnson and associates, 1967). For example, severe articulation disorders, whether organic or nonorganic, probably need intensive, individual work. Possibly clients who are unintelligible or otherwise very conspicuous in their speech and those who must learn compensatory articulation movements should receive individual treatment (McDonald, 1964). However, in many instances group treatment is quite effective. Sommers (1969) cited two studies that found group treatment to be as effective, if not more so, than individual treatment with school-aged articulation-deviant children. Group work saves time for the clinician, does not always sacrifice advantages of individual treatment, and has some distinct advantages over individual work (Powers, 1971). Unique advantages of group work include: (1) clients tend to stimulate and motivate each other, (2) many opportunities are provided for realistic social speaking situations or interactions, (3) clients realize that others also have speech problems, (4) a broader variety of materials and activities can be used, (5) opportunities are provided to listen critically, and (6) clinician time can be used more economically (Johnson and associates, 1967; Powers, 1971; McDonald, 1964; Backus and Beasley, 1951). Naturally each client likely will receive less attention than in individual sessions, but the advantages probably counterbalance this disadvantage (McDonald, 1964). Perhaps a combination of group and individual treatment would be optimum. Certainly some individual work should be done with those who are not progressing as rapidly as other members of a group, yet McCabe and Bradley (1975) state that such differences can be handled effectively within a group framework. Where individual differences exist, 5 or 10 minutes of individual attention prior to or immediately following a group session—a preclinic or postclinic laboratory—may be required.

Of course group treatment is not effective if used inappropriately. All too often such an approach merely involves clients taking turns rather than all actively participating all the time. The speech-language pathologist's role is to keep several clients simultaneously and beneficially involved in the treatment process during the entire session. The following criteria should be met when conducting group sessions:

1. All clients are continuously active in participation.
2. Each client receives some individual attention from the clinician.
3. Clinical activities serve individual needs and goals for each client.
4. Motivation is centered around speech objectives rather than on winning.
5. The client is constantly aware of progress toward the objectives (Black, 1964; Van Riper, 1952).

Various techniques can be used for keeping all clients actively participating (Black, 1964; McDonald, 1964). One procedure is to present a stimulus and pause before calling on a client to respond. In this way all clients listen to the stimulus and prepare to respond since no one knows who will be called. Another technique involves clients listening to one another and then evaluating the response verbally or through a tracking procedure. Also clients can be instructed to respond in unison. One client can produce an articulation pattern for the others to repeat. Additionally various stations can be set up for individual clients using tape recorders, Language Masters, and so forth. Clients who are in advanced treatment stages can help those in earlier phases, similar to a "buddy" system. During the carry-over phase of treatment clients can participate in role-playing, dramatizations, putting on plays for classrooms, simulated telephone conversations, and other social activities involving connected speech. Whatever procedures are used, group activities should stimulate interest and be enjoyable for the participants.

Group sessions generally are conducted with two to six clients selected on a homogeneous basis. Length of sessions ranges from 20 to 40 minutes. Bases for grouping include articulation proficiency, age level, and similarly misarticulated sounds. Sommers (1969) believes that articulation proficiency should be the primary consideration so that a group can concentrate on any one of such activities as auditory training, sound production, and carry-over. The age spread should be limited to 2 or 3 years because intellectual and social maturity and interests are significant factors for group interaction. Last, misarticulation of the same sound(s) may be considered, although it is quite feasible and appropriate for different group members to be working on different sounds. Backus and Beasley (1951) recommend heterogeneous grouping, but most other approaches prefer homogeneous grouping as described previously. Whichever approach is considered, it should be differentially applied to the specific etiologies (Appendix P).

Groher (1976) experimented with group situations in which older students (14 to 17 years of age) worked with younger students (6 to 8 years of age) on their articulation skills. The clinician met with the group of older students weekly. Each older student met with a younger student twice a week for ½-hour sessions for 4 months. One group of older students had articulation deviancies and received treatment from the clinician once a week, and another group had articulation disorders but did not receive treatment. The younger clients who worked with the former group improved the most. Both groups of older students also improved in their articulation skills. Subjectively speech-language pathologists noted that the older students who were receiving and providing treatment were more receptive to their own individual sessions. Thus the procedure of grouping an older client with a younger one was quite effective. All in all, group remediation seems to be an efficient and useful method of administering articulation treatment.

BLOCK SCHEDULING

Another method of administering treatment—block or intensive scheduling—is effectively utilized by school speech-language pathologists. Block scheduling refers to intensive scheduling so that each school and consequently each client for which the clinician is responsible is scheduled more frequently for shorter periods of time. In traditional scheduling the clinician visits each school the same number of days per week throughout the school year. For example, a particular school may be visited four times a week for three 6-week periods in block scheduling rather than twice a week for 36 weeks in traditional scheduling. Much research has been conducted to determine if block or traditional scheduling is more efficient (Ausenheimer and Irwin, 1971; Sommers, 1969; Weston and Harber, 1975). Results have generally shown the block approach to yield higher dismissal rates for nonorganic articulation clients. Other advantages are that more children receive services, students and teachers do not forget sessions, transporting of equipment and supplies is reduced, and teachers and principals tend to prefer block schedules. A major disadvantage is that it is not as successful as traditional scheduling for organically involved clients, who usually need intensive treatment over a longer period of time than block scheduling allows. Ideally the two scheduling options should be combined, with a block approach being used at the beginning of the school year when establishing production of target sounds and traditional scheduling used later during the carry-over phases of treatment. Block scheduling also is used in clinics and private practice.

COMMUNICATION AIDES

More and more, speech-language pathologists are utilizing communication aides, also referred to as supportive personnel, to help alleviate the problem of insufficient time to provide all needed speech-language pathology services. Sometimes aides are paid, and sometimes they are volunteers. The qualifications to become an aide vary depending on the tasks to be performed. Aides are not allowed to diagnose speech and language disorders, plan treatment, or confer with parents and teachers. They can carry out treatment programs, record responses, and perform clerical duties. Relative to articulation treatment, supportive personnel generally are not expected to undertake the initial tasks of providing stimuli to elicit sounds relative to correcting error sounds, but they can implement the drill work needed to stabilize sound production. We recommend that the guidelines for the role and task of communication aides developed by the American Speech Language and Hearing Association be followed (Appendix O). It must be kept in mind at all times that the speech-language pathologist is responsible for the work that aides perform with clients; therefore, the work done by aides needs to be supervised closely.

Several journal articles have been published relative to training and using aides to assist in articulation treatment. Results have shown communication aides to be effective in helping to conduct articulation programs that have been devised by professional speech-language pathologists (Alpiner, Ogden, and Wiggins, 1970; Braunstein, 1972; Costello and Schoen, 1978; Galloway and Blue, 1975; Gray and Baker, 1977; Scalero and Eskenazi, 1976; Strong, 1972). Criteria for selection of communication aides have varied considerably and include such qualifications as plans to remain in the geographic area, completion of high school, normal speech and hearing, good speech discrimination ability, 18 years of age or older, an expressed desire to work with children, access to transportation, driver's license, ability to follow directions, willingness to study, enthusiastic supportive involvement with children, and ability to type. Such criteria generally are used to select paid aides, but other types of personnel have also been utilized.

A rather unique program was developed and used by a school system in southern Oregon. Low-achieving, rather than high-achieving, high school students were selected as aides. Stringent requirements were set up for them to maintain their aide positions. Two benefits were derived: (1) the articulation skills of clients improved, and (2) the school attendance of the aides and their attitudes toward school improved dramatically. Possibly the training and the programming of aides is more critical to success than prerequisite requirements. Hall and Knutson (1978) reported on a public school program in which undergraduate speech-language pathology students functioned as communication aides on a limited basis. The program was found to be beneficial to both the school speech-language program and to the students. It seems to us that potentialities and resources for the use of communication aides are extensive.

Training of aides has also varied considerably. Some projects spend much time providing general background information relative to organization of the school, professional responsibilities, speech and language development, behavioral principles, phonetics, anatomy and physiology of the speech mechanism, and description of various disorders, whereas others devote time only to explaining and practicing the techniques that will be utilized in the treatment process. We tend to believe that training need not devote too much time to lectures on general information and introductory material. Instead the training time probably can be used more profitably in explaining articulation programs and in tracking and recording procedures, as well as practicing the actual carrying out of the programs, tracking and recording client responses, and discriminating between correct and incorrect productions. Sometimes published treatment programs, such as those described in Chapter 8, are used, or the clinician devises relevant programs. Whichever is the case, the aide must know

exactly what to do. Training also involves observation of clinical sessions conducted by the speech-language pathologist. After the aide begins working with clients the clinician should frequently observe the sessions. Later a gradual decrease in frequency and length of observations may be possible. Some form of flexible system needs to be devised so that the aide can confer with the clinician whenever the need arises. Communication aides can be extremely valuable in articulation treatment if they are well trained and well supervised. Otherwise they are of minimal benefit.

PARENTS

Parents also assist the clinician in the implementation of articulation treatment programs in addition to the ways they help in the carry-over process as discussed earlier in this chapter. Research has shown that it is worthwhile to train parents to assist in treatment (Carrier, 1970; Fudala, 1973; Van Hattum, 1969; Wing and Heimgartner, 1973). Care must be taken in selecting parents to provide articulation treatment to their child, since it seems that those who willingly assist will probably produce better results (McCroskey and Baird, 1971). Fudala (1973) found that clients whose parents attended clinical sessions and subsequently worked with their children at home showed three times as much progress as those children whose parents did not attend the sessions. Two training sessions were held with the parents. Parents then observed clinical sessions and were given assignments to complete at home with their child. This procedure was effective probably because the parents expressed willingness to participate and observed the clinician using techniques they were to use later in the home assignments.

A slightly different approach was used by Fudala, England, and Ganoug (1972). No specific training was done with the parents, but they attended and observed their children's clinic sessions. The children whose mothers attended made greater gains in articulation skills than those whose mothers did not attend. The teachers reported similar results. Principals and teachers, as well as parents, expressed overwhelming approval of the program. They noted benefits in areas other than speech. The results show that parents can be involved effectively with a minimum of extra clinician effort.

A simple, clearly written program was devised by Carrier (1970) to be implemented by parents after the speech-language pathologist trained the clients to imitate the target sound in isolation. Mothers participating in the study effectively administered the program, and at the end of the program the clients were beginning to use the standard sound in conversation. Carrier (1970) believes that it was successful because the speech tasks were simple and clearly stated. Carrier (1970) lists the specific lessons used in the program.

SUMMARY

Articulation treatment poses some special problems that can be dealt with by implementing certain techniques. The lack of carry-over is a major source of frustration in articulation management. Numerous techniques have been developed for both in-clinic and outside-of-clinic activities to aid in carry-over. Often traditional articulation treatment approaches are not effective with childhood and adult dyspraxia, mental retardation, cerebral palsy, cleft palate, hearing impairment, and multiple educational handicaps; therefore, specialized techniques need to be used. Another problem area is insufficient time to handle the needs of all potential clients. Group treatment, block scheduling, and employment of communication aides and parents function to alleviate this problem. It is believed that children whose parents are supportive of them experience more success in the articulation treatment program. Counseling of parents helps in enlisting such support. There are no "sure" solutions to all the problems, but many have been developed. The clinician must be aware of the different possible solutions and practice a differential approach to treatment (Appendix P) rather than routinely using the same approach for different problems.

STUDY SUGGESTIONS

1. Name the special skills necessary for effective counseling and establish a rationale for the speech-language clinician to be trained and competent in these skills.
2. Differentiate among the terms carry-over, transfer, generalization, automatization, habituation, maintenance, and retention and relate these to overall management of articulation disorders.
3. For a child with an articulation problem caused by impaired hearing, what are several procedures that could be used to achieve carry-over? How would these procedures differ from those used for a child with mental retardation? Other special problems?
4. Discuss the pros and cons of involving parents and others close to the child in articulation treatment and show how best these individuals can be used in the carry-over process.
5. Since the speech-language clinician often does not have time to treat all clients individually, what other measures can be used to include more clients in the treatment program?
6. Compare differences among articulation problems caused by cleft palate, cerebral palsy, hearing impairment, dyspraxia, and mental retardation and suggest the most appropriate treatment approaches for each.

REFERENCES

Alpiner, J., Ogden, J., and Wiggins, J.: The utilization of supportive personnel in speech correction in the public schools: a pilot project, ASHA **12:**599-604, 1970.

Ausenheimer, B., and Irwin, R.: Measures of articulatory proficiency, Lang. Speech Hear. Serv. Schools **5:**43-51, 1971.

Backus, O., and Beasley, J.: Speech therapy with children, Boston, 1951, Houghton Mifflin Co.

Bankson, N., and Byrne, M.: The effect of a timed correct sound production task on carryover, J. Speech Hear. Res. **15:**160-168, 1972.

Barbara, D.: The art of listening, Springfield, Ill., 1958, Charles C Thomas, Publisher.

Black, M.: Speech correction in the schools, Englewood Cliffs, N.J., 1964, Prentice-Hall, Inc.

Bloodstein, O.: Speech pathology: an introduction, Boston, 1979, Houghton Mifflin Co.

Braunstein, M.: Communication aide: a pilot project, Lang. Speech Hear. Serv. Schools **3:**32-35, 1972.

Byrne, M., and Shervanian, C.: Introduction to communicative disorders, New York, 1977, Harper & Row, Publishers.

Bzock, K., editor: Communicative disorders related to cleft lip and palate, Boston, 1972, Little, Brown and Co.

Carrier, J.: A program of articulation therapy administered by mothers, J. Speech Hear. Disord. **35:** 344-353, 1970.

Chappell, G.: Childhood verbal apraxia and its treatment, J. Speech Hear. Disord. **38:**362-368, 1973.

Costello, J., and Bosler, S.: Generalization and articulation instruction, J. Speech Hear. Disord. **41:**359-373, 1976.

Costello, J., and Schoen, J.: The effectiveness of paraprofessionals and a speech clinician as agents of articulation intervention using programmed instruction, Lang. Speech Hear. Serv. Schools **9:**118-128, 1978.

Crickmay, M.: Speech therapy and the Bobath approach to cerebral palsy, Springfield, Ill., 1966, Charles C Thomas, Publisher.

Dabul, B., and Bollier, B.: Therapeutic approaches to apraxis, J. Speech Hear. Disord. **41:**268-276, 1976.

Darley, F., Aronson, A., and Brown, J.: Motor speech disorders, Philadelphia, 1975, W. B. Saunders Co.

Deal, J., and Florance, C.: Modification of the eight-step continuum for treatment of apraxia of speech in adults, J. Speech Hear. Disord. **43:**89-95, 1978.

Dublinske, S.: PL 94-142: developing the individualized education program (IEP), ASHA **20:**380-393, 1978.

Dublinske, S., and Healey, W. C.: PL 94-142: questions and answers for the speech-language pathologist and audiologist, ASHA **20:**188-205, 1978.

Eisenson, J., and Ogilvie, M.: Speech correction in the schools, ed. 4, New York, 1977, Macmillan Publishing Co., Inc.

Engel, D., and Groth, L.: Reinforcing postarticulation responses based on feedback, Lang. Speech Hear. Serv. Schools **7:**93-101, 1976.

Engel, D., and associates: Carryover, J. Speech Hear. Disord. **31:**227-233, 1966.

English, R. L., and Lillywhite, H. S.: A semantic approach to clinical reporting in speech pathology, ASHA **5:**547-650, June 1963.

Ferrier, E., and Davis, M.: A lexical approach to the remediation of final sound omissions, J. Speech Hear. Disord. **38:**126-130, 1973.

Finnie, N.: Handling the young cerebral palsied child at home, New York, 1975, E. P. Dutton & Co., Inc.

Fudala, J.: Using parents in public school speech therapy, Lang. Speech Hear. Serv. Schools **4:**91-94, 1973.

Fudala, J., England, G., and Ganoug, L.: Utilization of parents in a speech correction program, Except. Child. **38:**407-412, 1972.

Galloway, H., and Blue, C.: Paraprofessional personnel in articulation therapy, Lang. Speech Hear. Serv. Schools **6:**125-130, 1975.

Garcia, E., Bullet, J., and Rust, F.: An experimental analysis of language training generalization across classroom and home, Behav. Mod. **1:**531-550, 1977.

Garrard, K. R.: The changing role of speech and hearing professionals in public education, ASHA **21:**91-98, 1979.

Gerber, A.: Goal: carryover an articulation manual and program, Philadelphia, 1973, Temple University Press.

Gray, B., and Baker, K.: Use of aides in an articulation therapy program, Except. Child. **43:**534-536, 1977.

Griffiths, H., and Craighead, W.: Generalization in operant speech therapy for misarticulation, J. Speech Hear. Disord. **37:**485-494, 1972.

Groher, M.: The experimental use of cross-age relationships in public school remediation, Lang. Speech Hear. Serv. Schools **7:**250-258, 1976.

Hall, P., and Knutson, C.: The use of preprofessional students as communication aides in the schools, Lang. Speech Hear. Serv. Schools **9:**162-168, 1978.

Hartbauer, R., editor: Counseling in communicative disorders, Springfield, Ill., 1978, Charles C Thomas, Publisher.

Ingram, D.: Phonological disability in children, London, 1976, Edward Arnold.

Irwin, J., and Weston, A.: The paired stimuli, ASHA Monogr. **6:**1-76, 1975.

Johnson, W.: People in quandaries, New York, 1946, Harper & Row, Publishers.

Johnson, W., and associates: Speech handicapped school children, ed. 3, New York, 1967, Harper & Row, Publishers.

Johnston, J., and Johnston, G.: Modification of consonant speech-sound articulation in young children, J. Appl. Behav. Anal. **5:**233-246, 1972.

Knepflar, K. J.: Report writing in the field of communication disorders, Danville, Ill., 1976, The Interstate Printers & Publishers, Inc.

Leonard, L.: Referential effects on articulatory learning, Lang. Speech **16:**44-56, 1973.

Lewis, T. T.: The semantics of psychiatric labels, Etc. **35**(2):180, June 1978.

Ling, D.: Speech and the hearing-impaired child: theory and practice, Washington, D.C., 1976, Alexander Graham Bell Association for the Deaf.

Lowell, E., and Stoner, M.: Play it by ear, Los Angeles, 1960, John Tracy Clinic.

Manning, W., Keappock, N., and Stick, S.: The use of auditory masking to estimate automatization of correct articulatory production, J. Speech Hear. Disord. **41:**143-149, 1976.

Marquardt, E.: Carry-over with "speech pals," J. Speech Hear. Disord. **24:**154-157, 1959.

McCabe, R., and Bradley, D.: Systematic multiple phonemic approach to articulation therapy, Acta Symbol. **6:**1-18, 1975.

McCroskey, R., and Baird, V.: Parent education in a public school program of speech therapy, J. Speech Hear. Disord. **36:**499-505, 1971.

McDonald, E.: Articulation testing and treatment: a sensory-motor approach, Pittsburgh, 1964, Stanwix House, Inc.

McDonald, E., and Chance, B.: Cerebral palsy, Englewood Cliffs, N.J., 1964, Prentice-Hall, Inc.

McLean, J.: Extending stimulus control of phoneme articulation by operant techniques. In A functional analysis approach to speech and language, ASHA Monogr. **14:**24-47, 1970.

McLean, J.: Introduction: developing clinical strategies for language intervention with mentally retarded children. In McLean, J., Yoder, D., and Schiefelbusch, R.: Language intervention with the retarded: developing strategies, Baltimore, 1972, University Park Press.

McLean, J., Yoder, D., and Schiefelbusch, R.: Language intervention with the retarded: developing strategies, Baltimore, 1972, University Park Press.

Mitcham, S.: Location of dyspraxic characteristics in children with severe "functional" articulation disorders, A thesis completed at Portland State University, 1975.

Morley, M.: Cleft palate and speech, Edinburgh, England, 1970, E. & S. Livingstone.

Mowrer, D.: Transfer of training in articulation therapy, J. Speech Hear. Disord. **36:**427-446, 1971.

Mowrer, D.: Methods of modifying speech behaviors, Columbus, 1977, Charles E. Merrill Publishing Co.

Nation, J. E., and Aram, D. M.: Diagnosis of speech and language disorders, St. Louis, 1977, The C. V. Mosby Co., pp. 159-174.

Newby, H.: Audiology, New York, 1972, Appleton-Century-Crofts.

Nichols, R.: Ten components of effective listening, Education **75:**292-302, 1955.

Oyer, H., and Frankmann, J.: The aural rehabilitation process, New York, 1975, Holt, Rinehart and Winston, Inc.

Patton, B., and Griffin, K.: Interpersonal communication: basic text and readings, New York, 1974, Harper & Row, Publishers.

Philips, B.: Stimulating language and speech development in cleft palate infants. In Bzoch, K., editor: Communicative disorders related to cleft lip and palate, Boston, 1972, Little, Brown and Co.

Powers, G.: Cleft palate, Indianapolis, 1973, The Bobbs-Merrill Co., Inc.

Powers, M.: Clinical and educational procedures in functional disorders of articulation. In Travis, L., editor: Handbook of speech pathology and audiology, New York, 1971, Appleton-Century-Crofts.

Raymore, S., and McLean, J.: A clinical program for carry-over of articulation therapy with retarded children. In McLean, J., Yoder, D., and Schiefelbusch, R.: Language intervention with the retarded: developing strategies, Baltimore, 1972, University Park Press.

Rogers, C.: Client-centered therapy, Boston, 1951, Houghton Mifflin Co.

Rosenbek, J., and associates: A treatment for apraxia of speech in adults, J. Speech Hear. Disord. **38:**462-472, 1973.

Rosenbek, R., and associates: Treatment of developmental apraxia of speech: a case study, Lang. Speech Hear. Serv. Schools **5:**13-22, 1974.

Sanders, D.: Aural rehabilitation, Englewood Cliffs, N.J., 1971, Prentice-Hall, Inc.

Scalero, A., and Eskenazi, C.: The use of supportive personnel in a public school speech and language program, Lang. Speech Hear. Serv. Schools **7:**150-158, 1976.

Schiefelbusch, R.: Language of the mentally retarded, Baltimore, 1972, University Park Press.

Schlanger, B.: Speech measurements of institutionalized mentally handicapped children, J. Speech Hear. Disord. **19:**339-343, 1954.

Shelton, R., Johnson, A., and Arndt, W.: Monitoring and reinforcement by parents as a means of automating articulatory responses, Percept. Mot. Skills **35:**759-767, 1972.

Shelton, R., and associates: Monitoring and reinforcement by parents as a means of automating articulatory responses. II. Study of preschool children, Percept. Mot. Skills **40:**599-610, 1975.

Skinner, P., and Shelton, R.: Speech, language, and hearing: normal processes and disorders, Reading, Mass., 1978, Addison-Wesley Publishing Co., Inc.

Sommers, R.: Factors in the effectiveness of articulation with educable retarded children, Final report of project number 7-0432, U.S. Department of Health, Education and Welfare, 1969.

Sommers, R., and Kane, A.: Nature and remediation of functional articulation disorders. In Dickson, S., editor: Communication disorders: remedial principles and practices, Glenview, Ill., 1974, Scott, Foresman and Co.

Spriestersbach, D., and Sherman, D., editors: Cleft palate and communication, New York, 1968, Academic Press, Inc.

Strong, B.: Public school speech technicians in Minnesota, Lang. Speech Hear. Serv. Schools **3:**53-56, 1972.

Tennov, D.: Psychotherapy: the hazardous cure, New York, Abelard-Schuman, Limited, p. 18.

Turnbull, A., and Schulz, J.: Mainstreaming handicapped students, Boston, 1979, Allyn & Bacon, Inc.

Van Hattum, R.: Clinical speech in the schools, Springfield, Ill., 1969, Charles C Thomas, Publisher.

Van Riper, C.: The revision of public school speech correction: an unpublished paper, 1952.

Van Riper, C.: Speech correction principles and methods, ed. 6, Englewood Cliffs, N.J., 1978, Prentice-Hall, Inc.

Webster, E.: Counseling with parents of handicapped children, New York, 1977, Grune & Stratton, Inc.

Weiss, C. E., and Lillywhite, H. S.: Communication disorders: a handbook for prevention and early intervention, St. Louis, 1976, The C. V. Mosby Co.

Wells, C.: Cleft palate and its associated speech disorders, New York, 1971, McGraw-Hill Book Co.

West, R.: The neurophysiology of speech. In Travis, L., editor: Handbook of speech pathology, New York, 1957, Appleton-Century-Crofts.

Westlake, H., and Rutherford, D.: Speech therapy for the cerebral palsied, Chicago, 1961, National Society for Crippled Children and Adults, Inc.

Weston, A., and Harber, S.: The effects of scheduling

on progress in paired-stimuli articulation therapy, Lang. Speech Hear. Serv. Schools **6**:96-101, 1975.

Wing, D., and Heimgartner, L.: Articulation carryover procedure implemented by parents, Lang. Speech Hear. Serv. Schools **6**:182-195, 1973.

Winitz, H.: From syllable to conversation, Baltimore, 1975, University Park Press.

GLOSSARY

automatization The process of making the use of new or corrected sounds "automatic," used without conscious effort, outside the clinic as well as in the clinic.

CMR Custodial mental retardation, IQ below 25. A classification of a level of mental retardation recommended by the American Psychological Association to indicate that an individual in this range is not capable of self-management but needs "custodial" care.

carry-over Refers to capabilities of a client to use new sounds or sounds corrected in the clinic in situations outside the clinic. Other terms used for carry-over or different stages of it are automatization, generalization, habituation, maintenance, and retention.

EMR Educable mental retardation, IQ 50 to 75. A classification recommended by the American Psychological Association to indicate that an individual falling within this range is "educable" in a scholastic sense but will learn at a slower rate.

generalization *See* Carry-over. Has the same basic meaning as carry-over but may refer to broader, more general usage outside the clinic.

habituation *See* Carry-over.

maintenance *See* Carry-over. May refer to more long-term, continuing usage outside the clinic.

meaningful Used here in a special sense to refer to stimulus material used in the clinic that has meaning, as distinguished from nonsense, unmeaningful material.

nonsense material Sequences of sounds that have no meaning, used as stimulus material to elicit sound responses in the clinic.

punishment Has special meaning as a process in behavior modification in which mild negative reinforcement, "punishment," is used for incorrect response to stimuli.

retention *See* Carry-over.

TMR Trainable mental retardation, IQ 25 to 49. A classification recommended by the American Psychological Association to indicate that an individual falling in this category is trainable for certain tasks but is not educable in a scholastic sense.

tracking A clinical process of locating, identifying, and following a target sound in different contexts.

transfer *See* Carry-over.

CHAPTER TEN

Writing clinical reports

"Hold fast the form of sound words."
FIRST EPISTLE TO TIMOTHY

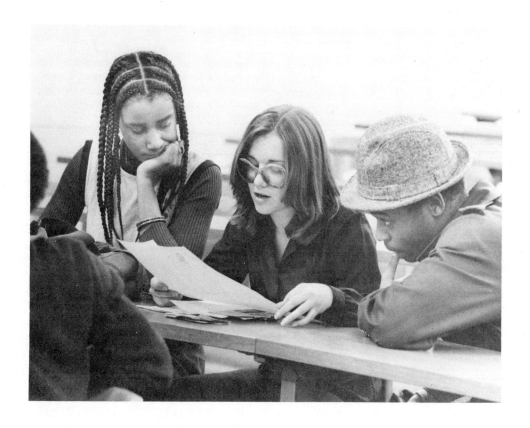

GENERAL CONCEPTS OF CLINICAL REPORTS

The clinical report, regardless of the kind and purpose, is tremendously important in the overall management of a communication disorder but is perhaps even more important in representing the speech-language pathologist, audiologist, clinic, training program, or school clinic program. Unfortunately judgment of the quality of clinical work done is based as much on the reports received as on the results of treatment, because the results often are not as visible to the referring source.

In spite of the importance of reports, many students manage to graduate and enter the field without learning the key role that good reports can play and often without acquiring the knowledge and skill of writing good reports. Knepflar (1976) believes that most of the members of our profession probably regard report writing as a necessary evil or an unpleasant responsibility and, because of this, reports often are unclear, sketchy, poorly written, and monotonous. Often the speech-language pathologist feels overburdened with report writing and believes that reports interfere with other clinical activity thought to be more important. In other cases the individual is "turned off" by report writing, as Knepflar suggests.

Our experience has demonstrated that one of the major tasks in training student clinicians is to help them to realize the importance of good reports and the need to write them conscientiously as soon as possible after the clinical activity being reported has taken place. To many students working with communicatively disordered persons is much more interesting and exciting than writing about the work that has been done or will be done with them.

This attitude seems to carry over into full-time clinical activity. Over the years we have observed many excellent clinicians who cannot seem to bring themselves to write the necessary reports until it is too late to do a good job or the reports are no longer of value to the referral sources. They keep notes of diagnostic or treatment sessions for months, with reports unwritten, while eagerly accepting any new clients for diagnosis or treatment. As a result, the reports, when they finally are written, often are incomplete and poorly prepared because they have been left so long. Part of the discipline for student training in speech-language pathology and audiology and part of the discipline that must be maintained throughout practice is to hold oneself rigidly to the prompt writing of good reports as near to the time of the end of the clinical activity as possible.

To write a good clinical report is difficult because it is essential that the report accurately represent the entire situation being reported. To borrow an analogy from general semantics, the map (report) must represent a wide territory, including the client, the disorder, the situation, and all relevant matters. Weiss and Lillywhite (1976) discuss the "map-territory" relationship as it applies to clinical speech-language pathology and audiology.

We have recommended elsewhere that assessment and management of articulation disorders make use of the scientific method insofar as possible. Others (English and Lillywhite, 1963; Johnson, 1946; Nation and Aram, 1977) are in agreement with this approach. This recommendation includes reporting. To demonstrate how this can apply to report writing, we shall use the Ladder of Communication Levels (Weiss and Lillywhite, 1976), which is an adaptation of Johnson's (1946) levels of abstraction. In fact the student in clinical practice doing report writing is referred to Chapter 1 in the Weiss and Lillywhite book (1976), which deals with the semantic aspects of clinical procedures.

The Ladder of Communication Levels, as can be seen in Fig. 10-1, shows four levels of communication, beginning with the very concrete, largely nonverbal level 1 (observation and information gathering) up the ladder through three other increasingly abstract verbal levels. Level 2 (reporting and describing) is only one level above the most

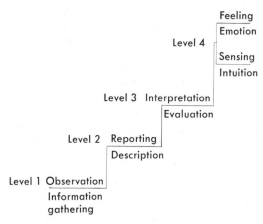

Fig. 10-1. Ladder of communication levels ascending from most concrete, objective, largely nonverbal (level 1) to verbal levels of increasing abstraction and subjectivity (levels 2 to 4). (From Weiss, C. E., and Lillywhite, H. S.: Communicative disorders: a handbook for prevention and early intervention, St. Louis, 1976, The C. V. Mosby Co.)

concrete, largely nonverbal level 1. As applied to clinical reporting, level 2 is concerned with reporting and describing what has been observed and what other information has been gathered from whatever source at level 1, including examination and testing. Level 3 is interpretation and evaluation of the information gathered in level 1 and reported in level 2. Level 4 (clinical intuition and sensing) should be used sparingly in clinical procedures and reporting, but every good clinician develops an intuitive sensitivity that is invaluable in clinical activity. This should not be discounted, but one should realize that biases, personal motivations, and value judgments can easily distort function at this level and can creep into reports. The task of report writing is largely confined to level 2 (reporting and describing), although all of the other levels may have been part of the clinical processes leading to the report.

DETERMINING FACTORS IN CLINICAL REPORTS

Purpose, style, format, content, and sometimes language of the report may be largely or in part determined by the setting in which the clinical activity takes place. For example, two of the authors of this book have been involved in clinical work in a medical setting. Reports, especially the major ones, became part of the entire medical record of the patient. Style and format were largely determined by the medical record, and the terminology and language were strongly influenced by that setting. In the matter of terminology, for instance, the term "patient" was used exclusively, whereas the term "client" or sometimes the misused term "case" is to be found in many other settings. Another co-author functions in a university clinic where reports serve other purposes and where "client" rightfully replaces "patient."

The school clinician is in still another kind of setting that calls for different kinds of reports to fit different purposes. Even from one school system to another and from one clinic to another there are wide differences in some aspects of clinical reports. In private practice reports may serve many kinds of purposes and may be more critical to the report writer than in any of the other settings because the person in private practice should be more visible than one in a clinic or a school and may be represented more directly by written reports. In private practice, community clinics, and to a lesser extent college and university clinics and schools, reports may be needed for Medicare, Medicaid, private insurance purposes, legal testimony, health maintenance organizations (HMOs), and other rare special purposes.

Because of the many purposes various kinds of reports must serve, a word of caution is important. Every precaution should be taken to avoid misunderstanding in light of the recent freedom of information movement and the rightful insistence on the part of clients, parents, and some others that they be informed and have access to reports and records. Unfortunately we are living in a time of "instant" lawsuits, and the speech-language pathologist, audiologist, agency, school, or clinic dealing with people with communication disorders and with their parents is no more immune to a lawsuit than is the physician, psychologist or other professional or institution dealing with people with problems. Written reports of any kind can be used to the detriment of the client and the person or institution engaged in diagnosis and treatment because reports of any kind can become available to lay persons. For this reason the writing of a clinical report requires very careful preparation.

Related to this danger are such recent developments as health maintenance organizations and the related requirements for peer review and accountability regarding quality care. In 1972 Public Law 92-603 and in 1975 Public Law 94-142 created the necessity of directly evaluating the quality of care being provided patients. This led to establishment of professional standards review organizations (PSROs), all ostensibly pertaining to medical care but encompassing all health-related fields such as speech-language pathology and audiology. This led to such procedures as retrospective review, concurrent review, continued stay review, and patient care audit, the latter of which seems to be a term covering all the others. All of this has affected our profession to such an extent that the American Speech and Hearing Association conducted workshops throughout the country to train members in the techniques involved.

The passage of PL 94-142 also relates significantly to reports and records as well as to other aspects of the role of the speech-language clinician. Called The Education of All Handicapped Children Act, this new law makes it mandatory that all handicapped children must be educated in the least restrictive environment possible. That is, if a handicapped child can possibly be educated with normal children, such provision must be made by the schools to do so. The law also stipulates that all handicapped children receive *total* education according to their capabilities. This means that many handicapped children previously in special programs will be in the main-

stream with normal children and that many handicapped children not previously provided special services, such as treatment for communicative disorders, now are to receive them. "Failure to provide adequate services to communicatively handicapped children is considered a violation of the law" (Garrard, 1979). Several speech-language pathologists have discussed the implications of this law and the vastly changing role it will mean for speech-language clinicians, especially those in public schools, including high level of competence, team treatment, and many other aspects (Garrard, 1975; Dublinske, 1978; and Dublinske and Healey, 1978).

These developments have attached importance to records and reports that we have not known before. Perhaps "in-house" records may be of primary importance to a peer review panel, but written reports of all kinds are subject to inspection, even in court. The diagnostician's records and reports are more available to many more people than ever before, so skill and care in their preparation become paramount.

ELEMENTS OF REPORT WRITING

To be able to write good reports the clinician needs to know and use efficiently five elements of a report: (1) terminology, (2) language, (3) format, (4) content, and (5) style. As used here *terminology* refers to the specialized vocabulary used in the health professions but applying specifically to speech-language pathology and audiology. *Language* refers to the syntactic structure in which this terminology is couched. Language in the report is closely related to style, but they are not synonymous. *Format* as used here refers to the sequential order of items discussed in the report, the form in which the report is laid out. *Content* is the material or subject matter the diagnostician or clinician elects to put in the report. *Style* is the manner in which information, interpretations, and recommendations are expressed.

Comments will be made about each of these elements as they relate to different kinds of reports and settings, but since style can be so critical to the report, a special note is made here. Knepflar (1976) has listed twelve "basic rules" of style in report writing. These will not be discussed in detail here, but they are listed, paraphrased, and sometimes expanded.

Avoid ambiguous terms

The report writer can easily fall into the trap of using many words to say very little, especially if one is inclined to be overly verbose. The report is not a place to expound, to demonstrate vast knowledge of the field, or to create a literary masterpiece. Specific, simple terms couched in brief, clear language should be used.

Avoid jargon

Terms that may not be readily understood by the reader should be defined, or they should not be used.

Avoid abbreviations

Even though clinicians may use abbreviations in their own notes, such as C.P. for cerebral palsy, artic. for articulation, and so on, they should not be used in clinical reports.

Avoid using stereotyped words and phrases

This is difficult when one is dealing with many similar problems and reports, but it makes for tiresome reading.

Avoid long, complicated sentences

One of the most serious faults of professional writing is the tendency to report simple concepts in unneeded verbiage, that is, to make simple ideas complicated. The converse—striving toward simplicity and directness—is recommended. Short, uncomplicated sentences and the simplest terminology that will serve the purpose should be used.

Avoid flippancy, superiority, or condescension in report writing

Sometimes there is the temptation to use slang or colorful terms to be a little "smart" in describing the behavior of a client or parent. The description should be professional, serious, and sincere, and needless words and phrases should be omitted.

Avoid contractions and misuse of hyphens as much as possible

Such terms as "didn't," "couldn't," and "won't" may be acceptable in a letter, but a professional report is somewhat more formal and such usage generally should be avoided. Hyphens also provide a trap for many. The hyphen should not be used in place of more legitimate punctuation such as, "David had been seen by an orthodontist—no dental irregularities were reported." A period after orthodontist is the correct punctuation. Hyphens should be used as they are meant to be used, such as in "2-hour intervals" or "4-year-old child," to link two or more words together to create a particular meaning, whereas if the words are used separately they have an entirely different meaning.

Generally avoid qualifiers and noncommittal language

Terms such as "it would seem," "it is believed," "it appears," "probably," "somewhat," and "apparently" are used all too frequently in written reports, giving the reader the impression that the report writer is unsure. There is a place in report writing for tentative, qualified statements, but there should be clear reason in the report for such statements. For example, a client's behavior may be such that a definite diagnosis cannot be made, yet the examiner has a distinct impression that at the time of the examination dental abnormalities, for example, appeared to be causing sibilant distortion, or whatever the impression was. In such instances the reason for not being more positive should be stated. Perhaps the child would not allow adequate examination, as is often the case. The possibility of being too positive may be present without enough evidence, to cover up lack of adequate assessment, or because of an inability to make the assessment.

Avoid awkward circumlocutions

Phrases such as "it is believed" instead of "I believe" and "David responded readily to this examiner" for "David responded readily to me" should be avoided. The report writer should not hesitate to take responsibility for what is written. The active voice and personal noun or pronoun should be used where appropriate, and nonparallel construction should be avoided.

Avoid exaggeration and overstatement

The use of superlatives has become part of our culture but should be avoided in clinical reporting as well as in clinical thinking. There is little or no use for such terms as "perfectly," "extremely," "totally," "completely," and "absolutely." Terms such as "always," "never," "entirely," and "obviously" should be used sparingly. The report writer should be direct and omit embellishment.

Avoid misusing words

Knepflar (1976) lists a number of words that frequently appear incorrectly in professional reports. They are those words that have meanings very much like other words in some cases or sound like other words but have entirely different meanings. Some of these words are listed below in pairs: ability and capacity, accept and except, affect and effect, among and between, amount and number, apt and likely, fewer and less, good and well. The list can be expanded considerably, but these examples should give the student a start in attending to vocabulary. The beginning professional particularly, but all of us generally, should consult a dictionary more frequently in order to use the precise term for the precise meaning. All of us become careless in the use of many terms, and some habitually misuse them because they do not know they are doing so.

Avoid passive verb construction as much as possible in favor of active verb construction

Often this means a different construction, but whenever possible active construction should be used because it shortens the statement and adds vitality and directness. For example, the passive voice construction, "inability to produce the /r/ phoneme was observed" carries the same meaning but not as directly and vigorously as the active voice form "she did not produce the /r/ phoneme correctly." Perhaps the passive voice construction is one of the lesser of our report-writing faults, but anything that will make the report more direct, alive, and readable should be practiced.

BASIC IDENTIFYING INFORMATION NEEDED IN ALL REPORTS

There is room for difference in most aspects of clinical reports, but all must contain the following information about the client: name; birthdate; age; address; telephone number; date of assessment, treatment, or other clinical activity; date of report; referral source; reason for referral; if client is a minor; names of parents or guardian with address and telephone number; if the client is in school or some other institution; name of the school or institution, address, and telephone; name and identification of report writer; and name of clinic or school, if the report is not written on a letterhead. Other basic information is needed in some kinds of reports and not in others. This will be considered under content as different kinds of reports are discussed.

KINDS OF REPORTS

When we consider report writing, too often we think in terms of only one type of report, the one that is prepared after diagnostic procedures have been completed. Actually there are several different kinds of reports that most clinicians and diagnosticians must write at different times in different settings. These include (1) preliminary or initial report, (2) diagnostic or assessment report, (3) consultation report, (4) progress report, and (5) final or summary report. Included in Appendix N are outlines of an individualized educational program and of goals and procedures. Each of these reports has different purposes, is prepared at different stages of the management process, and requires different contents and somewhat different style, format, and language, but all should include statements on how the information was obtained. Reports can serve at least three purposes: (1) as a guide for further services, (2) as a means of communicating our findings with others, and (3) for research purposes (Emerick and Hatten, 1979).

There are other specialized reports, such as those required by some schools, insurance agencies, Medicare and Medicaid, Veterans Administration, and other agencies. Many of these special reports have forms or checklists and can be completed by using information that will comprise one or more of the five previously named major reports, so they need not be discussed here. The number and variety of reports will differ with the setting, the problem, and the clinician. Some settings require several kinds of reports, perhaps too many and too frequently. This may be why some clinicians are turned off by report writing, but that cannot be used as an excuse for not writing reports when they are due or not writing them as efficiently as possible. When a professional accepts a position, he or she also accepts the responsibility of working within the policies and operating procedures of that situation. In other words report writing is here to stay, for better or worse, and the professional must strive to make it "for better."

WRITING THE PRELIMINARY REPORT

The preliminary report can also be called an initial report, and there are many and varied purposes for it. In some situations such a report may never need to be written, but in many it is important. Perhaps the most common purpose for this kind of report, especially in clinical situations and private practice, is the necessity of responding to a referral source shortly after initial contact with a client. For example, it may become obvious to the speech-language pathologist or audiologist soon after early contact with a client that other examinations or treatment should precede speech or hearing diagnosis or treatment, such as might be provided by a psychologist, otologist, otolaryngologist, plastic surgeon, orthodontist, or other specialist. Such a recommendation would be made in an initial report with a copy sent to the referral source.

In such a report the contents should include: identifying data, pertinent information gathered during the first interview, related background information, initial impressions of the problem, and reasons for the recommendation being made. Often a referral by another professional is made to obtain the initial impressions of the speech-language pathologist or audiologist. A school official, physician, or agency representative, for example, may want an opinion about how to proceed with a particular kind of problem. Of course the preliminary report may include a recommendation that a complete speech, language, and hearing workup is indicated, but unless a complete workup is requested with the referral, preliminary impressions may be all that are required. If there is doubt as to what is wanted, the question probably can be answered quickly by telephone and no report will be required at that time.

The essential aspect of this kind of report is its design for the user, which means that the report writer must know the user and what the needs are insofar as possible. Many clinics, school systems, and private practitioners will have a fairly standard style and format for such reports, but these can be so impersonal that they give the impression of lack of attention to the referral, especially since this is an initial report. Such forms should be reviewed frequently to see that they fit the needs of referral sources or other uses of the report.

Another purpose of the preliminary report, particularly in schools, is to provide information for classroom teachers, administrators, supervisors, or other school personnel. In such cases these persons may not be considered referral sources because the problem usually has been discovered in the clinician's initial survey of the classroom. However, the classroom teacher is frequently a referral source aside from the clinician's survey. In some school systems the only children seen for assessment by the speech-language pathologist are those referred by a teacher. The preliminary report for the teacher or other school personnel may be primarily for the purpose of providing information about the nature of the disorder and plans for further management.

The preliminary report may also include a request for further information or participation of the teacher or someone else. Content can be brief and to the point but should be extensive enough to provide a full picture of the situation. Technical terminology should be avoided as much as possible. For example, the clinician may see what appears to be dysarthria and will use such a term in personal notes, but describing the organic articulation disorder without any label is more meaningful to the teacher. If technical terms seem necessary, they should be defined and described in the report.

A final purpose of a preliminary report is sometimes to provide parents or guardians with information concerning initial findings. This may be necessary if the problem seems to be a complicated one that may require extensive measures for diagnosis and treatment. In such cases the contents of the report may well include, in addition to the clinician's initial findings and impressions, recommendations for measures that should be taken prior to a diagnostic workup and treatment, such as those mentioned previously. The report might outline procedures for overall management of the child or simply for the next steps in management, depending on how much is known of the problem at this time.

Language in this kind of report must be very explicit, clear, and direct yet not be abrupt, alarming, or subject to misinterpretation. This information usually has been given to the parents in an initial or subsequent interview, but a follow-up report or letter often is necessary to avoid misunderstanding. We, and probably most others in speech-language pathology, have had the frequent experience of having explained information as thoroughly as possible to parents, a caseworker, or someone else accompanying a client, only to find gross misinterpretations later. In some instances these misinterpretations can result in serious problems in the management of the disorder. At the very least they can cause confusion and waste of time. This is primarily the reason for a written follow-up preliminary report to parents or whoever is responsible for the child. If the client is an adult, the chances of misunderstanding may also be as great and the written follow-up may be as important.

Before writing any report, a signed release of information form should always be obtained from the parents or whoever is responsible for the client. Parents, adult clients, and others who may be responsible, including referral sources, should know and approve who is to see the report and what its outside distribution might be. With this knowledge those persons responsible should sign the release of information form. In light of what has been said previously about the danger of misinterpretation and even lawsuits, obtaining a signed release becomes extremely important. Certain personnel in clinics and other institutions usually take care of obtaining a signed release of information, but the person in private practice and others in any setting should make sure that a release has been obtained.

WRITING THE DIAGNOSTIC REPORT

The diagnostic report is the major and sometimes the only report relative to a particular client that is necessary. For this reason the report must be written carefully and thoroughly. The diagnostic report may have several purposes, depending on the setting, the referral source, and other factors. Often the same report will go to several different readers at one time, such as a referring speech-language pathologist in a school, the classroom teacher, possibly parents or guardians, and the family physician, as well as being included in the clinical chart. For this reason the content, language, style, and format must be adequate for all of them.

Making a report serve several purposes at once is difficult. In the medical setting the diagnostic report often is used primarily as a basis for further clinical intervention to be integrated with a number of different disciplines. If the referral source is a physician, the report, as written for the medical chart, is adequate in most cases. If the referral source is a school or lay agency, the report may need to be altered or rewritten or a cover letter written to meet the different needs; however, if carefully done the same report could serve these multiple needs most of the time.

Diagnostic reports prepared by the school clinician usually serve still different purposes. Certainly such a report becomes part of the child's permanent school record. Its most important use, however, is likely to be as a basis for management of the problem. Public Law 94-142 now requires school staff specialists to meet jointly to plan for the management of whatever problems the child presents. In such cases the diagnostic report of the speech-language clinician serves a valuable purpose in the group decisions.

In the past a full diagnostic report usually was not made available to parents or other responsible nonprofessionals. As pointed out previously, however, the time has arrived when parents and other lay persons generally have access to reports and records; these documents will have to be written so that they are understood by both lay persons and professionals and still convey the needed information. As mentioned previously in discussing initial reports, terminology and language are critical when the reports are to be read by nonprofessionals or professionals not in the field of speech and hearing. These aspects are most critical in diagnostic reports because more specific terminology is needed. Even so, we tend to use too much technical terminology that could be avoided. Lewis (1978) quotes Tennov (1975) in reference to terminology in

psychiatric diagnosis, "Technical jargon is a kind of inner-sanctum code system, meant, quite deliberately, to keep others out and to impress." A great many reports in speech, language, and hearing lead one to the conclusion that the report writers too often indulge in the same practices. Readers must be let in rather than kept out, and it is possible to write meaningful reports and accomplish this, but report writing takes practice.

If technical terms are needed, they should be defined in the report in nontechnical language. Even the seemingly innocent term, "retarded speech," can alarm parents, because "retarded" is likely to be associated immediately with the frightening thought of mental retardation. "Speech delay" may be less frightening, but even that expression need not be used. To make the statement more meaningful to both professional and lay persons, the label can be avoided altogether and the child's speech described in terms of existing norms and functioning age levels, for example, "This 5-year-old child's articulation is at a 3- to 3½-year level, according to performance at this time. Substitutions include /w/ for /r/ and /l/ and /θ/ for /s/." If phonetic symbols are used, the regular letter might be placed beside it in parentheses.

Because of the multiple uses of diagnostic reports, contents become all-important. After the basic *identifying data,* other *background information* needed in a good report includes purpose of the referral; pertinent information from the differential client history, such as previous diagnostic speech or hearing assessment, previous treatment and the results, pertinent medical and dental history, psychologic examinations and treatment, and current treatment of any kind; and pertinent information regarding family, home, school, and other environmental aspects. Here again caution is advised in reporting this kind of information. Whereas the diagnostician's impressions and interpretations are useful and necessary at this point, prudence dictates describing these verbally to the parents, or others if necessary, and including a bare minimum in the report.

The report should include what *procedures* have been followed in the diagnostic workup, what tests have been given, and what these tests are designed to measure, observations made, conditions during testing and examination, and behavior of the client and parents, if pertinent, other individuals present, and other information relating to the testing situation. If examination and testing could not be completed or if results were not valid because of the client's resistance or other reasons, this should be noted and described, not in negative terms, but simply reported.

With the preceding information in the report, the remainder should be devoted to *results* of speech, language, and hearing tests given, speech mechanism examination, and other assessment procedures. This section should include a careful, specific description, with scores from tests, if included at all, embedded in terminology to fit the users of the report. Generally numeric test scores should be interpreted or avoided, if possible, in favor of descriptive behavior and comparisons with norms. The amount of detail can vary greatly in this section depending on the setting and the uses of the report.

Reporting the results of articulation testing involves attention to aspects that are different from other types of disorders. Pannbacker (1975) points out that results should be reported in a manner consistent with the theoretic construct of whatever test was used. The traditional manner is to test for phonetic errors, in which case defective phonemes and types of errors are elicited. However, results should be recorded and reported in terms of distinctive feature errors or phonologic rules if testing was done within the framework of either of these constructs. How much detail is provided varies with the uses of the report, but detailed results need to be recorded as a basis for treatment and baseline, although they may be summarized in the report.

Not all procedures can or should be re-

ported, and all responses may not be pertinent. Much must be omitted in the interests of specificity and brevity. Most users of diagnostic reports are more interested in results of procedures than in the procedure themselves. For example, the articulation inventory or the audiogram would be of little interest to anyone except possibly another speech-language pathologist or audiologist, but the results would be. Too much detail can discourage the reader from attending to important information in the report and can be a waste of time.

The next part of the report is a *statement of the diagnosis,* if the results are quite clear-cut and a specific diagnosis can be made. Here technical terminology often is used and may or may not need to be explained, depending on the users of the report. Often a tentative diagnosis is made, pending more testing, examination, or information. Many prefer to state the diagnosis in terms of "impression," which is more tentative than a definite label. Others make an operational description in terms of what the problem is or seems to be. Regardless of the form in which the diagnosis is stated, the diagnosis should be as specific as the data will allow and should be a solid basis for stating a prognosis and plan of management (see Appendix N).

Statement of prognosis is the next part of the report. The statement is the diagnostician's evaluation of the possibilities of success of a treatment program. Often the prognosis is simply a statement such as, "prognosis for normal speech is good," "prognosis for improvement is favorable," or, to use a medical expression, "prognosis is guarded" or "prognosis is poor." This may be all that is written under the heading, or the writer may want to explain some of the reasons for the stated prognosis. The explanation might include such factors as client motivation, parent understanding and cooperation, client stimulability, limitations or lack of a management program for the client, and other such factors. The statement reflects an interpretation and evaluation of a number of aspects of the entire situation and as such should be made with care and freedom from personal bias and value judgments. Such statements often are made under "comments" rather than under "prognosis."

Many diagnosticians like to include a section in the diagnostic report titled *comments*. This section often is useful to explain many of the judgments mentioned previously in determining prognosis, thus allowing for flexibility and clarity, and providing a section in which a number of extraneous matters can be brought together. This section may also be useful in some of the other kinds of reports.

After the section on comments, or sometimes preceding it, a section appears that is variously called *plan of management, treatment plan,* or in some settings *recommendations;* this section outlines a plan for intervention. We prefer the latter, because often the plan of management or treatment plan can be only a recommendation for someone else to carry out. The specificity of statements in this section will vary with the purposes of the report. Presenting a detailed treatment plan may not be in good taste if someone else is to carry out the treatment, unless this is requested. Often a school makes a referral to a clinic for help with a diagnosis but with the intention of carrying on from there in the school. In a clinical or medical setting the recommendations might be quite specific as to treatment because they likely will be carried out in that setting. In private practice and often in clinics a fairly detailed and specific plan of management will be included for the information of the person or agency who made the referral, even though treatment is to be carried out by the writer of the report.

Recommendations for a treatment plan should consider other pertinent factors and events involving the client, such as treatment being given for reasons other than speech, language, or hearing disorders, the school situation, the home, availability of treatment to the client, and many others. Language in this section should be as simple and direct as possible and should leave no possibility for misunderstanding.

Finally the diagnostic report should note at the bottom where copies are to be sent. Sometimes sending a cover letter with the report is necessary, particularly if the report is to serve several purposes. Explanations can be made in a cover letter that may not be suitable in the report. The report should be signed by the diagnostician with appropriate identification, and if a student wrote the report, it should be signed by the student, indicating the student status, and then countersigned by the staff member who supervised the student, with identification of the status of the staff member.

Attention is called here to the article previously mentioned by English and Lillywhite (1963), which deals with the language of clinical reports and also discusses terminology, content, and style. Study of this article and others (Pannbacker, 1975; Jerger, 1962) should assist in developing the skills and techniques of report writing.

WRITING THE CONSULTATION REPORT

Any referral could be considered a consultation, and the resulting report a consultation report. As used here, however, a consultation report is one that is needed when one speech-language pathologist refers a client to another for assistance with a special kind of problem, such as a difficult diagnosis, what direction treatment should take, or why a client is not responding to treatment being given. This kind of referral is most common among private practitioners but also occurs among clinics or between a public school and clinic.

A complete diagnostic workup usually is not requested in a consultation referral because the referrer probably has already done that, but a full workup may be requested because of special expertise or equipment available to the individual being asked for help. The person who has received this kind of referral should be careful to do what has been asked, and the report should be directed specifically toward these requests. For this reason the format may be more varied than in other types of reports. A report in the form of a letter may be suitable, or a more formal report may be needed. The important factor is that format, style, content, language, and terminology should be designed specifically for the referral source and may be quite different from reports to other referrers who are not speech-language pathologists. Usually there is only one specific purpose for this kind of report, which is limited by that purpose. Specificity of purpose should not pose problems if this is kept in mind and if the diagnostician does only what is asked.

WRITING THE PROGRESS REPORT

Progress reports have several purposes and may be quite brief or rather detailed, depending on the situation in which the treatment is being done. In any kind of setting, however, regular progress reports should be made, if only to chart what has been done and as a guide to what remains to be done. In many cases progress reports are required at the end of a specific period, such as the end of a school term, semester, year, or other designated period. In schools, especially, this kind of report usually is required regularly. Often this report is used by a different clinician when the child passes from one grade or school to another. The report also may be written for a supervisor, teacher, administrator, and sometimes parents. Periodic brief progress reports may be particularly helpful to parents and can do much to promote understanding between parents and clinician. If parents have been involved in the treatment process, written reports to them may not be necessary.

Not uncommonly in clinics and in private practice, periodic progress reports are submitted to the referral source, especially if treatment extends over a fairly long period of time. If the client's treatment is covered by private insurance, Medicaid, Medicare, or other sources of funding, progress reports most likely will be required as a basis for continued funding. Standard reporting forms often are provided by such agencies but may not be.

Progress reports as considered here should not be confused with the clinician's *daily*

log, or working notes that are important to maintain continuity and to give a detailed running account of goals set and goals achieved. Many other kinds of information are recorded in the daily log, usually written as soon as possible after each clinical session. These include notes on such aspects as the client's behavior, the parents and their behavior, new information that often becomes apparent as treatment progresses, and sometimes a revision of short- and long- term treatment plans whenever a change in direction is indicated. This log then serves as source material for the periodic progress reports and the final report as they are needed. If the log is conscientiously kept, the progress report becomes something of a summary and is easy to prepare, as is the final report.

Contents of the progress report will be quite varied according to the purpose it is to serve. Basic information needed includes number, length of time, and frequency of treatment sessions, both scheduled and kept; initial and succeeding goals that have been set; and progress toward these goals based on comparisons between baseline behaviors and terminal behaviors. Statements on progress should be made in quantifiable terms. Changes in goals and reasons for the changes should be noted, and some kind of prognostic statement and recommendations may at times be included in the report. Other information that may or may not be needed is types of treatment procedures used, the effectiveness of these procedures, motivation of the client and parents and their cooperation or lack thereof, environmental factors influencing management of the problem, and other treatment such as medical, psychologic, or dental care. The more specific the progress report can be, the better. Progress should be based on whatever kinds of measurements were made from the starting base at the beginning of treatment.

Language of the progress report should suit the purposes, but certainly it should be primarily reporting and describing. Interpretation and evaluation will be needed in order that assessment of progress can be stated and recommendations made, but reporting of these should be primary, with enough interpretative statements to substantiate the conclusions and recommendations. Even intuitive statements may be included, but they should be used carefully. Personal reactions and value judgments should be used sparingly, if at all. Progress usually can be stated quite briefly and concretely to suit the purposes.

Style in progress reports, because they usually are quite brief, may not be an important consideration, but the rules for good style discussed previously should be observed. A specific format may determine style and language and to some extent content. Standard progress report forms are frequently required in certain settings, thus predetermining many of these aspects. The individual speech-language pathologist often will develop a relatively standard format, style, and language for most kinds of reports based on experience in a particular setting, but in doing so care must be taken not to develop stereotypes and inflexibility.

WRITING THE FINAL REPORT

The final report is perhaps second to the diagnostic report in importance and is required as often in most situations. This report usually has three principal purposes: (1) made at the conclusion of treatment to indicate that the problem has been corrected; (2) made when the client leaves the jurisdiction of the clinician involved to indicate that the problem still remains and the client is going into another treatment program; and (3) made to indicate that treatment has been terminated for some other reason, such as the client withdrawing, moving, or being dismissed because of lack of progress, lack of willingness to cooperate, or other such reasons.

In each of these purposes, the final report may well be largely a summary of progress reports or of daily logs when progress reports have not been necessary. When the problem has been corrected and no further treatment is anticipated, progress, procedures, and such details may be at a minimum in the final report. The report then may be only a summary and whatever concluding statements might be necessary. Inclusion of recommendations for follow-up checkups is usually wise and necessary, even when the disorder appears to have been eliminated. Not uncommonly a problem may resurface after a client has left treatment with seemingly adequate speech. A parent-counseling or client recheck and counseling program may be needed, particularly when reappearance of the problem is anticipated. Such recommendations should be a part of the final report.

When the client leaves the management program before the problem is corrected, for whatever reason, the nature of the report will be quite different. In such cases a thorough progress summary should be included, with recommendation for further treatment in the event that intervention will be available for the client at some later time and place. This consideration is even more important if the client is moving to another location. In this circumstance the client or parents probably should be given a summary report suited to their understanding. With this report should be the assurance, in the report and to the parents, that more detailed information will be supplied to another clinician if the client enters some other program.

If the client has been dismissed from treatment for some negative reason, the writing of the final report becomes more complicated. However, even though the reason for dismissal is a negative one, there need not be negative feelings involved and no unpleasantness in relation to the dismissal. If the clinician has been careful to refrain from showing negative feelings toward the client and has based the decision for dismissal on demonstrable evidence that is presented to the parents and client in friendly, positive terms aiming at the good of the client, there should be no unpleasantness. Besides, dismissal for negative reasons should not preclude consideration for additional treatment in the future.

If the client is a child, the dismissal and

the report will be much less difficult if the parents have been closely involved in the treatment program from the beginning and understand the problems, if they center around the child. However, the parents or the environment they provide might be the problem. In this situation great care must be taken to report accurately, yet not make statements that might be considered libelous or at least might be cause for ill feeling and loss of confidence in treatment of the disorder by anyone. If the family has confidence in the clinician, even though they may be blocking progress, reporting the situation will be much easier. A reminder again may be necessary as to the importance of obtaining a signed release of information form from the parents or client, if an adult, at the beginning of the program and to be aware of other safeguards in the use of terminology, evaluative judgments, and conclusions. The following discussion may be of considerable help in this regard.

HOW TO AVOID SOME SEMANTIC PITFALLS IN REPORTING

As mentioned earlier, the task of the writer of any report is to make the word-map (report) accurately represent the client (territory) and yet not create more problems for the client, clinician, clinic, or

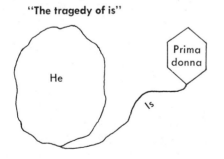

Fig. 10-2. Large "territory" (he) does not balance on the fulcrum "is" with the small, rigid concept (prima donna) of the "he." (From Weiss, C. E., and Lillywhite, H. S.: Communicative disorders: a handbook for prevention and early intervention, St. Louis, 1976, The C. V. Mosby Co.)

agency in which the clinical activity took place. Accurate representation becomes critical when assessment leads to a diagnosis of a problem of unusual severity, if the client or parents are unwilling or unable to accept the diagnosis or if the client has been in treatment and has been dismissed for some negative reason.

One of the best safeguards is to avoid, as completely as possible, making evaluative statements and judgments without careful explanation, documentation, and qualification. In other words what is called in General Semantics "The Tragedy of Is" should be avoided. This expression designates the fallacy of trying to make the map represent the territory by the simple expedient of a noun or pronoun, a verb, and an adjective or adjective phrase, such as is shown in Fig. 10-2 from Weiss and Lillywhite (1976).

This kind of expression is one of the most frequently used in the English language, and it probably leads to the most trouble. All through our waking hours most of us make interpretive, evaluative, or judgmental statements such as, "She is charming," "He is a bore," and "The people are unfriendly." Clinically we make such statements as, "Those parents are overprotective," "She is overanxious," "Johnny is uncooperative," "Jane is hostile," "They are good parents," and "This child is spoiled." The problem with such statements is that trying to make such a word-map as "hostile," "uncooperative," "anxious," "good," or any of the many other one-word or one-phrase maps represent the whole territory is impossible. The person making such a statement may think the meaning is clear, but a human being represents so much territory that the person can never be even closely described by a limited word-map, especially to another person hearing or reading such a remark.

To avoid "The Tragedy of Is" in report writing, functional or operational descriptions of behavior or situations are preferred. An objective description of how a child behaves may require more words and time than a flat judgmental statement, but the description will more nearly represent the territory. This approach also will run much less risk of being misinterpreted or of arousing apprehension. Instead of the statement, "Harry was quite hostile during the diagnostic session," an operational statement, such as, "Harry struck out at his mother on several occasions, stuck his tongue out at the clinician when he was unhappy about something, and hit other children" lets the reader know how Harry behaved rather than how the clinician reacted to and labeled the behavior. The clinician should practice and refine techniques for using operational descriptions in reports. A stark statement that a child *is* hostile not only fails to give much of a clue as to how the child behaved but also requires a label that can lead to misinterpretation and mismanagement unless the reader of the report is aware that the map does not represent the territory; sad to say, very few readers are aware of this.

Another technique for avoiding "The Tragedy of Is" in reports is to use more conditional or tentative statements and fewer positive ones. Even though we previously suggested avoiding qualifiers, their occasional use can prevent the report from sounding too positive in the absence of adequate supportive evidence. Absolutism should be avoided in most clinical endeavors. Qualifications such as, "At this time . . . ," "On the basis of performance during this testing period . . . ," "Test results indicate . . . ," and "Mary's performance during treatment sessions leads me to believe . . . " can and should be used liberally. Such statements may appear to be hedging or to be too indirect and unsure, but they more accurately represent a small portion of the territory by specifying time and the activity leading to the evaluative statement. This leaves room for possibly differing behavior and test results at another time or in another situation.

One can rarely be positive about anything, and thinking or writing in absolutes can lead to endless trouble. Such often is the language of persons who are bigoted,

ignorant, and opinionated but also often is the language of persons who are unsure, fearful, and incompetent or who use language to cover up, to reassure themselves, or to impress others. The secure, competent professional can afford not to know, or to be tentative, and to write reports that leave room for other possibilities, if such exist, and they usually do. Language and style should demonstrate confidence yet leave room for differences.

Another semantic pitfall that almost universally entraps most of us is the categorizing and labeling of individuals according to their disorders and crippling conditions. This process is so routine that we rarely are aware of it. We speak of "the blind," "the deaf," or "he is a stutterer," "an aphasic," etc., as if the person and the handicap are the same. The map "stutterer" does *not* represent the boy, Richard, who stutters. Richard is a very "normal" person, much like the rest of us who do not stutter, but by labeling Richard with the name of a speech deviation we equate all of Richard with that deviation. Worse yet, we put Richard in a category that we have made that includes all persons who stutter (stutterers), and by the common label we give to all who stutter, we imply that they are different from the rest of the human race, as fish are different from birds and birds from rabbits. Perhaps we know that this is not true when we apply this label, but is Richard aware of this?

Probably Richard does know that we know we do not mean what we say, but more than likely he thinks we do mean what we say, so he comes to regard himself as different in terms of the label we have given him and others who stutter. Once he accepts the label that has been attached to him, he begins to behave as if the label represents him, just as those of us who labeled him do. Thus the labeled and the labeler make the speech deviation the most important characteristic about the person or group labeled. In doing this we are helping to alter the individual's self-image and to detract from that person's sense of individuality, personal worth, and dignity. The simple expedient of thinking, speaking, and writing in language such as, "Richard stutters" rather than "Richard is a stutterer," "Mary has an articulation problem" rather than "Mary is an articulation case," and "This child is deaf" rather than "This is a deaf child" would change this process of degrading people. The distinction may seem slight to us but important to those persons who come to us with problems. If we would make the distinction, much would be done to channel our behavior and that of our client toward the territory rather than concentrating on the map and forgetting the territory.

SUMMARY

We have described and discussed five different kinds of reports that many clinicians are called on to write, and we have related the different purposes for these reports and the different needs according to various settings. Format, style, content, language, and terminology have been considered according to each kind of report. Legal aspects and the need for caution in writing reports have been stressed, along with the relatively recent requirements of federal law for quality review, accountability, audit of clinical activity, appropriate treatment, and related matters. These factors have added elements of a new vocabulary, along with new responsibilities. We have stressed the need for a disciplined approach to report writing and record keeping, the aspects of clinical work that can too easily be set aside for another time. To allow these kinds of clinical work habits to develop will be detrimental to all concerned. For that reason we stress self-discipline and a conscious, continuing effort toward not only competent reports, but prompt reports, remembering that report writing takes practice. Finally we have offered a number of suggestions and techniques for avoiding semantic pitfalls in clinical thinking and report writing.

Several clinical reports of various types are included in Appendix N. The student is invited to examine these carefully. They are selected from several different settings and are reports of actual clinical activity written by experienced speech-language pathologists.

STUDY SUGGESTIONS

1. Compare content and purpose in the five different kinds of reports that might be required in any of several different settings.
2. Define "style" as used in this chapter. How might style differ from one kind of report to another?
3. Relate Knepflar's twelve suggestions concerning style to different kinds and purposes of reports.
4. What are some of the implications for report writing of Public Law 94-142, the establishment of professional standards review organizations, and other such measures?
5. Describe how the "map-territory relationship," as used in this chapter, relates to report writing.

REFERENCES

Dublinske, S.: Planning for child change in language development/remediation programs carried out by teachers and parents, Lang. Speech Hear. Serv. Schools **5:**225-237, 1974.

Dublinske, S.: PL 94-142: developing the individualized education program (IEP), ASHA **20:**380-393, 1978.

Dublinske, S., and Healey, W. C.: PL 94-142: questions and answers for the speech-language pathologist and audiologist, ASHA **20:**188-205, 1978.

Emerick, C., and Hatten, J.: Diagnosis and evaluation in speech pathology, ed. 2, Englewood Cliffs, N.J., 1979, Prentice-Hall, Inc.

English, R. L., and Lillywhite, H. S.: A semantic approach to clinical reporting in speech pathology, ASHA **5:**547-650, June 1963.

Garrard, K. R.: Consideration of the speech pathologist's role in early childhood education for the handicapped, ASHA **17:**90-92, 1975.

Jerger, J.: Scientific writing can be readable, ASHA **4:**101-104, 1962.

Johnson, W.: People in quandaries, New York, 1946, Harper & Row, Publishers.

Knepflar, K. J.: Report writing in the field of communication disorders, Danville, Ill., 1976, The Interstate Printers & Publishers, Inc.

Lewis, T. T.: The semantics of psychiatric labels, Etc. **35**(2):180, June 1978.

Nation, J. E., and Aram, D. M.: Diagnosis of speech and language disorders, St. Louis, 1977, The C. V. Mosby Co., pp. 159-174.

Pannbacker, M.: Diagnostic report writing, J. Speech Hear. Disord. **40:**367-379, 1975.

Tennov, D.: Psychotherapy: the hazardous cure, New York, 1975, Abelard-Schumann, Limited, p. 18.

Weiss, C. E., and Lillywhite, H. S.: Communicative disorders: a handbook for prevention and early intervention, St. Louis, 1976, The C. V. Mosby Co.

GLOSSARY

concurrent review A procedure used by professional standards review organizations (PSROs) having to do with cost containment and reduction.

continued stay review A procedure used by PSROs to document continued treatment related to federal payment for a patient's continued stay in a hospital. It may apply indirectly to the speech-language pathologist if such patient is receiving treatment for a communication disorder.

patient care audit A procedure of PSROs that is an objectively structured, sequential analysis of patient care, pertaining originally to medical and hospital care but relating to and sometimes required for care of patients (clients) under treatment for communication disorders.

professional standards review organizations (PSROs) Mandated by Public Law 92-603 necessitating the establishment of professional peer review procedures throughout the United States to assure appropriate and adequate care being provided persons receiving Medicare and Medicaid. Originally designed for medical care but pertaining to care by all health-related professions.

retrospective review A PSRO procedure for retrospectively assessing the quality of care delivered to a specific category of patients. Pertains to medical and all health-related professions.

CHAPTER ELEVEN

Different employment settings

"Speak the speech, I pray you, as I pronounced it to you."
SHAKESPEARE

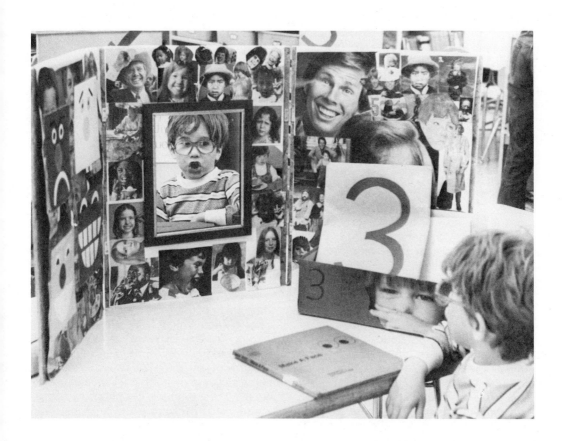

The speech-language pathologist provides diagnosis and treatment of articulation disorders in a wide variety of settings. Such diversity among clients and environments requires the clinician to possess a number of skills and traits (Ainsworth, 1948; Eisenson and Ogilvie, 1977; Van Hattum, 1969). To function effectively, the clinician should have maturity, understanding, humility, a sense of independence, honesty, empathy, controlled permissiveness, a sense of humor, patience, imagination, resourcefulness, and dependability (Chapman, 1969). These characteristics, as well as the ability to relate to administrators, teachers, children, parents, adult clients, colleagues, and professionals in other health and allied health disciplines, are all part of the requirements for becoming a successful speech-language pathologist.

This list of desired qualifications, although not exhaustive, may seem overwhelming. Can, or should, one person realistically be expected to possess all of them? Certainly the bachelor's or master's degree and the training they represent do not guarantee all, or even most, of the skills and characteristics listed. This is not expected, but it is expected that the clinician work diligently to develop them. Fortunately, given the dedication and comprehensive training of most clinicians, they do eventually meet a majority of these requirements as they gain experience, but they need to work at it.

Possessing all or most of these characteristics and skills enables the clinician to function effectively in most of the varied settings in which employment possibilities exist. These are: (1) public and private schools, (2) public and private clinics, (3) private, state, and federal hospitals, (4) college and university clinics, (5) private practice in a clinician's office, a physician's office, or at home, (6) state crippled children's service programs, (7) Head Start programs, (8) nursery schools, (9) medical schools, (10) state departments of health and education, (11) convalescent homes, and (12) research settings (Van Riper, 1972).

Treatment in any of these settings may be (1) individual and intensive, (2) groups that are homogeneous or heterogeneous, (3) a combination of individual and group, (4) intermittent or sporadic, (5) indirect or consultative, and (6) team. Additionally some treatment settings may be primarily diagnostic in nature. In order to assist the prospective clinician in knowing what to expect, some diagnostic, treatment, organizational, and management requirements and procedures for each of these settings will be discussed.

PUBLIC AND PRIVATE SCHOOLS

Nearly all public schools now provide some kind of speech-language service, although unfortunately some schools in some isolated localities provide little or none. The service usually emanates from a central city school district or county office and is free to children. Clinicians are hired by the district or county rather than by individual schools and receive direction and assignments from that source. The programs are coordinated by a speech-language supervisor or director located in the central school office. Private schools are not so fortunate in that many offer no service to communicatively handicapped children. Many, however, refer such children to various available clinics or private practitioners in the community. Expenses are usually born by parents for such treatment. Some private schools do provide such services at school by hiring a clinician to come to the school on a periodic basis. In some cases parents are asked to pay for this service even when it is provided in the school. We do not know of many private schools that hire full-time clinicians.

Van Hattum (1969) has discussed at some length the responsibilities of the school clinician. These include cooperation and interaction with teachers and administrators and assignments that are peculiar to educational settings, such as attending teachers' meetings, parent-teacher meetings, and open houses. The responsibilities involve educating teachers about speech-language problems and establishing rapport that will enable interaction with them.

Obviously the responsibilities go far beyond the actual working with clients. The clinician must be able to assume the roles of a diagnostician, consultant, counselor, educator, resource person, team member, community activist, and member of the public relation team. The responsibilities are diverse and many, but the challenge can be stimulating, be exciting, and give great rewards.

One of the most challenging aspects of this kind of setting is the interaction with so many diverse specialists and personalities concerning specific children and their problems, as well as the treatment program in general. These other professionals include psychologists, nurses, teachers, special educators, administrators, and many more. In this setting a clinician must also become familiar with school protocol, such as children's records or files, reports, individual educational plans, classroom sessions, recesses, all-school programs, vacations, field trips, and the chain of authority. Further the clinician must be aware of specific timetables for all manner of functions and individuals, procedures, priorities, and rules indigenous to a school. Within all of these limiting factors the clinician must be able to devise some rather ingenious and intricate treatment schedules, be they traditional, block, or some combination of both. In some settings schedules may already be in effect, such as time allocated per school, per session, for report writing (particularly the ubiquitous individual educational plans), and counseling. In these cases the clinician must be able to fit into these and adapt as necessary.

Because of the itinerant nature of most school clinicians' activity, efficiency and independence are key requisites. The clinician must be able to select and schedule children in several schools. This requires consulting with a number of different teachers, principals, and parents. The necessity of traveling among several schools and coping with numerous interruptions, such as pupils' illnesses, turnovers, classroom field trips, assemblies, and other scheduled and unscheduled events, requires consider-

able efficiency, patience, and understanding. However, not all school situations require itinerant care. In very large schools a clinician may work full time. Also in special settings, such as a school for children who are retarded, have cerebral palsy, or other problems requiring intensive treatment, usually in individual sessions, one or more clinicians may be needed full time.

A time-consuming responsibility in public schools is screening. Some clinicians spend up to 3 or 4 months screening children for potential enrollment or placement on a waiting list. At this time there does not appear to be an acceptable solution to reducing the amount of time spent in screening. However, if the situation is fairly stable, that is, if a clinician is to be working with the same schools for a fairly long time, in-service training of the classroom teachers by the clinician will enable some of the teachers to do some of the screening. After selection has been made, obtaining parental and teacher approval can take considerable time. Teachers are not a major problem if scheduling is consistent with classroom routine, but parents can present many problems. Usually they are willing to have the child receive treatment but are surprised that there is a problem with the child's speech, and sometimes they are alarmed, doubtful, and in need of considerable counseling and information about the disorder and the nature of the treatment.

One final responsibility in most settings is accountability. The time is with us when we must present solid evidence of the need for treatment, but, more important, we must set specific, understandable plans as to the expected time that treatment will take and then we must be accountable for the time, effort, and expenditure of funds required in the treatment. Thus the clinician must have or must develop a system for collecting, storing, and retrieving information about each client. Records must be complete, and reports on each client must be understandable, not only to school personnel, but to lay persons as well. They must be objective, quantifiable, and complete. If data are not communicable, the records have little relevance, applicability, and accountability. We suggest that the student review Chapter 10 for a more complete discussion of reports, records, and accountability.

All work situations are different, and clinicians must be prepared to adapt to them; however, certain generalizations can be made about speech-language diagnosis and treatment in schools. First the majority of the clinician's client load consists of children having nonorganic articulation disorders, although organic disorders are not uncommon, such as those caused by cleft palate, dental malformations, and paresis. Only a few, if any, children with severe multiple-handicapping conditions will be seen in the regular school, although with Public Law 94-142 the number of multiply handicapped children in the classroom is increasing. Many city and county school districts provide separate classes or schools for severe handicapping conditions, and speech-language clinicians nearly always are assigned to them. Second most of the client load will be made up of young children, unless the clinician has been assigned to middle schools and high schools, which is far less frequent because of fewer problems in older children. Third most of the treatment will be short term. Only a few of the children will be treated for as long as a year; however, some do require longer periods. Fourth most of the treatment sessions will be relatively brief, 30 minutes or less, and usually not more than three times a week, often less. An exception to this is block scheduling mentioned earlier. These sessions could be scheduled daily. Fifth the majority of the sessions will include more than one child. Group size may range from one to three or four children, depending on the type, severity, etiology, age, stimulability, and homogeneity of the children and their disorders and the philosophy of the administration and the clinician.

Scheduling can also consume considerable time. It involves obtaining parental approval, determining which children might best fit with other children, working around the daily school activities, such as class time, recess, lunch, and assemblies, consulting with teachers regarding preferred times when children can be seen, and sometimes consulting with parents about when they would prefer that their children be seen for treatment. Determining the most appropriate client load in the most efficient manner is difficult. Allowing for travel time between schools and giving each school its fair share of the clinician's time are other important factors.

PUBLIC AND PRIVATE CLINICS

By public clinic we mean such agencies as community clinics, usually named for the community, such as San Francisco Speech and Hearing Center, Portland Center for Hearing and Speech, etc. These clinics usually are supported partly by community funds, such as United Good Neighbors, partly by donations, and partly by fees charged clients. By private clinic we mean one involving several speech-language pathologists and audiologists, operating their own clinic in the same manner as medical and dental clinics. These persons are private practitioners usually, although some might be attached to a college, university, or medical school. For this reason we have chosen to discuss them as members of clinics, since they work with a group.

The speech-language clinician's functions and responsibilities in a clinic are quite different from those in schools and some other settings. Although the clinical environment is challenging and stimulating, clinical activities are dictated, to some extent, by the need for generating money. The clinician must "produce" in order to exist, especially in the private clinic that receives no outside funds. This does not mean that clinicians in other settings need not produce effective and efficient results, but the pressures of time and effectiveness must obviously be greater where the sole revenue is from clients' fees.

Interrelated with fees and successful clinical results is word-of-mouth advertising. The most effective way of generating more referrals is by providing excellent service.

Satisfied customers inform potential future customers of the quality of the service, and thus the word is spread. So in a sense, pressure is on the clinician to produce good results effectively and without any waste of time.

The client load in a clinic may be somewhat different than in a school or other settings. The clients may tend to have more severe communication problems, there may be a greater incidence of multiple problems, the parents may be more concerned, and the attendance may perhaps be more consistent. Depending on the clinic, the clinician may interact with specialists from a number of health and health-related disciplines who practice in the community or sometimes in the same building. The clients may tend to be preschool children or post-school adults.

Since time is a critical factor in this setting, the clinician must schedule carefully, write concise reports, and utilize the most efficient and effective procedures available. Vacations and other off-time activities must be thoughtfully planned, because unlike some other settings, when the clinician is not in the clinic, funds are not being generated or accumulated for retirement. High ethics and standards are most important in this setting because the clinician and results of treatment are highly visible and open to judgment from many sources.

PRIVATE, STATE, AND FEDERAL HOSPITALS

The speech-language pathologist who works in a hospital setting sees most clients in the hospital as inpatients, although some are seen as outpatients who return to the hospital for treatment by one or more specialists. Sometimes the clinician may even go to the home to treat a patient. Since treatment for patients in the hospital usually is short term, treatment must be quite intensive, perhaps for a matter of only a few days, weeks, or months. Sometimes all there is time for in the hospital is an assessment of the disorder, which then may be treated elsewhere by another clinician.

Although the disorders exhibit a wide range of severity, the majority probably have organic etiologies. In a large majority these patients will have articulation problems along with other kinds of disorders. Some hospitals operate children's wards that may retain patients for longer periods of time; some of these are residential and some are outpatient. Another type is the hospital devoted entirely to crippled children, such as the many excellent Shriners' hospitals, and the ever-expanding special hospital centers or wings in which a wide variety of functional as well as organic children's disorders are treated.

Other hospitals maintain wards for adults, many of which are elderly persons suffering from stroke, cardiac problems, senility, and other problems. Some of the patients in these wards are convalescent, and some are terminal. Veterans Hospitals, located in all parts of the country, treat adults of all ages with all types of disorders. All, or most, of these hospitals employ speech-language pathologists, as well as audiologists, on a full- or part-time basis. They have been especially consistent in providing diagnosis and treatment for communication disorders.

Patient mortality obviously is higher in a hospital setting than in most other settings. If the patient survives, preoccupation with the illness, chances for recovery, and death often is detrimental to treatment. Counseling, giving encouragement, and listening to the concerns of the patient and family may be a part of the overall management. The clinician should also have adopted an attitude encompassing the possibility of the patient's becoming more seriously ill or dying. Sometimes the patient may be progressing well with treatment of the communication disorder only to have the progress terminated suddenly by death or additional serious illness. Intensive treatment helps take the patient's mind off these concerns, as does significant improvement in communication. This improvement need not be great, but it could be dramatic in the thinking of the patient.

Family needs and concerns are also important considerations. Because of the often sudden trauma of the illness, the family may have experienced emotional devastation. Members are likely to be concerned about possible death of the patient, chances for recovery, lasting effects, financial matters, guilt, and lack of knowing what to do. The clinician must be able to empathize and provide support and still be concerned mainly with the patient's communication. Family involvement in treatment can be beneficial to the family as well as to the patient.

Accountability, maintenance of clear, accurate records and reports, and completion of hospital, state, and federal forms, usually in great quantity, are most important and often quite time-consuming. In most settings of this type, rigorous guidelines and protocol will have been established that the clinician must follow. Suggestions in Chapter 7 on records and reporting should help in this regard.

COLLEGE AND UNIVERSITY CLINICS

Although the overall responsibilities of the speech-language pathologist in a college or university setting may be somewhat similar from one institution to another, certain procedures and policies may vary. Some schools have highly structured clinical programs, whereas others have more flexibility; some have comprehensive guidelines for all clinicians to follow, whereas others encourage more individualistic approaches. Similarities are assured by the fact that all accredited programs must meet ASHA standards, and most reputable college and university programs are accredited.

Another similarity among college and university clinics is the clientele. There is a tendency toward a greater number of adults than in some other settings; many of these have articulation disorders, often as the only problem, but also frequently as part of a larger deficit. Foreign dialects are not uncommon in these clinics. Conversely school-aged children are less common, although most clinics offer summer programs for school-aged children and most treat a few such children after school hours. The apparent lack of variety is not typical of all university clinics, some having considerable variety among their clinical populations. Severely multiply handicapped clients are not uncommon to many such clinics. Other clinics are not so fortunate. Since exposure to different types of communication disorders is necessary for adequate student training, externships are commonly provided to give access to a wider variety of disorders. These externships may be taken in any of the other settings discussed in this chapter, depending on what is available in a certain locality.

The clinician in this setting is nearly always a full-time staff member, perhaps teaching some classes but spending most of the working time supervising student clinicians. Some programs have full-time clinic supervisors; in others that responsibility is given to different staff members as a major responsibility but several other staff members may also supervise student clinicians as well as teach courses. Supervision of student clinicians, whether full- or part-time, should also include demonstrations of diagnostic and treatment procedures for students. This would apply to anyone supervising students in clinical practice. Some college and university clinics employ full- or part-time clinicians to work directly with clients as one of the services offered by the institution. In either situation the clinician must be knowledgeable, competent, and capable of providing exemplary care to persons with communication disorders.

A position in this setting is demanding, but rewarding. The clinician has the opportunity to interact with many different personalities among students, staff, and community. The excitement of helping student clinicians develop competence and experience success in a clinical setting is doubly rewarding because not only is the client helped, but so is the student. The speech-language pathologist in this setting must be able to get along with people at many levels and at the same time aggressively maintain high standards of clinical competence and scholarship.

Employment in a college or university usually offers many advantages for a clinical working situation. Clinics usually have an ample supply of materials and equipment. An abundance of resources and the availability of colleagues combine to facilitate stimulating and rewarding working conditions. The number of clients supervised or seen for treatment is likewise more ideal than in some other settings. Accreditation standards recommend that the clinician supervise no more than twenty-four students a semester as a full-time load (ASHA, 1978). Each student probably would not be treating more than two clients per semester. In many nonaccredited institutions, however, shortage of staff often causes an overload and clinic supervision suffers as a result.

Unlike working in private practice, employment in a university setting alleviates some of the financial concerns the clinician might otherwise have. Income is not dictated by the number of clients seen. Because clients are seen for the express purpose of student training, except in the case of direct service, the clinician is free to emphasize quality of care without too must concern for quantity. The same should be true in public and private clinics, but pressure for quantity is always present.

One final aspect of the clinician's responsibilities in a college or university clinic is planning, record-keeping, and reporting. The clinician must be able to assist the student clinician in planning thoroughly, creatively, and effectively. This is accomplished partly through showing the student where to go for ideas and resources and partly through exemplary client care. The important factor is to help the student learn good habits in regard to planning and carrying out treatment. Besides planning, the supervisor must also be able to report student progress and all clinic activities clearly and objectively. This requires a thorough knowledge of all clinic activities, especially student clinicians' functions and progress,

fairness, objectivity, and effective recording and writing. In turn these skills must be taught to students through a combination of didactic instruction, demonstration, close supervision of student records and reports, and good counseling and help.

PRIVATE PRACTICE IN A CLINICIAN'S OFFICE, A PHYSICIAN'S OFFICE, OR AT HOME

More and more speech-language pathologists and audiologists are going into private practice, either on a full- or part-time basis. This movement toward more private practice is related partly to convenience and partly to necessity.

A common type of private practice is that in which an individual equips and opens an office and offers services to communicatively handicapped persons on a full- or part-time basis, as do other professionals in psychology, medicine, and dentistry. The speech-language pathologist in private practice often is with a group of other professionals who operate a private practice clinic for treatment of communicative disorders, but since this kind of setting is discussed elsewhere, the present concern is with the individual alone in private practice.

Persons in private practice may do their work in a medical clinic or, less often, in a dental clinic. A few practice in an individual physician's office. Regardless of the location of the private practitioner, the level of training usually is high and the service must meet ASHA standards. When private parties are paying directly for service, they demand positive results. If these results do not meet their expectations, negative publicity may follow. This problem is especially serious when the clinician's sole support is dependent on private practice, that is, if the practice is a full-time occupation.

Part-time practice may be slightly less demanding, especially if it can take place in the kind of situation in which a college, university, or other agency employs the speech-language clinician on a part-time basis and private practice outside that setting occupies the rest of the clinician's time.

Some colleges, universities, and medical schools will allow a full-time speech-language pathologist to use facilities within the institution after hours and on weekends to carry on a part-time private practice. Usually in such cases a percentage of the clinician's fees from the private practice are paid to the institution for this privilege.

Another type of private practice sometimes is found in a clinician's home. Over 80% of the members of this profession are females (ASHA, 1978). Of this percentage a substantial number are living with their husbands and families in communities where employment in schools, clinics, and other settings is difficult to obtain and in which it does not seem feasible to equip and open an office in the downtown area. So, as a substitute for employment in one of the more common settings, the female clinician, and occasionally a male clinician, does private practice in the convenience of the home. The derogatory term "kitchen therapy" sometimes has been attached to this kind of practice, and it is looked on by many in this profession with disapproval because of the likely lack of facilities for proper diagnosis and treatment of communication disorders in a home. There is good reason for disapproval in some cases, but if great care is taken to meet ASHA standards and to stay within the limitations of such a setting when accepting clients, this kind of practice can be adequate.

Any of the preceding situations require the clinician to be competent in virtually all aspects of speech-language pathology as well as a good business person. Another important asset is that the clinician be able to establish and maintain good working relationships with key referral individuals and agencies, because these are the sources from which clients come and funds are generated.

The clinician in private practice frequently functions quite independently and in the absence of other speech-language clinicians. The advantage of having independence is offset by the disadvantage of not having colleagues with whom to interact.

This lack of interaction with colleagues on a regular basis underscores the importance of the clinician in private practice having a strong background in all the areas of speech-language pathology. For the individual with this strong background who prefers to work independently, private practice can be very rewarding.

As mentioned previously, the clinician in private practice must realize that the report is both a mode of communication and an advertisement. The report reflects the clinical expertise of the clinician as well as pertinent information about the client. The clinician should develop a style and format that is efficient and concise, that will fit into the situation in which the work is being done, and that will carry the information necessary for the referral source. To repeat, attention must be paid to legal aspects of the reports, because the private practitioner is particularly vulnerable.

STATE CRIPPLED CHILDREN'S SERVICE PROGRAMS

All states provide services for crippled children through agencies set up specifically to administer the programs. They are partly state and partly federally financed. Service to the children usually is free, but sometimes small fees are collected from those who can pay. In all or nearly all of these programs communication disorders are considered crippling conditions, so speech-language pathologists and audiologists are employed, along with specialists from several other disciplines. Most crippled children's programs are administered by independent state agencies, but some are under state health departments, some are divisions of medical schools, and a few are connected with universities.

In an agency such as this the speech-language clinician usually needs to be competent to work with multiple-handicapped and severely handicapped children. Services are offered to clients aged birth to 21 years, but a preponderance of the clients are quite young, many being infants and babies. Inasmuch as services are provided in an interdisciplinary setting, cooperation with other highly trained professionals is essential. This requires that the clinician have an understanding of the roles of the different specialists and how they relate to diagnosis and treatment of communicative disorders. The clinician usually will function as a member of an interdisciplinary diagnostic team, including staffings, where plans are made for treatment. Often the clinician will also be part of a treatment team, working very closely with other professionals on the team. This requires multiple skills of the clinician but can be a most stimulating, exciting, and rewarding situation in which to work.

In some of the programs we have known, the cancellation rate of clients' appointments is quite high. Clients do not always keep their appointments, and they do not always inform the clinician that they will not be attending. Although only an impression, absenteeism appears to be higher when services are free to clients than when they pay. This may be the reason that many programs charge at least a token fee. Frequent absences sometimes interfere with providing a systematic, successful treatment program for the client.

Another characteristic of the clinical population in this setting is the long-term nature of many of the disorders. Because the clients usually have some severe physical, mental, or psychologic crippling condition and often a combination of two or all of these, treatment generally takes longer than for clients who have less severe disorders. These programs typically include such conditions as cerebral palsy, cleft palate, mental retardation, schizophrenia, autism, and many others. In all or most of these conditions communication disorders are present, most of which are severe and almost always include a major component of articulatory malfunction.

Because of the typically long-term nature of treatment, the clinician must be able to create a variety of different activities and approaches in order to maintain interest over a treatment period that may extend into several years. A child cannot be expected to maintain interest for such a long period if treatment sessions lack variety and creativity. However, we have seen many such children, especially the more severe orthopedically handicapped, such as those with cerebral palsy, who look forward eagerly to their treatment sessions in speech-language, physical, and occupational therapy, because coming for treatment is a diversion for them and because the professionals are expert at making the sessions pleasant and rewarding to the children.

In many crippled children's programs the clinician might expect a major portion of clinical activities to be diagnosis rather than treatment. The speech-language pathologist must be a capable diagnostician, as well as being able to formulate a viable treatment program that can be integrated with treatment by other specialists, if such is necessary. This means that the clinician must understand a great deal about the crippling problems that bring children to such programs. This is no minor requirement, because such conditions as cerebral palsy, cleft palate, mental retardation, and many others are complex and nearly always multiply crippling. The effect of these conditions on the communication structures and processes must be understood, and the clinician must be able to detect the intricacies of these effects and place them in the proper perspective in regard to the whole child and the multiple problems.

Because these programs are state and federally funded, records, forms, and reports are very important, numerous, and often time-consuming. The matter of accountability is carefully scrutinized. Protocol and agency procedures must be understood and carefully followed, and since several persons from other disciplines may be involved with care of the same client, the clinician's awareness of their procedures is most important.

HEAD START PROGRAMS

A number of years ago there was a proliferation of federally funded Head Start programs for preschool children. These programs were designed for "deprived" children who often lack many of the basic skills, language and speech included, common to average children of preschool ages. Therefore, the purpose of these programs is to provide ample stimulation, enriched environment, and instruction to help them "catch up" with their peers before entering schools. The development of these programs has provided another setting in which speech-language pathologists may function.

Children in Head Start programs usually are below the age of 5 years, although older children with considerable developmental delay may also be found. Obviously a major type of communication problem in such a population is delayed language and speech. In fact the majority of problems might best be described as communication delays rather than "disorders," but the delays in such a population often are serious enough to require treatment if the child is to be able to communicate adequately by the time he enters school.

In addition to delayed speech this population often has more serious speech disorders, especially articulation distortions caused by imitation, malformations of the articulators, and transient hearing loss. There is a noticeably higher than normal prevalence of hearing problems in this population, usually related to untreated upper respiratory infections and poor ear and nasal hygiene. This condition contributes to the articulation delay but may also account for many of the more serious articulation disorders. Fortunately most of these disorders are functional and may be alleviated during the time the child is in the program. Because the delayed functioning and problems such as the hearing losses are usually related to environmental deprivation, these children often make rapid progress in an enriched setting provided the upper respiratory problems are eliminated or controlled.

In this setting part of the clinician's responsibilities, besides working with children, are record-keeping, reporting, and completing federal forms. Such tasks are necessary in many settings, but in federally funded programs they are numerous and time-consuming. The clinician must also be able to interact with Head Start staff, such as teachers, early childhood specialists, and others, in order to bring about maximal changes in the children. An awareness of service resources for parents and children outside the programs and how to obtain these services is necessary for the clinician to have and to share with those who need the information. In some situations the clinician serves only as a consultant and resource person to staff of the program and to parents of the children in it. In others the clinician works directly with children, generally as a part-time staff member. Unfortunately many Head Start programs do not employ speech-language clinicians since this is not a requirement but is left to the discretion of the local head of the program.

NURSERY SCHOOLS

Nursery schools rarely employ full-time speech-language clinicians, but some of the very large ones may. Others employ part-time clinicians who may work directly with the children or who may work with the teachers to help them with identification of problems and whatever remedial procedures they can carry on with their teaching. Many nursery schools refer children with problems to clinics or private practitioners. As a result the speech-language clinician is likely to deal with children from nursery schools in any of several different settings.

Nursery schoolchildren usually are between the ages of 2 and 5 years, and, although similar in age, they may present somewhat varied types of disorders. Etiology and characteristics of the disorders are varied, but usually children with severe disorders are not enrolled in nursery schools. For this reason the disorders are often rather mild, perhaps predominantly articulation deviations with occasionally delayed speech and language development. The degree of severity, however, may vary with the nursery school admission policies and with the procedures used in detecting problems in the school population. If a speech-language clinician does the screening, both severe and mild problems are probably in the client load, but if teacher referral is relied on, only the more obvious problems may surface. These may include children with developmental deviations that do not require treatment and may omit some who should have help, depending on the greatly varied philosophy, alertness, and training of teachers.

A position in this setting might require travel, because, as pointed out previously, a single setting usually does not provide enough clients for full-time employment. If the clinician is itinerant, thought must once again be given to scheduling, travel time, and relating to several different administrators and a number of different teachers and their aides. Record-keeping, reporting, and accountability probably are not overburdening in such settings, but what is required should be undertaken with care.

In addition to nursery school personnel the speech-language clinician may need to interact with specialists from a few other disciplines. These disciplines include psychologists, psychiatrists, social workers, and child-development specialists, any of which might be acting as consultants to the school or actually carrying out some type of treatment or other help to the children. The speech-language clinician will need to integrate with these specialists in whatever manner is required for the best good of the children. This means that the clinician may not be isolated from professionals of other disciplines, but isolation from other speech-language and hearing professionals may be a factor and, if it is, may be one of the disadvantages of such settings. This need not be the case, however, because association with professionals in this field nearly always is possible in most locations.

MEDICAL SCHOOLS

Another exciting setting in which the speech-language pathologist can work is a medical school, or health sciences center, as some medical schools are now called.

Certain qualifications are necessary for this setting, perhaps more stringent than in some others. The clinician must be able to interact with a number of different specialists from other disciplines and with a wide range of different persons and types and severity of communication disorders. The clinician must be knowledgeable and competent in order to demonstrate to specialists from such disciplines as neurology, otology, pediatrics, psychiatry, psychology, and many others that diagnosis and treatment of communication disorders is a necessary part of patient care, when indicated, and that the speech-language pathologist is capable of providing it. This must be accomplished at the same time that the speech-language pathologist or audiologist makes clear the fact that this is an independent profession and that we do not work under orders from any others in the management of persons with communication disorders, although we will work as closely as possible with others for the best good of the patient.

Many professionals, especially in medicine, still view the speech-language pathologist and audiologist as "paramedical" workers who should function only under the orders from a physician, as do nurses, occupational therapists, and physical therapists. One very important reason for this is that too many in this profession call themselves "therapists" and allow others to do the same, thereby implying subservience to the medical profession. Another reason is that some clinicians have lacked the confidence, and sometimes the competence, to be worthy of independent functioning. This means making one's own diagnosis of communication disorders and carrying out treatment according to one's own best judgment, while at the same time working with other professionals without friction and fitting management of the communication disorder into the overall care of the patient. This is no easy task in a medical setting because of the many other specialists usually involved with the care of any one patient.

The actual clinical population includes

many multiple-handicapped and severely handicapped persons, but there are many degrees of severity of communication disorders among these persons. The clinician will be exposed to rare and unusual problems as well as to terminal patients. These, and others, may be seen on an inpatient or an outpatient basis, depending on the nature, purposes, and philosophy of the institution. A major emphasis for the speech-language pathologist in many medical settings is diagnosis, but others may carry on extensive treatment programs, often requiring close integration with persons from many disciplines.

An understanding of the basic functions of the different disciplines is essential. Integrating diagnosis and treatment with other specialists can be most helpful in managing communication problems. In fact this availability of help from so many other specialists is partly what makes working in such a setting so desirable and exciting. A medical school can provide an excellent environment for additional learning, especially about health care and health-related professions.

In many medical settings the speech-language pathologist is involved in "staffings." These are group meetings in which all specialists who have examined a patient come together to present their findings, arrive at a diagnosis, perhaps of several problems, and make plans for treatment. Staffing presupposes good diagnostic skills on the part of the different specialists. In addition the specialists must be able to relate and communicate effectively during the staffings. This includes the speech-language specialist, who must understand and be able to discuss aspects of the overall welfare of the patient, as well as problems specifically related to communication disorders. The ability to write pertinent, concise, meaningful reports and present them in the same manner in staffings is important. Counseling families and other professionals often is very important in this setting.

In staffings and in all other activities in this setting, there is a strong temptation for the clinician to adopt some of the vocabulary, and occasionally the functions, of other specialists, as well as to make our own professional vocabulary complicated in order to appear erudite. In this setting professional jargon often is rampant, some of it needed and some not, but often tempting others to do the same. This temptation must be resisted at all costs in our conversation and our written and oral reports. At the same time every effort should be made to understand the vocabularies of other specialties as well as their functions.

STATE DEPARTMENTS OF HEALTH AND EDUCATION

All states have departments of health and education. Some of these are single departments, but most are separate. Many of these agencies, especially departments of education, employ one or more speech-language specialists as consultants and resource persons to schools and county health departments in the state. Employment in these agencies usually requires considerable travel. The clinician may be located at the state capital or in a major city of that state and will be responsible for a particular region or all of the state. Responsibilities include consultation, counseling, and in other ways acting as a resource person for health and education programs throughout the state concerning communicatively handicapped persons. Part of the speech-language consultant's work is with speech-language personnel in schools, particularly in rural communities, and part of it is with nonspeech and hearing personnel in health departments, providing them with information as to where they might refer a person with a communication handicap for help. They may also participate actively in the diagnosis of a problem and perhaps staffing it with other health department personnel. Rarely is the clinician directly involved in treatment but will find outside sources for this help.

In most states the same consultant does not serve both the department of education and the department of health. Usually each department has its own consultant, but since the children seen in health departments usually are in school, they are educational problems and often are referred through the educational consultant for help. Many health departments do not hire a full-time consultant for communication disorders but refer children to speech-language clinicians in private practice or from a nearby clinic or university.

The job of the state consultant for either education or health departments may become fatiguing and lonely because of the travel. Isolation from other clinicians also may be felt, but there are compensations, such as a variety of activities, opportunity to plan and control most of one's own activities, and ability to interact with a great variety of people at all levels. Administrative record-keeping, completing forms, and accountability procedures are important although time-consuming functions. In many of these situations there is often a great deal of public speaking to parent groups, teachers, nurses, colleagues, and others. The individual in this kind of setting is more in the public view than in many other settings, so one should be prepared for this or else should not seek such a position. It is obvious that skills in working with a wide variety of people and interacting on many different levels are required. Many do not have these skills to the extent needed in such a position, so one should assess individual assets before seeking employment in such a setting. Employment opportunities in these settings are limited.

CONVALESCENT HOMES

This type of facility often is called a nursing home as well as a convalescent home, and work in it involves older persons. Problems peculiar to this setting are lack of motivation of the client, progressive illnesses, limited opportunities or desire to communicate, preoccupation with illness and death, and sometimes just a depressing environment. The clinician working in this setting may function both as a consultant and as a clinician providing direct services to patients. Employment opportunities are limited at present, but interest is growing from several sources, including our own profession.

Communication problems common to persons in nursing homes typically are dysphasia, dysarthria, dyspraxia, voice disorders, and hearing loss. The majority of these disorders are almost always accompanied by a large component of articulation problems. Besides being competent to deal with these severe disorders, the clinician must be able to work with families, nurses, and nursing aides. Programmed instruction and self-instruction usually are needed as part of a treatment program.

Work in this setting is generally itinerant because one facility usually does not have sufficient numbers of clients to employ a full-time clinician. Thus travel and scheduling problems must be considered if one individual gives service to several such facilities. Service in a convalescent home commonly is done as "moonlighting" rather than as the clinician's primary job; that is, a clinician may hold a full- or part-time position in some other setting and give service to one or more homes part time or outside of regular working hours of the permanent setting.

Records and reports in this setting are becoming a more important responsibility as federal and state regulations multiply. Careful notations in patient's charts and sometimes full reports are required on each patient, making clinical accountability an important aspect. Records are often subject to inspection and audit.

RESEARCH SETTINGS

There are few employment opportunities for an individual to do research only, but more of these positions are developing. For the most part research in this field, particularly clinical research, is being done by individuals who teach college or university courses or work in clinics or other settings full or part time. They devote part of the time to research or do the research outside of regular working hours. Unfortunately too often the latter is the case. Actually any of the situations in which speech-language pathologists work could be considered research settings because research is done in all of them.

We believe that all speech-language clinicians should be research oriented. That is, they should view all communication problems from the eyes of the researcher as well as the clinician, because there is the potential for adding to one's knowledge about communication disorders while working with them. Obviously the clinician cannot set up an experimental design, carry out the necessary measurements, and write the results on every client, but thinking in that direction makes for more objective clinical processes and also keeps the clinician aware of current research being done and making clinical application of it when appropriate.

Some important qualifications for doing research are self-discipline, order, imagination, creativity, patience, the ability to recognize researchable problems, the knowledge and skill to use the tools of research to do the job, and many others. The research situation may be an isolated one, but more often it involves two or more persons working together on the same problem.

The researcher needs the ability and patience to keep meticulous records and be able to synthesize these into a readable report of the research. Since research is pointless unless it can be utilized, usually by publication, the researcher must possess writing skills beyond those needed for records and reports. Research often is exciting and rewarding, but it can also demand many hours, months, or years of painstaking, exhausting, and sometimes disappointing work. One must have the temperament demanded by these requirements, and not all of us do, especially if we are absorbed in clinical work. But all clinicians can become research oriented and capable of using results of research in clinical endeavors.

SUMMARY

Responsibilities and competencies of speech-language pathologists have been dis-cussed in relation to the different employment settings. Each setting has its unique characteristics, advantages, and disadvantages. Some settings are quite similar in terms of the clinician's responsibilities and competencies, whereas others are quite different. An awareness of the similarities and differences by the clinician should facilitate clinical management of articulation disorders.

STUDY SUGGESTIONS

1. Compare and contrast work settings in college and university clinics, medical schools, and community speech and hearing clinics regarding types of clients, speech-language pathologist responsibilities, competencies needed, and related aspects.
2. What are the major qualifications and characteristics for work as a school clinician? Which of these are unique to this situation?
3. Discuss the changing roles of the school clinician in the past decade. What has brought about some of the major changes? Consider legislation, school populations, and other factors in your discussion of causes of changes.
4. How have the changes mentioned in No. 3 influenced the responsibilities and competencies needed by the speech-language pathologist?
5. Compare full-time private practice with other types of settings. What especially unique aspects are found in private practice that are not found in other settings?
6. Discuss the terms speech-language pathologist, clinician, and therapist relative to various settings. Why are the terms therapist and therapy not in the best interests of the individual or the profession?

REFERENCES

Ainsworth, S.: Speech correction methods, a manual of speech therapy and public school procedures, Englewood Cliffs, N.J., 1948, Prentice-Hall, Inc.

ASHA, 90-30 Section, **20:**90-996, 1978.

Chapman, M.: The speech clinician—as a professional person. In Van Hattum, R., editor: Clinical speech in the schools, Springfield, Ill., 1969, Charles C Thomas, Publisher.

Eisenson, J., and Ogilvie, M.: Speech correction in the schools, ed. 4, New York, 1977, Macmillan Publishing Co., Inc.

ETB manual accreditation of professional education programs in speech pathology and audiology, Rockville, Md., 1977, American Speech and Hearing Association.

Van Hattum, R., editor: Clinical speech in the schools,

Springfield, Ill., 1969, Charles C Thomas, Publisher.

Van Riper, C.: Speech correction principles and methods, ed. 5, Englewood Cliffs, N.J., 1972, Prentice-Hall, Inc.

GLOSSARY

autism A condition in which an individual is out of touch with reality, preferring material objects to people. Often this person does not relate to people at all but seems to withdraw into an internal life. Usually there is no speech.

block scheduling Clients are scheduled for intensive treatment in concentrated blocks of time, usually of fairly short duration. When a block period is ended, treatment is discontinued but may be resumed later in another block of time if needed.

clinical setting Used here to refer to a situation in which several communication specialists function in a single setting, agency, or building as one unit, as opposed to a private practitioner or public school clinician who usually works alone.

externship Student clinicians are assigned to settings outside the clinic, such as crippled children's programs, centers for the mentally retarded, rehabilitation centers, etc., in order to gain experience with persons with a wide range of types of disorders.

screening Used here to refer to brief testing of clients, usually in a school classroom but may be individualized, to see if there is evidence of communication disorders that should be assessed more thoroughly to determine if treatment is needed.

schizophrenia A common type of mental disturbance in which the individual often is withdrawn from, uninterested in, and detached from the world around him. Perception and thinking may be distorted. This person may at times seem normal without any of these symptoms, thus the term "split personality" often is attached to the condition. Speech is often present but may be distorted, and language may be confused and inaccurate.

traditional scheduling Clients usually are scheduled two to three times a week for 15-, 30-, or 60-minute sessions over an extended period of time.

Relationship between cranial nerves and production of specific phonemes

Cranial nerve V is related to the production of /æ/, /a/, /ɔ/, and the diphthongs including these vowel components. This nerve is partly responsible for producing the following consonants and the consonant blends that they are a part of: /f/, /v/, /m/, /p/, /b/, and /ð/. Because this nerve innervates the muscles of mastication, it is important in modifying movements.

Cranial nerve VII is partly responsible for the production of /t/, /ɪ/, /u/, /ʊ/, /ɛ/, /o/, and the diphthongs including these vowel components. This nerve is also partly responsible for producing the following consonants and the consonant blends that they are a part of: /f/, /v/, /p/, /b/, /m/, /w/, and /j/. This nerve is very important in the cosmetic aspects of contextual speech.

Cranial nerve VIII is partly responsible for every phoneme, voiced and nonvoiced. It monitors articulation and, as such, is part of the feedback servosystem. It is especially important in learning articulation.

Cranial nerve IX provides motor supply to the pharynx and, as such, is important to velopharyngeal closure for all the phonemes except the three nasal phonemes. This nerve also relates to resonance.

Cranial nerve X, assisted by cranial nerve XI, is primarily responsible for breathing and phonation. Although partly related to the production of most phonemes because it provides motor impulses to the back of the tongue, it is most directly related to all voiced phonemes. Cranial nerve XI also provides motor supply to the lower pharynx, making it indirectly related to resonance.

Cranial nerve XII is also related to the production of nearly all phonemes because it is responsible for tongue movement and proprioceptive or kinesthetic feedback. It is especially important to /t/, /d/, /l/, /n/, /s/, /z/, /ʃ/, /ʒ/, /tʃ/, /dʒ/, /k/, /g/, /θ/, /ð/, vowels, and diphthongs.

Sequence of diagnostic procedures

STEPS IN SEQUENCE

I.
Obtaining case history data

Case history form Clinical reports Interview or other procedures

II.
Observing

III.
Diagnostic testing

IV.
Scoring test results

V.
Synthesizing information

VI.
Analyzing test results

VII.
Interpreting test results

Possibly recommending additional evaluations*

Possibly deferring diagnosis and treatment*

VIII.
Determining treatment plan

IX.
Conveying findings and counseling

X.
Reporting and distributing diagnostic information

*These considerations may or may not be necessary, depending on the specific client.

Children's case history form

CONFIDENTIAL

(information not to be released without special permission)

Please return to the speech-language pathologist

IDENTIFYING INFORMATION

Child's name: _____

Sex: _____

Birthdate: _____ Age: _____

School: _____

Grade: _____ Teacher: _____

Referred by: _____

_____

_____

Date: _____

Parent: _____

Telephone: _____

Address: _____

_____

Name of person completing this form:

_____

Relationship to child: _____

Please attach a recent photograph of your child (any snapshot will do) (optional)

Nature of the problem (describe your child's problem as fully as possible): _____

_____

_____

_____

_____

_____

_____

_____

_____

_____

_____

_____

_____

_____

FAMILY INFORMATION

a. Mother's occupation: _____   Father's occupation: _____

b. Education: _____ Age: _____   Education: _____ Age: _____

c. Child lives with: ☐ Both parents ☐ Father ☐ Mother ☐ Other: _____

d. Other adults living in the home: _____

e. Who usually takes care of your child? _____

FAMILY INFORMATION—cont'd

f. Children in family:

Name	Age	Sex	Special problems

CHILD'S DEVELOPMENT
Birth history

a. Mother's health during pregnancy: _____

b. Pregnancy duration: _____ Birth weight: _____

c. Length of labor: _____ Complications (please check): ☐ Rapid ☐ Prolonged
   ☐ Breech ☐ Cesarean ☐ Other (explain): _____

d. Baby's health (color, jaundice, bruises, breathing problems, incubator, abnormalities): _____
   _____

e. Feeding problems? _____
   _____

Speech and hearing

a. Describe crying during first year (type, amount): _____

b. First words—what were they? _____ Age: _____

c. Two-word phrases: Age: _____ Examples: _____

d. What percent of the time is the child's speech understood by: Mother: _____ Father: _____
   Brothers and sisters: _____ Playmates: _____ Strangers: _____
   Teacher: _____ Relatives: _____

e. Does your child customarily communicate by use of: ☐ Gestures: Pantomime _____
   Sounds _____ One or two words _____ ☐ Phrases ☐ Complete sentences

f. Does your child understand and/or speak another language besides English? _____ Explain:
   _____
   _____
   _____
   What percent of the time is each language spoken in the home? _____

g. Vocabulary: How many words can your child say? (check) ☐ 1-10 ☐ 10-50 ☐ 50-100 ☐ 100-300
   ☐ 300-500 ☐ Over 500
   If he has more words than you can count, how does his vocabulary compare with that of other
   children of the same age (friends, brothers, sisters)? _____
   _____

h. Give a few examples (if any) of phrases and/or sentences that your child typically uses at this time:
   _____
   _____
   _____

i. Do you think your child has a hearing problem? _____ Explain: _____

j. Has your child's hearing been tested? _____ By whom? _____
   Findings: _____

Continued.

Motor development

a. At what age did your child:
   Sit without support _____
   Walk, holding on to furniture _____
   Walk alone _____
   Drink from cup, no help _____
   Eat with utensils _____
   Finish toilet training _____
   Remain dry during the day _____
   Remain dry at night _____

Health history

a. Child's physician: _____ Address: _____
   Others consulted: _____   _____
                     _____   _____

b. Have child's eyes been examined? _____ By whom? _____
   Findings: _____

c. Is child receiving any medication or physical or occupational therapy at present? _____ What
   kind? _____
   Why? _____

d. Childhood illnesses (note age and severity)

   Measles _____   Tonsillectomy _____
   Rubella _____   Adenoidectomy _____
   Mumps _____   High fevers _____
   Chickenpox _____   Allergies _____
   Asthma _____   Frequent headaches _____
   Bronchitis _____   Frequent colds _____
   Pneumonia _____   Ear infections _____
   Seizures (convulsions) _____   Other infections _____
   Other health problems or injuries _____
   _____

e. Child's dentist: _____
   Did child's primary teeth erupt normally? _____ When did permanent teeth begin to come in?
   _____ Unusual oral conditions (finger-, thumb-, or tongue-sucking)? _____
   _____ Dental problems? _____

Social development

a. Describe your child's personality. _____
   _____

b. What are his favorite activities? _____
   _____

c. Describe any social problems your child has with friends or family. _____
   _____
   _____

ADDITIONAL QUESTIONS

a. Check *any* of the following that may have contributed to your child's present problem(s).

- ☐ Brain injury
- ☐ Negativism
- ☐ Neglect by mother
- ☐ Neglect by father
- ☐ Cultural differences
- ☐ Brother/sister rivalry
- ☐ Environmental factors
- ☐ Behavioral problems
- ☐ Developmental slowness
- ☐ Lack of playmates

- ☐ Hearing problem
- ☐ Temper tantrums
- ☐ Feeding/eating problems
- ☐ Parental rejections
- ☐ Mental retardation
- ☐ Emotional problems of child
- ☐ Too much protection by mother
- ☐ Too much protection by father
- ☐ Inconsistent parental handling
- ☐ Emotional problems of parents

- ☐ Sleeplessness
- ☐ Cerebral palsy
- ☐ Epilepsy
- ☐ Laziness
- ☐ Stubbornness
- ☐ Thumb-sucking
- ☐ Strong fears
- ☐ Visual disturbance
- ☐ Others: _____
_____

b. If your child attends school, check any of the following that apply:

- ☐ Doesn't like school
- ☐ Learning problem
- ☐ Poor reader
- ☐ Math problems

☐ Other: _____
_____
_____
_____

c. Does your child receive special help at school? _____
_____

d. What do you consider to be your child's greatest problem(s) now? _____
_____

e. Do you have any other comments that you feel might be helpful to us? _____
_____
_____
_____

f. Do you have any particular questions you would like to ask us? _____
_____
_____
_____

Adult case history form

INSTRUCTIONS: Please provide as much information as you can recall for each of the categories below.

IDENTIFYING INFORMATION

Name _____ Sex _____
     (First)   Nickname   Middle   Last)

Address _____ Telephone _____

Birthdate _____ Referred by _____

Age _____ Address _____

FAMILY INFORMATION

A. Adults in home

    Husband's (wife's) name _____ Age _____

    Occupation or former occupation _____

    Education _____

    Health _____

    Previous marriages _____

B. Children in home

Name	Age	Sex	Special problems

NATURE OF THE PROBLEM

In your own words describe your speech or hearing problem as you see it. _____

_____

_____

_____

BACKGROUND INFORMATION

History of the problem

A. When and by whom was the speech and/or hearing problem first noticed? _____

_____

_____

B. What do you think caused, or is causing, this speech or hearing problem? _____

_____

_____

History of the problem—cont'd

C. What have you done, if anything, to help the speech or hearing problem? (Give names, dates, and places if you have received any professional help in the past.) _____

_____

_____

_____

Developmental history

Describe any difficulties in your birth or early development. _____

_____

_____

Do you know of any difficulties you might have had when first learning to talk? _____

_____

Does anyone have difficulty understanding your speech? _____

_____

Health history

A. Medical care

Physician _____ Address _____

Others consulted: _____

Medical findings:

Has your hearing been tested? _____ By whom? _____

Findings: _____

Have your eyes been examined? _____ By whom? _____

Findings: _____

Are you receiving any medication or treatment at present? _____ What kind? _____

_____

B. Illnesses and health problems (give age and severity)

Measles _____	High fevers _____
Rubella _____	Allergies _____
Mumps _____	Frequent colds _____
Chickenpox _____	Frequent headaches _____
Asthma _____	Ear infections _____
Bronchitis _____	Other infections _____
Pneumonia _____	Seizures _____

Other health problems _____

Have you had serious injuries or accidents? _____

Have you ever been hospitalized? _____

Other surgery _____

C. Dental history

Dentist _____ Address _____

Social and emotional development

Describe any other problems you are having at this time. _____

_____

_____

_____

Continued.

Social and emotional development—cont'd

List your interests and leisure activities. _____
_____
_____

ADDITIONAL QUESTIONS

A. What do you consider to be your greatest problem right now? _____
_____
_____

B. Do you have any other comments that you feel might be helpful to us? _____
_____
_____

C. Do you have any particular questions you would like to ask us? _____
_____
_____

Guidelines for confidential parental questionnaire

GENERAL INFORMATION

Patient _____ Birthdate _____ Sex _____ Race _____
Address _____ County _____ Telephone _____
Father's name _____ Mother's name _____
Address _____ Address _____
Father's occupation _____ Age _____ Mother's occupation _____ Age _____
Father's education _____ Mother's education _____
Referred by _____
     (Name)   (Address)
Family physician _____
     (Name)   (Address)
Name of school child attends _____ Grade _____
Name of person filling out questionnaire _____
    (Relation to patient)
Address _____
Other children in family

Name	Age	Grade

BIRTH AND PRENATAL HISTORY

During this pregnancy, did mother experience any unusual illness, condition or accident, such as German measles, false labor, RH imcompatibility, etc.? _____ If so, describe. _____

Length of pregnancy _____ Duration of labor _____ Birth weight _____
Conditions at birth: ☐ Cesarean ☐ Breech birth ☐ Anesthetics ☐ Forceps
Was infant blue? _____ Jaundiced? _____ Other unusual conditions? _____
Conditions immediately following birth. Did infant have: Feeding problems _____
Seizures _____ Swallowing or sucking difficulties _____ Scars or bruises _____
Was birth weight quickly regained? _____

DEVELOPMENT

When did the child first hold up his head alone? _____
When did the infant first crawl? _____
When did the infant sit alone without support? _____
When did the infant pull himself to a standing position? _____

Continued.

DEVELOPMENT—cont'd

When did the infant walk unaided? _____

When did the infant gain bowel control? Day _____ Night _____

When did the infant gain bladder control? Day _____ Night _____

Weight of infant at age 6 months? _____ Height at age 6 months? _____

Weight of infant at age 1 year? _____ Height at age 1 year? _____

Weight of child at present? _____ Height at present? _____

Does child prefer right or left hand? _____

Does child fall or lose balance easily? _____

Does child seem awkward or uncoordinated? _____

Does child have difficulty chewing or swallowing? _____

Comments: _____

_____

_____

MEDICAL

Check diseases patient has had, giving age, degree of severity, and aftereffects.

Disease	Age	Mild	Average	Severe	Disease	Age	Mild	Average	Severe
Measles	___	☐	☐	☐	Croup	___	☐	☐	☐
Diphtheria	___	☐	☐	☐	Pleurisy	___	☐	☐	☐
Chickenpox	___	☐	☐	☐	Tonsillitis	___	☐	☐	☐
Typhoid	___	☐	☐	☐	Tuberculosis	___	☐	☐	☐
Mumps	___	☐	☐	☐	Paralysis	___	☐	☐	☐
Dysentery	___	☐	☐	☐	Bronchitis	___	☐	☐	☐
Whooping cough	___	☐	☐	☐	Otitis (earache)	___	☐	☐	☐
Influenza	___	☐	☐	☐	Goiter	___	☐	☐	☐
Scarlet fever	___	☐	☐	☐	Rickets	___	☐	☐	☐
Meningitis	___	☐	☐	☐	Cerebral palsy	___	☐	☐	☐
Cleft palate	___	☐	☐	☐	Rheumatism	___	☐	☐	☐
Heart disease	___	☐	☐	☐	Hay fever	___	☐	☐	☐
Convulsions	___	☐	☐	☐	Asthma	___	☐	☐	☐
Nervous trouble	___	☐	☐	☐	Frequent colds	___	☐	☐	☐
Skin disease	___	☐	☐	☐	Kidney disease	___	☐	☐	☐
Eczema	___	☐	☐	☐	Enlarged glands	___	☐	☐	☐
Chorea	___	☐	☐	☐					

Others: _____

Describe aftereffects: _____

_____

Is the patient in good health at this time? _____ State any physical handicaps: _____

_____

Does the patient have a learning problem? _____ Describe: _____

_____

How is the health of other family members? _____

SOCIAL

Does the child fear? ☐ Often ☐ Sometimes ☐ Rarely   What does he fear? _____

Is the child "nervous"? _____ How does he show it? _____

_____

Has he been harder to manage than other children? _____

Is the child a follower or a leader of his age-group? _____

Describe any eating problems: _____

_____

SOCIAL—cont'd

Describe any problems of elimination: _____

Circle any of the following that have been observed frequently enough or to a degree to warrant consideration:

Lying	Preference for younger	Bed wetting
Begging	children	Snoring
Stealing	Sluggishness	Convulsive attacks
Smoking	Boastfulness	Sex misbehavior
Rudeness	Showing off	(masturbation)
Swearing	Disobedience	Sleepwalking
Fighting	Destructiveness	Night terrors
Jealousy	Temper displays	Fainting
Selfishness	Acts of violence	Face twitching
Excitability	Quarrelsomeness	Indications of not hearing
Skipping school	Daydreaming	plainly
Nose picking	Thumb-sucking	Tongue-sucking
Nervousness	Nail biting	Strong fears
Mouth breathing	Sleeplessness	Strong hates
Easily depressed	Nightmares	Shyness
Easily discouraged	Constipation	Worrying
Suicidal inclinations	Preference for older children	Sensitiveness
Running away from home	Failure to adjust to older	Drugs
Associating with bad company	children	

Discuss any of the listed items in more detail if you think they are important. _____

_____
_____
_____
_____

COMMUNICATION

During the first year, did the child make much sound other than crying? _____
Other than crying, would you say he was: ☐ A silent baby ☐ A very quiet baby
☐ An average noisy baby ☐ A very noisy baby
At what age did he first say words? _____ What were they? _____

Did he: ☐ Say one or two words and then go a long time before adding other words
☐ Keep on adding words once he started to talk
At what age did he begin to name people and objects? _____
At what age did he have a name for everything? _____
At what age did he combine words into small sentences like, "Want drink" or "Me out"? _____
At what age did he use more complete short sentences? _____
Did speech learning ever seem to stop for a period? _____ Describe: _____

Does the child seem to be aware of a speech difference? _____ Describe: _____

What efforts have been made to help the child talk better? _____

Has there been a change in the child's speech in the last 6 months? _____ Describe the change:

Has the child ever talked better than he does now? _____

_____

Continued.

SCHOOL

At what age did the child start school? _____ Were grades repeated? _____ Why?
_____

With what subjects has the child had particular difficulty? _____

How does he get along with others at school? _____
_____

What are his usual grades (excellent, above average, average, below average, or failing)? _____

How far in school did he go? _____ Reason for stopping (if not still attending): _____
_____

OTHER INFORMATION

When, why, and by *whom* was the communicative problem first noticed? _____

Is the child teased about his communicative problem by others? _____

What is the child's reaction to his communicative problem? _____
_____

Comments: _____
_____
_____
_____

Has the child had a communicative examination prior to this time? _____ Where? _____

Has the child had a hearing test prior to this time? _____ Where? _____

Has the child had a neurologic examination prior to this time? _____ Where? _____

Has the child had a psychologic examination prior to this time? _____ Where? _____

Has the child had a recent medical examination? _____ Where? _____

Describe, in your own words, your or your child's communicative problem. _____
_____
_____
_____
_____
_____

Grid for diagnosing intelligibility

	1	2	3	4	5
Articulation					
Redundancy					
Syntax					
Mean length of utterance					
Juncture					
Rate					
Prosody					
Pronunciation					
Intensity					
Rhythm					
Voice quality					

(The diagnostician might also include morphology, stress, inflection, resonation, semantics, pitch, dysfluency, and morphophonemics.)

SCORING KEY: **1** = Excellent—within normal limits
          2 = Good—does not interfere with intelligibility
          3 = Fair—slightly interferes with intelligibility
          4 = Poor—moderately interferes with intelligibility
          5 = Inadequate—severely interferes with intelligibility

Adapted from Casteel, R.: Grid for diagnosing intelligibility (unpublished), 1970.

Phonetic symbols*

Consonants	Vowels		Diphthongs
/ŋ/ is ng as in ri*ng*	/i/ is e as in s*ee*	/o/ is o as in h*o*pe	/aɪ/ is uy as in b*uy*
/j/ is y as in *y*es	/ɪ/ is i as in h*i*t	/ʊ/ is oo as in b*oo*k	/aʊ/ is ow as in c*ow*
/θ/ is th as in *th*umb	/ɛ/ is e as in m*e*t	/u/ is u as in r*u*de	/ou/ is o as in *ow*es
/ð/ is th as in *th*at	/e/ is a as in r*a*te	/ʌ/ is accented u as in h*u*t	/ɔɪ/ is oy as in b*oy*
/tʃ/ is ch as in *ch*ur*ch*	/æ/ is a as in *a*t	/ə/ is unaccented a as in *a*bout	/eɪ/ is ay as in s*ay*
/dʒ/ is j as in *j*ud*ge*	/a/ is o as in g*o*t	/ɝ/ is accented r as in bi*r*d	/ju/ is u as in *u*se
/ʃ/ is sh as in *sh*oe	/ɔ/ is o as in d*o*g	/ɚ/ is unaccented r as in mothe*r*	/aɚ/ is ar as in f*ar*
/ʒ/ is z as in a*z*ure			/ɔɚ/ is or as in f*or*
			/ɛɚ/ is air as in p*air*
			/ɪɚ/ is ear as in f*ear*
			/uɚ/ is oor as in p*oor*

From Weiss, C. E.: Weiss Comprehensive Articulation Test, Hingham, Mass., 1978, Teaching Resources Corp. Reproduced by permission of the publisher. All rights reserved.

*For phonemes requiring symbols other than the traditional graphemes.

Hierarchy of treatment levels*

Level I. Perceptual training
   Division 1. Auditory memory
   Division 2. Speech discrimination of correctly and incorrectly produced target phonemes
   Division 3. Speech discrimination of maximally contrasting distinctive features
   Division 4. Speech discrimination of target phonemes in contextual speech
   Division 5. Speech discrimination of self
Level II. Establishment of phonemes
   Division 1. Phonemes produced in isolation
   Division 2. Phonemes produced in nonsense syllables
   Division 3. Phonemes produced in words
   Division 4. Phonemes produced in phrases and sentences
   Division 5. Phonemes produced in monologue and dialogue
Level III. Transfer of phonemes
   Division 1. Transfer to all phonemic contexts
   Division 2. Transfer to all physical environments
Level IV. Maintenance of target phonemes (conceptualization mastery)
   Division 1. In all phonemic contexts
   Division 2. All of the time over a period of 3 to 6 months

---

*Training in self-monitoring should continue throughout the entire treatment process.

Motokinesthetic speech sound stimulations

CONSONANTS*

I. Voiceless consonants

/h/—Move jaw downward; push on diaphragm if necessary.

/wh/—Move lips from corner to midline; push air if necessary.

/f/—Move lower lip upward and down for next sound.

/θ/—Curve index finger above upper lip.

/p/—Move lower jaw up and then downward quickly and firmly.

/t/—Touch center of region above upper lip and quickly bring the finger downward.

/k/—Place thumb on one side of the throat under the back of the tongue externally and index finger on opposite side. Press upward then move away quickly.

/ʃ/—Thumb and forefinger outside upper jaw starting at corners and pressing against upper jaw moving the lips somewhat toward center.

/tʃ/—Same as /ʃ/ except firmer. Pull lower jaw down as upper hand is released.

/s/—Press above center upper lip with thumb and forefinger.

II. Voiced consonants

/v/—Same as /f/ but bring lower lip into firmer contact with edges of upper teeth.

/ð/—Same as /θ/.

/b/—Place forefinger and thumb of one hand above upper lip and those of other hand below lower lip and bring lips together with pressure and then separate immediately.

/d/—Same as /t/ only more firm.

/g/—Same position as for /k/. Press upward and inward, then release.

/z/—Press outside upper jaws with thumb and forefinger with more pressure than for /s/.

/ʒ/—Same as /ʃ/, only firmer.

/dʒ/—Same as /tʃ/ without quick release, move jaw downward or into vowel which follows.

/m/—With thumb and forefinger placed on lower jaw, move jaw until lower lip easily contacts upper lip. Place finger of other hand firmly on bridge of nose.

/n/—Press lightly at midpoint above upper lip while lips are kept apart. Place finger of the other hand firmly on bridge of the nose.

/ŋ/—Same position as /k/. Press gently upward while pressing on bridge of nose with other hand.

/l/—Move jaws slightly downward, lips drawn toward corners. Use thumb and finger of other hand on upper jaw at points ¾ to 1 inch apart equidistant from midline to press steadily inward. Then by a quick firm movement of hand on lower jaw, move it downward.

/r/—With fingers of one hand, move jaw slightly downward from closed position and press slightly inward on lower jaw. May also do same for upper jaw. If attempted /r/ is heard, move lower jaw downward while it is still sounding.

/w/—With finger and thumb of one hand placed above lips on upper jaw and

---

*Excerpted and adapted from Moto-kinesthetic speech training by Edna Hill Young and Sara Stinchfield Hawk, with the permission of the publishers, Stanford University Press. © 1955 by the Board of Trustees of the Leland Stanford Junior University.

other hand similarly on lower, bring lips from corners toward midline leaving an opening at the center. Then move into next vowel.

/j/—Start with stimulation for /i/, then move jaws quickly downward, separating tongue from dental arch in a quick movement.

VOWELS

I. Main stimulations
   A. Elevating or lowering jaw
   B. Stimulating movement of the tongue
   C. Moving the lips

II. Front vowels
   /i/—Lower jaw is slightly lowered from closed, bringing lips apart and toward corners. Incisors usually show. Place thumb and forefinger over dental ridge outside, somewhat removed from midline above upper lip. Press at these two points. May need to use a piece of tongue depressor wider than edge.

   /ɪ/—Lower jaw a little more than for /i/. Draw lips slightly toward corner. Press along midline of lower lip with narrow edge of tongue depressor, about ½ inch down in outside of jaw. Inside, dip midline of end of tongue with edge of tongue blade.

   /ɛ/—Lower jaw slightly more than /ɪ/. Use index finger to press at midline just below lower lip. Press two sides of end of tongue toward midline with two halves of tongue depressor while at same time dipping tongue end behind lower incisors.

   /æ/—Place thumb and forefinger at equal distances from midline, below lower lip; with medium pressure bring lower jaw downward a little lower than /ɛ/. Next thumb and forefinger separate, pressing against jaw as they move outward from midline. Place tongue depressor flat in surface of front of tongue, depressing and behind lower front teeth. Tongue depressor should rest on edge of lower teeth about ¾ inch from end.

III. Central vowels

/ʌ/—Lower jaw a little more than for /æ/.

IV. Back vowels
   /a/—Put thumb and forefinger at points halfway between midline and corners of mouth below lower lip. Pressing inward, move jaw straight downward, slightly lower than /ʌ/. With other hand, move upper lip outward slightly and a little to center.

   /ɔ/—Move jaw downward, not quite as far as /a/. Press lower lips slightly toward middle and outward.

   /ʊ/—Place thumb and forefinger of one hand or upper jaw toward corners of lips and similar position on lower jaw with other. Move toward midline with both hands simultaneously and bring lips outward in a scoop-like fashion.

   /u/—Move lips from corners toward midline.

V. Diphthongs
   /eɪ/—Place thumb and forefinger on lower jaw about ½ inch from midline to corners. Press against jaw and bring it downward at same time. Then immediately move jaw upward and move thumb and forefinger slightly toward corners without lifting them.

   /aɪ/—Lower jaw. Then move it up and move lips toward corners.

   /oʊ/—Move jaw downward with thumb and forefinger. Press toward midline bringing jaw upward again, moving part above upper lip into rounded position.

   /ju/—Stimulate /i/. Then with thumb and forefinger at corners above upper lip begin to move toward center pressing firmly against the upper jaw as they move. Continue movement toward center, without lifting fingers, until /u/ is heard.

   /aʊ/—Bring lower jaw downward. Then with both hands, move parts above and below lips outward and toward center.

   /ɔɪ/—Start with /ɔ/. Then move lips away from midline to make /ɪ/.

Unit II, Lesson 3

1. *Interpersonal situation:* obtaining and giving information
2. *Speaking aspects of situation:* asking and answering questions
3. *Particular speech patterns:*

"Yes." "No."	"Right here."
"Guess again."	"Is this right?"
Street addresses	"Can you find my birthday?"
Age	
Birthdate	"I'm thinking of a birthday."
Telephone number	"When is your birthday?"
	"Is that your birthday?"
	"Where is your birthday?"
	"Show me your birthday."

4. *Sounds emphasized:* s θ ʃ r ð k
5. *Equipment:* blackboard and chalk

Procedures	Notes
Therapist: If you go to the doctor or the dentist, or enroll in a new school, or ask for a package to be sent, what are some questions you are usually asked?	
Children: (*Individually*) They ask your name, your address, how old you are, when your birthday is, and sometimes what your telephone number is.	The speech therapist will usually have this data available in her records. She should have it accessible in this lesson in case a child needs help.
Therapist: Today you are going to be working on speech you use in getting information about other people, or giving information about yourself, particularly birthdays. Try the word "birthday." It has a "θ" sound in it like "thank you" and "think."	The word "birthday" (containing "r" and "θ") is more difficult phonetically for some children and should be stressed only with children able to handle it, but can be used by all.
Children: (*Individually*) "Birthday."	
(*Therapist gives help where it is indicated.*)	
Therapist: Do you like having a birthday? I'm going to ask you some questions about birthdays. Some of the questions will require "Yes" for an answer, some of them "No." Let's see how well you can make the word "Yes" today. It is getting easier for some of you.	The therapist may ask questions similar to those suggested. In many groups the children will be able to do the asking. A few leading words on the board as cake, spanking, presents, party, may give them ideas around which to construct their questions.
Children: (*Individually*) Yes. (*The therapist may require their giving this response fairly rapidly, singling out those who need help.*)	
Therapist: As I ask these questions, you may think of some questions to ask, too. "Do you *sometimes* have ice cream on your birthday?"	The word *sometimes* is essential in phrasing the questions.
Child: Yes.	

From Backus, O., and Beasley, J.: Speech therapy with children, Boston, 1951, Houghton Mifflin Co.

Procedures

Therapist: Do you sometimes have cake on your birthday?

Child: Yes. (*May continue by asking the next question.*)

(*Other suggestions:* Do you sometimes have presents, a spanking, a party, a surprise, a picnic, birthday cards, special fun, etc. on your birthday? Do you sometimes eat the cake, open the presents, hurt from the spanking, see friends at the party, get surprised, have fun, cut the cake, blow out the candles, read the birthday cards on your birthday?)

Therapist: Let's find out when your birthdays are. That is a question you often ask a new friend. Listen: "When is your birthday?" Try asking it, watching the "θ" especially.

Children: (*Individually*) When is your birthday?

Therapist: As you give us information about your birthday, I will write it with your name on the board. I'm going to suggest that we begin on this side of the circle and go straight around. It will be easier to keep the dates straight that way. I will ask the first question; you can go on from there.

Therapist: When is your birthday?

Child: On August seventh. (*Continues with questioning.*)

Therapist: Take a look at each of the birthdays that are listed here. I'm going to erase the names soon, and see if you remember whose birthday comes at each date. If you have difficulty, you can count around the group and figure it out that way. (*Erases names after children have studied list.*)

Therapist: Can you find my birthday?

Child: Yes. Is this right? *or* Right here?

Therapist: Yes.

Therapist: Before we go on, let's give the people who are having difficulty with "r" some work on the speech response "Is this right?" or "Right here?" (*Gives help as indicated.*)

(*Continue with above pattern guiding the children to check themselves on the "ð," "s," "r."*)

(*Other patterns which may be worked out in connection with the list on the board:*)

Child: Show me your birthday.

Child: That one. (*Continue*)

•   •   •

Child: Ann, is that your birthday?

Child: Yes. (*Continue*)

•   •   •

Child: I'm thinking of a birthday.

Child: That one?

Child: No. Guess again.

Child: That one?

Child: Yes. (*Continue*)

•   •   •

Notes

The therapist should guide this question and answer period so that chief emphasis is placed on the response "Yes." She may do it by stopping the conversation for a moment and asking, "Why are you asking each other questions? Yes, to get practice on the words 'Yes' and 'birthday.' Keep that in mind as you go along."

The response "your" may be utilized for work on the "r" if it is appropriate for the area in which the child lives.

The ordinals are somewhat difficult for children who have defective sounds. It is suggested that the therapist help individual children as they show a need for it, but not go on giving particular work on it at this time.

Continued.

Procedures	Notes
Therapist: Can you erase your birthday?	
Child: Yes.	A similar lesson can be worked out dealing with
Child: Should I erase my birthday?	street addresses and telephone numbers. Such
Child: I think so.	lessons can be utilized to help children with the
	ways in which they say numbers, important in
• • •	various phases of school work as well as in fur-
	nishing the above information.
Therapist: What have you worked on saying better today? Why?	

APPENDIX K

Bibliography of articulation programs

Ausberger, C.: Here's how to handle /r/, Tucson, Ariz., Communication Skill Builders.

Baker, R., and Ryan, B.: The Monterey Articulation Program, Monterey, Calif., Monterey Learning Systems.

Brown, I., Timm, K., and Evans, E.: Universal articulation program, Boston, Teaching Resources Corp.

Butt, D., and Peterson, D.: R-kit for articulation therapy, Albuquerque, N. Mex., Speech & Hearing Clinic, University of New Mexico.

Carrier, J., Jr.: A program of articulation therapy administered by mothers, J. Speech Hear. Disord. **35:**344-353.

Click, M., and Ueberle, J.: Lisp correction program, Danville, Ill., The Interstate Printers & Publishers, Inc.

Collins, P., and Cunningham, G.: /s/ /z/ Articulation management program, Gladstone, Oreg., CC Publications.

Collins, P., and Cunningham, G.: /l/ Articulation management program, Gladstone, Oreg., CC Publications.

Collins, P., and Cunningham, G.: /ʃ/ Articulation management program, Gladstone, Oreg., CC Publications.

Collins, P., and Cunningham, G.: /tʃ/ /dʒ/ Articulation management program, Gladstone, Oreg., CC Publications.

Collins, P., and Cunningham, G.: /θ/ /ð/ Articulation management program, Gladstone, Oreg., CC Publications.

Collins, P., Cunningham, G., and Bakke, S.: /r/ Articulation management program, Gladstone, Oreg., CC Publications.

Delbridge, L., and Larrigan, L.: Stimulus shift articulation kit, Tempe, Ariz., Ideas.

Jackson, M.: Programmed articulation therapy for the modification of /r/, Tempe, Ariz., Ideas.

Jackson, M.: Programmed articulation therapy for the modification of /ʃ/, Tempe, Ariz., Ideas.

Jacobs, K., and Sauer, J.: The /r/ program, North St. Paul, Minn.

Lubbert, L., and associates: Behavior modification articulation program for speech aides, Tempe, Ariz., Ideas.

Lundquist, R.: Speech Therapy Transfer Program, Las Vegas, Nev., Clark County School District.

McLean, J.: Extending stimulus control of phoneme articulation by operant techniques, ASHA Monogr. **14:**24-27, 1970.

Mowrer, D., Baker, R., and Schutz, R.: Programmed articulation control kit, Tempe, Ariz., Educational Psychological Research Associates.

Shriberg, L.: A response evocation program for /ɚ/, J. Speech Hear. Disord. **40:**92-105, 1975.

Strong, B.: Articulation program for technicians, Thief River Falls, Minn., Public Schools.

SWRL Speech Articulation Kit, New York, American Book Co.

Van Hattem, R., and associates: The speech improvement system, Lang. Speech Hear. Serv. Schools **2:**91-97, 1974.

Waters, B.: Articulation base program, DeKalb, Ill., Department of Communication Disorders, Northern Illinois University.

Weston, A., and Irwin, J.: Paired-stimuli in modification of articulation, Percept. Mot. Skills **32:**390-397, 1971.

Drexler's distinctive feature system

Initial (release) position

	Vowel	Nasal	Lateral	Glide	Fricative	Stop	Voiced	Bilabial	Labiodental	Linguadental	Alveolar	Postalveolar	Velar	Glottal
p						+		+						
b						+	+	+						
t						+					+			
d						+	+				+			
k						+							+	
g						+	+						+	
m		+					+	+						
n		+					+				+			
hw					+			+						
w				+			+	+						
j				+			+					+		
l			+	+			+				+			
r				+			+					+		
f					+				+					
v					+		+		+					
θ					+					+				
ð					+		+			+				
s					+						+			
z					+		+				+			
ʃ					+							+		
tʃ					+	+						+		
dʒ					+	+	+					+		
h					+									+

From Drexler, H.: J. Oreg. Speech Hear. Assoc. **15**:2-5, 1976.   *Continued.*

Final (arrest) position

	Vowel	Nasal	Lateral	Glide	Fricative	Stop	Voiced	Bilabial	Labiodental	Linguadental	Alveolar	Postalveolar	Velar	Glottal
p						+		+						
b						+	+	+						
t						+					+			
d						+	+				+			
k						+							+	
g						+	+						+	
m		+					+	+						
n		+					+				+			
ŋ		+					+						+	
l	+		+				+				+			
ɚ	+						+					+		
f					+				+					
v					+		+		+					
θ					+					+				
ð					+		+			+				
s					+						+			
z					+		+				+			
ʃ					+							+		
ʒ					+		+					+		
tʃ					+	+						+		
dʒ					+	+	+					+		

Distinctive feature method proposed by Drexler

Level	Stimulus	Response	Reinforcement schedule	Criterion for movement	
				Pass	**Fail**
Isolation	Say /k/.	/k/	100% token 100% social	19/20	5/20
	Say /k,t.../.	/k,t,k,k,t,k,t,t,t.../	75% token 100% social	19/20	5/20
Nonsense syllables					
1. Releasing position	Say CV combination (high back vowel).	CV combination (/ku/).	100% token 100% social	10/10	3/10
	Say CV, CV pairs (high back vowel).	CV, CV pairs (/ku,tu/).	100% token 100% social	10/10	3/10
	Say CV, CV pairs on signal (high back vowel).	2- to 4-second delay; CV pairs (/ku,tu/).	75% token 100% social	10/10	3/10
	Say CV combination (low back vowel).	CV combination (/ka/).	75% token 100% social	10/10	3/10
	Say CV, CV pairs (low back vowel).	CV, CV pairs (/ka,ta/).	75% token 100% social	10/10	3/10
	Say CV, CV pairs on signal (low back vowel).	2- to 4-second delay; CV, CV pairs (/ka,ta/).	50% token 75% social	10/10	3/10
	Say CV combination (low front vowel).	CV combination (/kæ/).	50% token 75% social	10/10	3/10
	Say CV, CV pairs (low front vowel).	CV, CV pairs (/kæ, tæ/).	50% token 75% social	10/10	3/10
	Say CV, CV pairs on signal (low front vowel).	2- to 4-second delay; CV, CV pairs (/kæ, tæ/).	25% token 50% social	10/10	3/10
	Say CV combination (high front vowel).	CV combination (/ki/).	25% token 50% social	10/10	3/10
	Say CV, CV pairs (high front vowel).	CV, CV pairs (/ki,ti/).	0% token 25% social	10/10	3/10
	Say CV, CV pairs on signal (high front vowel).	2- to 4-second delay; CV, CV pairs (/ki,ti/).	0% token 0% social	10/10	3/10

From Drexler, H.: J. Oreg. Speech Hear. Assoc. 15:2-5, 1976. *Continued.*

Level	Stimulus	Response	Reinforcement schedule	Criterion for movement	
				Pass	Fail
2. Arresting position	Repeat as for releasing position with VC order.				
Words	Show picture. Say "Word," /k/ releasing position, /t/ releasing position.	Word, /k/ releasing position and word, /t/ releasing position.	100% token 100% social	19/20	5/20
	Show pictures, /k,t/ releasing position. Say "Name these pictures."	Words, /k,t/ releasing position.	75% token 100% social	19/20	5/20
	Show picture. Say "Word," /k/ arresting position, /t/ arresting position.	Word, /k/ arresting position and word, /t/ arresting position.	50% token 75% social	19/20	5/20
	Show pictures, /k,t/ arresting position. Say "Name these pictures."	Words, /k,t/ arresting position.	25% token 50% social	19/20	5/20
Phrases	Show pictures. Say "Phrase," /k/ releasing position; say "phrase," /t/ releasing position.	Phrase, /k/ releasing position and phrase, /t/ releasing position.	75% token 100% social	19/20	5/20
	Show pictures, /k,t/ releasing position. Say "Tell me about this picture," or use what or where questions.	Phrases, /k/ and /t/ releasing positions.	50% token 75% social	19/20	5/20
	Show pictures. Say "Phrase," /k/ arresting position; say "phrase," /t/ arresting position.	Phrase, /k/ arresting position and phrase, /t/ arresting position.	25% token 50% social	19/20	5/20
	Show pictures, /k,t/ releasing position. Say "Tell me about this picture," or use what or where questions.	Phrases, /k/ and /t/ releasing positions.	50% token 75% social	19/20	5/20
	Show pictures. Say "Phrase," /k/ arresting position; say "phrase," /t/ arresting position.	Phrase, /k/ arresting position and phrase, /t/ arresting position.	25% token 50% social	19/20	5/20

Level	Stimulus	Response	Reinforcement schedule	Criterion for movement	
				Pass	Fail
Phrases— cont'd	Show pictures, /k,t/ arresting position. Say "Tell me about this picture," or use what or where questions.	Phrases, /k/ and /t/ arresting positions.	0% token 25% social	19/20	5/20
Sentences	Show pictures. Say "Sentence," /k/ releasing position; say "sentence," /t/ releasing position.	Sentence, /k/ releasing position and sentence, /t/ releasing position.	50% token 75% social	19/20	5/20
	Show pictures, /k,t/ releasing position. Say "Tell me a sentence about this picture," or use what or where questions.	Sentences, /k/ and /t/ releasing positions.	25% token 50% social	19/20	5/20
	Show pictures. Say "Sentence," /k/ arresting position; say "sentence," /t/ arresting position.	Sentence, /k/ arresting position and sentence, /t/ arresting position.	0% token 25% social	19/20	5/20
	Show pictures, /k,t/ arresting position. Say "Tell me a sentence about this picture," or use what or where questions.	Sentences, /k/ and /t/ arresting positions.	0% token 0% social	19/20	5/20

Report guidelines and sample reports

BEHAVIORAL GOALS AND PROCEDURES

The behavioral objectives and procedures should be specifically outlined for each client and should include both short- and long-term goals. A space reserved for reporting progress should be provided on this outline. Additional information such as baseline, measurement procedures, and criterion levels should also be included. All of this information should be part of the client's folder.

EXAMPLE:

Long-term goal: Normal articulation 90% of the time in conversational speech in all settings by the end of the school year.
Procedures:

1. Follow the hierarchical steps outlined in Van Riper's stimulus approach
2. Supplement the stimulus approach by employing operant procedures such as tangible rewards for correct productions of target sounds, and charting and displaying progress
3. Use 90% criterion levels for each level of treatment; that is, the client must achieve at or above this criterion level three consecutive sessions before advancing to the next more difficult task
4. Incorporating play and other interactive or experiential activities for establishing transfer and maintenance; for these activities, the client will be exposed to four different persons, five different environments, and a variety of different phonemic contexts
5. Self-monitoring activities will be included at every level of treatment by the use of counters and tape recorders; both the client and the clinician will count correct and incorrect productions for 5-minute segments of each session

Short-term goal: To produce /s/ and /z/ correctly 90% of the time in isolated words (twenty-five words per session)
Short-term goal: To produce /s/ and /z/ correctly 90% of the time in four-word sentences containing no more than two of the target sounds in each sentence; the client will repeat twenty-five sentences each session
Procedures: Twenty-five words will be jointly selected by the client and clinician; the words will be typed on 3 × 5 cards and presented to the child and said by the clinician and then repeated by the client 8 seconds after they are spoken by the clinician
Sample format of an individualized educational program

1. Current educational level of student (base line)
2. Long-term goals (for the entire school year)
3. Short-term goals (for every 2 or 3 months)
4. Special educational services needed (specific type of communicative disorders)
5. Beginning and ending dates of special educational services
6. Amount of time spent each week in special educational program
7. Justification for needing special educational program
8. List and specialization of persons responsible for implementing the individualized educational program
9. Evaluative procedures (administered twice a year) used for determining achievement of short-term and long-term goals
10. Recommendation regarding future status (to terminate or continue special educational services next year; include rationale)

DIAGNOSTIC REPORT GUIDELINES

The diagnostic report is the first report written in the following cases: (1) after a patient is seen for the first time in our clinic, (2) the previous diagnostic workup has been longer than 6 months ago, (3) the patient's communicative abilities or disabilities have changed from what were indicated in the previous report, or (4) the supervisor believes that another diagnostic report should be written. The contents should be as follows:

I. *Identifying information:* This is the information that goes across the top of the page and should include, in the following manner:

Name: _____
B.D.: _____
C.A.: _____
Sex: _____
Referral source: _____
Parents: _____
Address: _____
Telephone: _____
Date: _____
Sessions attended: _____

II. *History:* This paragraph includes all *pertinent* background information: medical, dental, psychologic, communicative, developmental, educational, environmental, social, cultural, etc.

III. *Speech:* This paragraph includes findings, status, test scores, age levels, etc. about articulation, voice, and rhythm.

IV. *Language:* This paragraph includes linguistic abilities and disabilities, test scores, and levels of functioning regarding all of the receptive and expressive parameters of language.

V. *Oral:* This paragraph discusses all the dimensions of the peripheral oral mechanism, movable and immovable: face, lips, teeth, tongue, palate, jaw, pharynx, larynx, etc. The structures as well as the physiology are to be discussed here. Also include rate, range, and precision of articulator movements, sensation-perception, and velopharyngeal closure. This paragraph should help in making a differential diagnosis regarding the type and extent of etiology.

VI. *Hearing:* This paragraph includes pure tone results, SRT, SD, impedance, auditory memory and auditory conceptualization (indicated here or under "language"), and amplification or amplification needs, if any.

VII. *Summary:* This paragraph summarizes all salient history and findings, along with impressions. This paragraph should include only the major characteristics and should contain no new information. A statement about prognosis can be made here. Scores need not be repeated here, just levels of functioning.

VIII. *Recommendations:* The last paragraph should include, in outline form, all of the recommendations: speech treatment, additional testing, hearing testing, psychologic testing, physical examination, dental consultation, plastic surgery consultation, etc., and *specific* recommendations regarding communication (additional diagnosis, treatment, or overall management—seen when, where, how often, by whom, individual or group setting, type of treatment approach, etc.).

IX. *Signatures:* This report should be signed by the student clinician and by the supervisor as follows:

_____
Typed name
Student clinician

_____
Typed name and degree
Speech and language pathologist

Indicate where copies are to be sent and addresses of persons receiving the reports.

cc: Name, title
    Address

PROGRESS REPORT GUIDELINES

This report is written and distributed at the end of the semester. It should be completed by the last day of the clinic and be ready for distribution and filing at that time. The purposes of this report are to summarize the current status of the patient, to report progress made or attempted, to report the principal procedures used that did and did not work well, to review the general goals, to summarize overall impressions, to educate professionals other than speech and language pathologists, to make specific recommendations concerning communication or other aspects of the patient, and to "sell" our abilities and services to others.

I. *Identifying information:* Same as for diagnostic report.
II. *History:* This paragraph should include a brief but salient *review* of the patient's background, not only in regard to communicative development and treatment, but also in regard to any and all related areas. The amount of information contained in this section should not be as much as it would be in the diagnostic report.
III. *Management:* This paragraph includes summarized and consolidated goals, procedures, baselines, and progress. It should stress the major aspects of management and exclude less important specific details. Progress should be reported in quantifiable terms, and management procedures should be critically evaluated.
IV. *Summary:* This paragraph includes various observations, comments, opinions, facts, and impressions. It should reiterate the most important points previously discussed.
V. *Recommendations:* In this section specifically *outline* what is recommended in regard to communication management and any other areas related to the overall management of the patient. Indicate if parents were or were not receptive to the recommendations.
VI. *Signatures:* Same as for diagnostic report. If the student does not or cannot sign this report, the supervisor may sign it and release it for distribution.

These reports are varied in form, format, style, content, and purpose in order to give the student a wide sampling. They are not meant to be ideal reports, but they are adequate and should give the student a starting point for writing the various types of reports needed. These are copies of actual reports from several different institutions and settings, with minor changes and with names and other identifying information deleted. In addition to the sample reports, an instruction sheet used in one clinic as a student guide for writing diagnostic and progress reports is included. Can you identify words or statements that might have been used inappropriately?

PRELIMINARY REPORT
(Informal)

Location
Address   Telephone

Date:

Robert _____ , M.D.   Re: Mary _____
                                          Address

Dear Dr. _____ :

   I saw Mary _____ yesterday for a brief evaluation of her articulation, resonance, and velopharyngeal mechanism, as you requested. Her articulation is
normal as to place and manner, but she lacks the necessary closure to eliminate nasal
airflow and hypernasality. Consequently she has an alar squint associated with the production of all pressure consonants. Additional speech treatment is not indicated.

   Although the pharyngeal flap improved her velopharyngeal functioning, closure is still
inadequate. As you know, velopharyngeal exercises and speech treatment are ineffective in
improving inadequate velopharyngeal closure. The only two effective procedures for
achieving closure are surgery and prosthesis, but both are contraindicated in her case. Mary
is doing remarkably well considering her history of inappropriate speech treatment and
frequent surgeries.

Sincerely,

_____ , CCC, M.S.
Speech-Language Pathologist

NOTE TO STUDENT: This type of informal report usually is all that is needed for a preliminary report, but if more information is requested, a more formal report may be necessary.
This type of report by letter often will suffice for the consultation report also.

DIAGNOSTIC REPORT
(Formal)

Location
Address   Telephone

Diagnostic Report
CONFIDENTIAL

Name: ___DeeDee___   Parents: ___Mr. & Mrs. DeeDee___
Sex: ___Female___   Address: ___000 First St.___
Date of Birth: ___3/11/74___   Telephone: ___123-4567___
Age: ___3-9___   Referral source: Dr. ___Concerned___
Date of Evaluation: ___11/17/77___   Informant: ___Mother___

STATEMENT OF THE PROBLEM

DeeDee _____ was seen at the _____
Speech and Hearing Center for a speech and language evaluation on November 17, 1977.
Mrs. _____ stated that she and her husband were extremely con-
cerned with DeeDee's lack of verbal communicative ability. She stated that DeeDee's vocabulary was less than ten words and that the only two-word combinations have been "me
here" and "right here." Mrs. _____ said that the immediate family
rarely understood what DeeDee was saying and that people outside the family never understood her verbalizations.

DeeDee is the youngest of five children and the only female. Mrs. _____
stated that DeeDee got along well with her brothers and that the entire family, on advice of
the pediatrician, attempted to encourage DeeDee to ask for things and to do things for
herself.

According to Mrs. _____, pregnancy was normal except for spot-
ting during the first trimester which required hospitalization for a brief period. Mrs.
_____ stated that she did not feel that this was a contributing factor
to any problems DeeDee might have. Developmental history has been normal; however,
DeeDee is not completely toilet trained. DeeDee received an attainment age of 2 years 8
months on the *Preschool Attainment Record* indicating an overall depression in developmental abilities.

CLINICAL EXAMINATION

Initial impressions—DeeDee and her mother were observed through a one-way mirror at
the beginning of the evaluation. DeeDee cried initially for a brief period but adapted quickly
to the new situation. She played appropriately with a barn and animals. Vocalizations were
confined to two-syllable, unintelligible utterances such as /mahi/ and /maha/.

During the evaluation, DeeDee was cooperative. However, because of her short attention
span and unintelligible verbalizations, standard testing was inappropriate.

SUMMARY OF TEST DATA

1. *Articulation*
   The Weiss Comprehensive Articulation Test (single-word portion) was attempted imitatively. DeeDee was unable to imitate any of the words and was stimulable on only the
   initial sounds /v/, /m/, /p/, and /f/.

2. *Receptive language*

The *Peabody Picture Vocabulary Test* (Form B), a multiple-choice recognition test of single word receptive vocabulary, was administered. A basal age was unattainable. Comprehension of body parts, colors, numbers, and simple commands was informally tested. DeeDee knew body parts, such as mouth and arm, and was able to follow simple commands. She correctly identified common farm animals, such as horse and chicken, but did not correctly identify the cow or the pig. She did not appear to have the concepts of colors or numbers or understand the spatial prepositions (in, on, and under).

3. *Auditory acuity*

DeeDee was given a hearing screening for the octave frequencies 250 to 4000 Hz at 20 dB. She responded appropriately at all test frequencies bilaterally.

4. *Expressive language*

Standardized tests were not administered because of depressed receptive language skills and unintelligible speech. DeeDee's expressive language skills were confined to unintelligible single utterances. Minimal changes in intonation and inflection were noted.

5. *Gross and visual motor skills*

The *Developmental Scale of Motor Performance* was administered. DeeDee was unable to perform all items at the 3-year level. On drawing tasks the palmar grasp was observed. DeeDee did not copy a circle or cross. She was able to copy a straight line, which places her approximately at the 2-year level.

6. *Oral motor examination*

Symmetry of structure of the face and lips was adequate. DeeDee was unable to round her lips and move them to the right or left adequately. Lateralization of the tongue both to the right and left was limited. She was also unable to imitate licking the lips using a circular motion.

CONCLUSIONS AND RECOMMENDATION

DeeDee demonstrated a severe articulation deficit as well as a severe delay in receptive and expressive language. Gross and fine motor skills appeared to be depressed, whereas auditory sensitivity was normal.

The restriction of tongue and lip movement noted in the oral peripheral examination may be contributing to her limited articulation skills. Her inability to imitate sounds seems to coincide with these findings.

We recommend that DeeDee be seen for communication treatment at the _____ _____ Speech and Hearing Center beginning as soon as possible. Mrs. _____ was informed that treatment would be directed toward increasing DeeDee's attention span, stimulating language skills, and training on imitative articulation tasks. Mrs. _____ was advised that if progress was not evident after a 3-month period of treatment, DeeDee would be referred for a more extensive communication evaluation.

_____
Student Clinician

_____
Clinical Supervisor, CCC, Ph.D.

cc: Dr. _____, title
    Address

CONSULTATION REPORT

Same identifying information as for diagnostic report.

GENERAL INFORMATION: Bill _____ , who is in the second grade at _____ School, was referred by the district speech consultant with a request for our assessment to determine the cause of an articulation problem. The speech clinician who has been working with Bill for about 7 months reports that he is not responding to conventional treatment procedures and suspects that there may be an underlying organic basis for the problem, although medical examination has failed to confirm this. Medical records accompanying the referral are essentially negative, except for some jaundice at birth and a slow start as an infant. The psychologic report shows a mental age commensurate with his chronologic age. Bill has been an average student in his classes.

ASSESSMENT: Because of the nature of the referral, examination at this center was limited to assessment of the articulatory mechanism and related factors. No structural abnormalities could be found. Articulatory function, however, showed several kinds of deviations. Oral stereognostic testing showed kinesthetic deficiency. Tactile sensitivity in the oral cavity was diminished. Diadochokinetic function was well below normal, and there was a general inability of the articulators to perform precise movements on demand and to achieve the degree of integrated movement necessary for adequate articulation. Range of motion and strength of the articulators and their strength were adequate, but not under control.

IMPRESSION: Results of this assessment confirm the school clinician's suspicion of organicity as a basis for the disorder. A rather pronounced verbal dyspraxia is indicated by the boy's performance at the time of this assessment. Jaundice at birth could account for the verbal dyspraxia. A thorough neurologic examination may be indicated but probably would not alter the course of treatment.

PROGNOSIS: Since the dyspraxia is not extreme, improvement may be expected with concentrated long-term treatment aimed at developing more precision of the articulatory movements through visual and rhythmic approaches. No quick gains can be expected with this kind of problem. Completely normal articulation is not likely to be attained, but it probably can become adequate for intelligible speech if Bill's motivation can be maintained.

_____ , Ph.D.
Examining Speech-Language Pathologist

cc: _____ , Speech-Language Consultant
    Address

PROGRESS REPORT

The only changes necessary for this identifying information from that included in the diagnostic report are to add the period covered, sessions scheduled, and sessions attended.

HISTORY: Joe entered the clinic in the fall semester of 1978 for treatment of a functional articulation disorder, characterized by a frontal lisping pattern resulting in distortion of sibilant phonemes [s], [z], and [d/ð], [f/θ], [w/r], and [w/l] substitutions. A previous evaluation at this clinic, 2/15/78, indicated a tongue thrust, but there was no evidence of this problem during a later evaluation. Joe's tonsils and adenoids had been removed prior to the second evaluation. This, combined with maturation, may have been responsible for eliminating the earlier noted anterior tongue posturing habit and possible tongue thrust. Joe had received previous treatment through the _____ Public Schools while attending kindergarten, but when he entered a parochial school, this service was no longer available. A report from the previous clinician stated that Joe had made excellent progress in the remediation of /s/, /z/, /r/, and /l/. Prognosis for the correction of other distorted sounds was good because of Joe's excellent stimulability.

MANAGEMENT: Treatment was initiated for remediation of the phonemes /s/, /z/, /r/, /θ/, and /l/, since all were readily stimulable and earlier success had been reported by the school speech-language pathologist. Management procedures began with production of each sound in words and progressed to sentences and carry-over into spontaneous speech. Pictures and functional items were used to provide stimuli for production during drills, board games, and card games at the word and sentence levels.

Successful techniques employed to stimulate responses in spontaneous speech included field trips, taking photographs of items in the environment that contained target phonemes, cooking, drawing pictures, playing with a tractor, and playing with puppets. Positive reinforcement based on a fixed interval schedule served to increase cooperation and motivation and proved successful in increasing correct production. Progress with each target phoneme was as follows:

/s/ 30% correct in words to 100% in spontaneous speech
/z/ 10% correct in words to 100% in spontaneous speech
/θ/ 40% correct in words to 90% in spontaneous speech
/r/ 50% correct in words to 100% in spontaneous speech
/l/ 65% correct in words to 100% in words (Treatment for this phoneme was started near the end of the semester)

SUMMARY: Joe exhibited excellent progress in the correct production of all target phonemes. Since treatment for correction of /l/ was initiated late in the semester, the criteria for sentences and carry-over were not met. However, informal testing at the final session indicated a level of 80% correct production in spontaneous speech. Joe was well-behaved and cooperative throughout the treatment program, although he occasionally exhibited signs of fatigue, which affected the number of correct responses elicited.

RECOMMENDATIONS: We recommend that Joe return to this clinic next semester in order to complete treatment for his misarticulations. However, because of transportation problems, this will not be possible. The parents wish to be contacted for the summer clinic.

_____
Student Clinician

_____
Clinic Supervisor

cc: Mr. and Mrs. _____, Parents
    Address

_____, Principal
    Address

FINAL REPORT

Identifying information should be the same as in the progress report.

GENERAL INFORMATION: Henry first entered the speech-language treatment program at _____ School in September 1976, at age 6 years, 4 months. He was referred by his classroom teacher with a report that his speech was "indistinct." The teacher also reported that he was an average student, was not a behavioral problem, interacted with his peers and adults appropriately, came from a stable home environment, and had cooperative parents.

ASSESSMENT: Examination of the speech mechanism showed no oral structural deviations except a minor overbite, which in itself was not cause for the speech problem. Articulator functioning was adequate except for a tongue thrust of moderate severity. Hearing was normal with no history of hearing or upper respiratory problems. Voice and resonation were also normal. Articulation testing revealed a strong interdental lisp affecting all sibilants and difficulty with /r/ in all positions. Blends involving /r/ and /s/ were consistently in error. Speech was usually 100% intelligible but somewhat difficult to understand in connected speech because of the frequency of occurrence of the misarticulated sounds. Henry was stimulable 90% of the time and cooperative, suggesting a favorable prognosis in treatment.

MANAGEMENT: Henry was placed with two other children in a phonetic placement articulation treatment approach and an antagonistic placement approach for tongue thrust consisting of three ½-hour sessions per week. These programs continued for the remainder of the school year. During that time the tongue thrust and resultant interdental lisp were corrected. The sibilant sounds were used accurately in all positions, and carry-over seemed to be successful. The /r/, however, was more resistant and still was in error most of the time at the end of the school year, so further treatment was recommended for Henry in the fall. The following September he was enrolled in an integral stimulation treatment approach with one other boy who was also having difficulty with the /r/. Henry had retained maintenance of the normal swallow and of accuracy in sibilant sound productions, so no further work was needed in these areas. Concentration on the /r/ resulted in correct usage of the sound in the treatment setting by midterm, when carry-over procedures were initiated. Since the parents had been so cooperative, the remainder of the carry-over treatment was turned over to them and Henry's school treatment sessions were discontinued. He was rechecked twice during the remainder of the 1977-1978 school year, and at the last check in spring successful carry-over was apparent, so Henry was dismissed from the program.

RECOMMENDATIONS: Because Henry's speech and tongue thrust treatment has been successfully concluded, he should not be enrolled for further treatment in the speech-language program.

_____ , CCC, M.S.
Speech-Language Pathologist, _____ School

cc: Supervisor, Speech-Language Program,
_____ School District

   Mr. _____ , Principal, _____ School

   Mr. and Mrs. _____ , Parents

ASHA guidelines for training and use of communication aides

A. ROLE AND TASK OF THE COMMUNICATION AIDE

1. The clinician with the Certificate of Clinical Competence awarded by the American Speech and Hearing Association is responsible for the direction of all client services provided by the Communication Aide and is responsible to the client for the performance of these services.

2. Communication Aides should not be responsible for making decisions regarding the diagnosis, management, and future disposition of clients.

3. Communication Aides should only be assigned to duties for which they have been specifically trained and qualified.

4. Prior to utilizing Communication Aides, the speech pathologist or audiologist who is responsible for his direction should carefully define and delineate the aide's role and tasks. The employing organization would understand and agree to these regulations. It shall be the responsibility of the speech pathologist or audiologist to:
   a. Define and maintain specific lines of responsibility and authority
   b. Assure that the aide is responsible only to him in all client-related activities
   c. Conduct ongoing evaluations of the role and of task experiences of the aide
   d. Reassess and redesign programs when either the task or environment change significantly

5. In the selection of Communication Aides due consideration should be given to

fair employment practices and to the general employment requirements of the agency. In addition, the aide should evidence the following:
   a. An ability to communicate effectively with adults and with children
   b. An empathy for people, particularly the communicatively handicapped individual
   c. An ability to understand and to sympathize with the cultural and linguistic heritages of the area from which clients may come

B. TRAINING OF THE COMMUNICATION AIDE

1. The training of the Communication Aide should be dictated by the tasks to be performed. Training in housekeeping or clerical duties, the maintenance of equipment and supplies, or other tasks not directly related to client services are likely to require specific training, but such tasks and training *do not* require policy statements by the American Speech Language and Hearing Association.

2. The selection of trainees should be at the discretion of the professional in the speech and hearing program. The selection should be based on those mental, physical, and emotional qualifications that are appropriate to the tasks to be performed and the populations to be served. Communication Aides should be trained by the speech and hearing program in which they are to be employed or in collaboration with the organization with which they are to be employed. Should a speech and hearing pro-

From ASHA Committee on Supportive Personnel: ASHA J. 12:78-80, February 1970.

gram choose to employ a Communication Aide whose training or experience has been obtained elsewhere, the new employing program should provide additional training as required by the new tasks and new environment.

3. It should be the responsibility of the organization to provide training in those skills that the Communication Aide is to apply in the performance of his duties. The duration of training should be sufficient to enable the training organization to determine either that the trainee is competent to perform the directed duties or that the duties are inappropriate for the trainee. On-the-job training prior to the beginning of work by the aide may extend from a few days to several weeks, depending on the nature of the work to be performed.

4. All training for client-related services shall be provided by speech pathologists or audiologists holding the Certificate of Clinical Competence in the appropriate specialty. Such training may not be delegated to auxiliary, preprofessional, or supportive personnel.

5. The employing organization has the continuing responsibility to provide in-service training for supportive personnel and to encourage self-improvement of the Communication Aide.

6. The training of Communication Aides shall be task-oriented. The training, therefore, will vary according to the task to be performed by the aide in the particular employment environment. The training may include orientation regarding the significance of human communication; ethical responsibilities to the professional clinician, client, and employing organization; administrative structure for the provision of the speech and hearing services; the kinds of tasks that may be performed by the Communication Aide; and the recognition of appropriate and inappropriate responses of the client.

7. Counseling and guidance may be needed for the improvement of the Communication Aide's language, speech, reading and writing, work habits, and professional decorum.

C. POLICIES AND GUIDELINES REGARDING THE DIRECTION OF COMMUNICATION AIDES

1. Communication aides should not work in any setting in an activity of speech and hearing diagnosis and treatment except under the direction of an ASHA Member holding the Certificate of Clinical Competence.

2. The legal, ethical, and moral responsibility for the welfare of the client with whom the Communication Aide works is the responsibility of his immediate ASHA-certified director.

3. In the utilization of the Communication Aide, recommended guidelines for the clinician are as follows:

a. He must ensure that a qualified professional initially evaluate each client

b. He must outline and direct the specific program for clinical management of each client assigned to an aide

c. He must maintain direct contact with each client during the course of clinical management

d. He must ensure that at the termination of clinical services the case is reviewed by the clinician responsible for the client

e. Should conditions arise in which any of the preceding guidelines cannot be adhered to, then continued clinical services provided by the Communication Aide alone must be terminated

4. It is strongly recommended that service programs that employ Communication Aides should be registered by the Professional Services Board of the American Board of Examiners in Speech-Language Pathology and Audiology.

5. The direction provided to the Communication Aide must clearly and continually preclude independence in clinical decision making since this may in any way directly influence clinical practice.

6. It is the responsibility of the program director to ensure that the assignment and use of Communication Aides to certified staff members is such that it is possible to meet the preceding guidelines. In general the ratio of Communication Aides to certified professionals should not exceed 4 to 1.

Differential application of treatment approaches

Etiology	Setting	Treatment option
Functional infantile perseveration	Individual or group	Stimulus approach
	Group	Heterogeneous approach
Other nonorganic delay	Individual	Programmed approach
	Group	Heterogeneous approach
	Individual or group	Integral stimulation approach
Cerebral palsy (dysarthria)	Individual or group	Sensory-motor approach
	Individual or group	Progressive approximation approach
	Individual	Motokinesthetic approach
Dyspraxia	Individual or group	Sensory-motor approach
	Individual or group	Visual approach
	Individual	Melodic intonation or prosodic approach
Cleft palate	Individual	Motokinesthetic approach
	Individual or group	Multiple phoneme approach
	Individual	Distinctive feature approach
Mental retardation		
Educable	Individual	Programmed approach
	Individual or group	Stimulus approach
Trainable	Individual	Programmed approach
Auditory		
Impaired acuity	Individual or group	Ling approach (not described in text)
	Individual	Motokinesthetic approach
Imperception	Individual or group	Integral stimulation approach
	Individual or group	Phonetic placement approach
	Individual or group	Visual approach
Psycholinguistic	Individual or group	Phonologic process approach
	Individual or group	Auditory conceptualization approach
	Individual	Distinctive feature approach
Psychoemotional	Individual	Programmed approach
	Individual	Nondirect approach

Continued.

Etiology	Setting	Treatment option
Multiply handicapped	Individual or group	Sensory-motor approach
	Individual or group	Motokinesthetic approach
	Individual or group	Stimulus approach
Foreign dialect	Individual or group	Auditory conceptualization approach
	Individual or group	Stimulus approach
	Individual	Programmed approach
Learning disability	Individual	Programmed approach
	Individual or group	Integral stimulation approach*

*Additional consideration should be given to whether the client is a child or an adult.

Index